# Diagnostic Ultrasound Imaging

# Diagnostic Ultrasound Imaging

Editor: Bradley Hayes

AMERICAN
MEDICAL PUBLISHERS
www.americanmedicalpublishers.com

AMERICAN
MEDICAL PUBLISHERS
www.americanmedicalpublishers.com

**Cataloging-in-Publication Data**

Diagnostic ultrasound imaging / edited by Bradley Hayes.
p. cm.
Includes bibliographical references and index.
ISBN 979-8-88740-061-7
1. Diagnostic ultrasonic imaging. 2. Diagnostic imaging. 3. Ultrasonic imaging.
4. Ultrasonics in medicine. I. Hayes, Bradley.
RC78.7.U4 D53 2023
616.075 43--dc23



American Medical Publishers,
41 Flatbush Avenue,
1st Floor, New York,
NY 11217, USA

ISBN 979-8-88740-061-7 (Hardback)

# Contents

# Preface

This book has been a concerted effort by a group of academicians, researchers and scientists, who have contributed their research works for the realization of the book. This book has materialized in the wake of emerging advancements and innovations in this field. Therefore, the need of the hour was to compile all the required researches and disseminate the knowledge to a broad spectrum of people comprising of students, researchers and specialists of the field.

Diagnostic ultrasound imaging is a type of imaging technique used to view the internal parts or structures of the body. It is a non-invasive diagnostic technique that examines body parts for detecting any kind of damage or problems with functioning. In the process of diagnostic ultrasound, a transducer is placed on the skin, vagina or rectum. There are different types of diagnostic ultrasounds including abdominal ultrasound, renal ultrasound, breast ultrasound, Doppler ultrasound, pelvic ultrasound, transvaginal ultrasound, thyroid ultrasound, and transrectal ultrasound. Renal ultrasound is an ultrasound used to gain information about the location, size and shape of the kidneys. It can also be used to assess information about related structures like ureters and bladder. The conditions such as cysts, tumors, and infections inside and around the kidneys are diagnosed with the help of renal ultrasound. Doppler ultrasound is used to analyze the flow of fluids like blood in the body. This book contains some path-breaking studies in the field of diagnostic ultrasound imaging. With state-of-the-art inputs by acclaimed experts of this field, it targets students and professionals associated with this field.

At the end of the preface, I would like to thank the authors for their brilliant chapters and the publisher for guiding us all-through the making of the book till its final stage. Also, I would like to thank my family for providing the support and encouragement throughout my academic career and research projects.

**Editor**

1

# Learning process and improvement of point-of-care ultrasound technique for subxiphoid visualization of the inferior vena cava

Mauricio Gómez Betancourt[1], José Moreno-Montoya[2], Ana-María Barragán González[2*], Juan Carlos Ovalle[1] and Yury Forlan Bustos Martínez[3*]

**Abstract**

**Background:** Medical residents' training in ultrasonography usually follows the recommendations of the American College of Emergency Physicians (ACEP), even though these do not provide specific technical guidelines. Adequate training is considered to require 25 practical iterations in the majority of ultrasound procedures. However, the effectiveness of this approach has not been verified experimentally. We set out to determine the number of repetitions required for an acceptable ultrasound procedure of the inferior vena cava (IVC), as an important and emerging ultrasound procedure in cardiology.

**Methods:** Using three human models, each of eight medical residents in the Emergency Medicine (EM) Program at the Universidad del Rosario performed 25 iterations of the recommended procedure, with image quality evaluation by an EM physician expert in the technique. Logistic regression analysis was used to determine the lowest number of repetitions required to achieve an adjusted probability of success of 80 and 90 %, respectively.

**Results:** We obtained 200 ultrasound images. The percentage success by each resident ranged from 52 to 96 %. There was no statistical significance in the relation between gender and success ($p = 0.83$), but there was an association between year of residency and success ($p < 0.001$). The average time taken for each procedure was 17.3 s (SD 8.1); there was no association between the time taken and either repetition number or image quality. We demonstrate that eleven repetitions are required to achieve acceptable image quality in 80 %, and that 21 repetitions are required to achieve acceptable image quality in 90 %.

**Conclusions:** This is the first study to formally evaluate the effectiveness of recommended training in ultrasound techniques. Our findings demonstrate that training comprising 25 procedural repetitions is easily sufficient to achieve optimal image quality, and they also provide empiric knowledge toward elucidating the times and minimum repetitions needed to acquire and improve ultrasonographic technique in novice operators to a level which fulfills quality requirements for interpretation.

**Keywords:** Learning curve, Ultrasonography, Inferior vena cava, Point-of-care, Residents, Colombia

*Correspondence: ana.barragan@urosario.edu.co; yury.bustos@urosario.edu.co

[2] Epidemiology, Biostatistics and Public Health Research Group, EPIBIOS_UR, Escuela de Medicina y Ciencias de la Salud (EMCS), Universidad del Rosario, Bogotá, Colombia

[3] Chief of the Department of Emergency Medicine and Director of the Simulation Center, Escuela de Medicina y Ciencias de la Salud (EMCS), Universidad del Rosario, Bogotá, Colombia

Full list of author information is available at the end of the article

## Background

Emergency Ultrasound, also known as "point-of-care" or "bedside ultrasound," is part of the essential training requirement for Emergency Medicine (EM) and intensive care programs in the United States and elsewhere [1–3]. Cardiac focused ultrasound is part of the compulsory recommendations of physician training in critical care. The assessment of the IVC, which is part of this cardiac focused study, has been gaining importance due to its implications for the management of patients in shock [4–8]. In Colombia, the use of ultrasonography by specialized physicians is now in its initial phase, because of the recent inclusion of this training in the curriculum of EM programs. In addition, against the massive adoption of this practice arises the limited availability of equipment in emergency services and competent operators [2, 9]. Early diagnosis and treatment of critical care patients in the developed and developing world is supported by the diagnostic performance of the point-of-care ultrasound technique for subxiphoid visualization of the IVC, which has been reported to be superior to invasive tools such as central venous pressure, and similar to arterial pressure curve methods [10–12].

The American College of Emergency Physicians (ACEP) recommends a minimum of 25 repetitions for developing competence in ultrasonography. The aforementioned was based on learning curves for different techniques and approach windows, as well as expert recommendations [1]. However, the guidelines are not specific for the subxiphoid visualization of the IVC, and the number and characteristics of the required studies for optimal performance are still unknown [11]. Available literature regarding the learning of ultrasonographic techniques, such as that reported by Gaddis et al., suggests that the accuracy of Focused Abdominal Sonography for Trauma (FAST) increases with repetitive experience [13]. Consequently, the appropriation of the procedure not only will be useful for its application as a monitoring and evaluation tool of effectiveness of novice physician's training programs in ultrasonography, but also as a practical device in diagnosis schemes. This paper was aimed to assess the learning and improvement process of point-of-care ultrasound technique for subxiphoid visualization of the IVC in EM residents according to the ACEP recommendations.

## Methods

### Population and operators

Students from all years' EM residency participated as operators in this study once they attended a 40-min conference by an expert in ultrasound on basic principles and techniques for performing IVC ultrasonography visualization through subxiphoid window. Operators with previous training in ultrasonography were excluded. We used three models for the simulation of the procedure considering healthy adult males, aged 29, 33, and 39, with BMI of 26.8, 18, and 25, respectively. The study was conducted at the Center for Clinical Simulation at the Universidad del Rosario in Bogota, Colombia. All residents and participants signed informed consent, and the protocol was approved by the ethics committee of the same university.

### Technique

The equipment used was the *Sonosite ultrasound*-EDGE C60 with a 2–5 MHz transducer [14]. Transducer was positioned in the epigastrium and directed toward the left shoulder where, with the indicator on the right, the cardiac view was obtained. Then, the transducer was rotated 90° until the indicator was cephalic, where the longitudinal view of the IVC was obtained. At this point, a six-second video was taken.

Success was defined as a score of three which, according to the ACEP guidelines [1], allows the minimum adequate identification of key structures needed to make clinical decisions; clear identification of the inferior vena cava with visualization of at least 2 cm distal to the entrance of the vena cava to the right atrium, where the measurement of a cross-sectional cut should be performed. It was not necessary for the images to be centered, nor to have the adequate image depth.

### Experimental design

We used a complete factorial experimental design, i.e., a set of all possible combinations between models and operators [15]. The sample size of the experiment was set at 25 repetitions per operator, according to the recommendations of the guidelines for emergency ultrasonography, and, in order to ensure the minimum number of observations per subject [16]. This type of experiment allows to examine simultaneously the effect of each level of observation (repetition and residents) on the dependent variable, as well as the effect of interactions among factors. Data collection was conducted in March, 2015.

Variables included year of residency, gender, and the duration of each repetition defined as the time in seconds elapsed from when the transducer touches the skin and the operator determines that the best image of the IVC through the subxiphoid window has been obtained, until the end of a 6 s recording of the image.

All data were stored electronically through anonymous records and were evaluated by the expert, using the scale for quality assurance proposed by the ACEP. Table 1 shows the ACEP suggested quality assurance grading scale, 2011 [17].

**Table 1 Suggested quality assurance grading scale ACEP, 2011**

| Punctuation | Definition |
|---|---|
| 1 | No recognizable structures, no objective data can be gathered |
| 2 | Minimally recognizable structures but insufficient for diagnosis |
| 3 | Minimal criteria met for diagnosis, recognizable structures but with some technical or other flaws |
| 4 | Minimal criteria met for diagnosis, all structures imaged well and diagnosis easily supported |
| 5 | Minimal criteria met for diagnosis, all structures imaged with excellent image quality and diagnosis completely supported |

The scale consists of five levels. *1* is the lowest grade: image fails to recognize anatomical structures and therefore does not allow a diagnosis. *2* recognizes anatomical structures but not enough to make a diagnosis. *3* image allows a diagnosis, but there are certain failures in the image's position or image gain and depth. *4* and *5*, diagnostic is supported by images of good and excellent quality, respectively

### Statistical analysis

The descriptive analysis of quantitative variables was carried out by calculating means and standard deviations (SD), whereas categorical variables were reported as frequencies and percentages. The homogeneity of the answers by subgroups conformed by residents, gender, and year of residency was assessed by means of $\chi^2$-like tests; the association between the time and the number of subxiphoid window ultrasound examinations was evaluated using Spearman's rank correlation coefficient [18]. To identify the learning curve, we developed a two-level repeated measures model [19, 20], considering the residents as clustering units. The model (with success/failure variable response) was based on the logistic function to estimate the adjusted probabilities of success [19, 20]. All analyses were performed using the STATA V.12 statistical package [21].

**Table 2 Percentages and mean time for subxiphoid visualization of the IVC by novice EM Colombian residents**

| Resident | Success[a] | | Time (seconds) | |
|---|---|---|---|---|
| | *n* | % | Mean | SD |
| 1 | 20 | 80 | 13.5 | 4.1 |
| 2 | 19 | 76 | 16.7 | 8.2 |
| 3 | 23 | 92 | 24.1 | 9.6 |
| 4 | 13 | 52 | 17.6 | 9.8 |
| 5 | 17 | 64 | 17.2 | 5.44 |
| 6 | 24 | 96 | 15.7 | 7.2 |
| 7 | 22 | 88 | 18.9 | 9.3 |
| 8 | 24 | 96 | 14.7 | 4.3 |
| Total | 200 | 81 | 17.3 | 8.06 |

First column represents the total of residents that participate in the experiment. Followed columns represent the number and the percentage of success defined as a grading equal or greater than 3 according to an expert fulfillment of ACEP criteria [16]. Finally, the table presents mean time and standard deviations in seconds used by each resident in performing the repetitions

[a] Expert grading equal or greater than 3, according to ACEP [16]

## Results

We collected information on eight operators: three first year, two second year, and three third year residents. We did not collect information on three more ones (two first year and one third year) because they had previous training in ultrasonography. The final four residents enrolled in the program left the experiment voluntarily. The sample size reached 200 repetitions.

The most of repetitions ($n = 114$) were graded as three [11]. Twenty-two repetitions obtained the highest score (11 %), and nine repetitions earned the minimum score. The percentage of success by resident was between 52 and 96 % (Table 2). No relationship was found between gender and success ($p = 0.83$), but there was a relationship between year of residency and success ($p < 0.001$).

The average total time per repetition was 17.3 s (SD 8.1) (Table 2), although there was no statistically significant association between length of the repetition and the number of repetitions ($p = 0.18$). In addition, no significant differences were found between length of repetition and outcome (success/fail) ($p = 0.2$).

Regarding the learning curve, we calculated the probability of success adjusting by repetition and resident (Fig. 1); we estimated a maximum probability of 0.8 for repetition 11 (range 0.54 a 0.92), and repetition 21 had a probability of 0.9 (range 0.75–0.96).

## Discussion

This work assessed the learning process and the improvement in proficiency of the point-of-care ultrasound technique in Colombian EM residents. For that, we built a learning curve in order to guarantee a proportion of success greater than 80 % in performing the point-of-care ultrasound technique for subxiphoid visualization of the IVC, with adequate quality according to the ACEP, in novice EM residents. The number of repetitions needed to achieve 80 % success was found to be eleven, and for 90 % success, twenty-one repetitions were needed. No differences were found between success percentages by

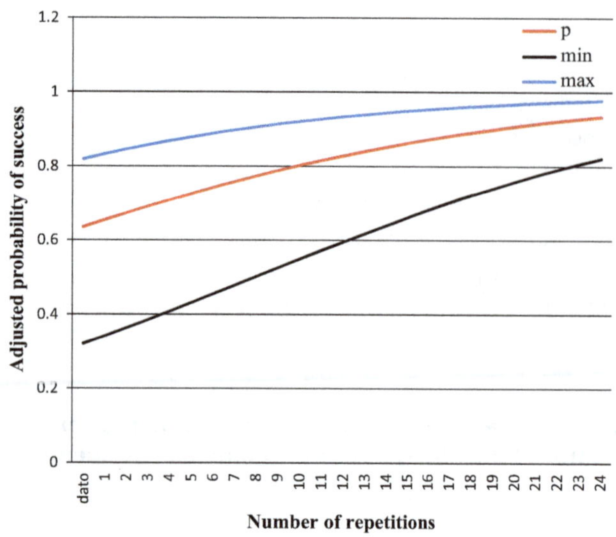


**Fig. 1** Learning curve for point-of-care ultrasound technique for subxiphoid visualization of the IVC by novice EM Colombian residents. The *y axis* shows the probability of success adjusted by repetition and resident. The *x axis* shows the repetition number. The *curve* shows how the probability of success increases with number of repetitions. The *red line* is the average probability, while the *blue lines* represent minimum and maximum values

gender, but there were differences by year of residency. However, due to the low number of residents, the multivariate model was not adjusted by year of residency. No statistically significant differences were found related to the time needed to acquire the image.

These results support the hypothesis that fewer than twenty-five repetitions are needed to achieve an acceptable quality ultrasonographic image of the IVC which is useful for decision making in clinical practice [17]. Previous evidence reported heterogeneous results about the number of repetitions [22–24] due to methodological or context variations of each scenario. Some authors have reported 10 repetitions as the optimal number needed to visualize anatomic structures in the right upper abdominal quadrant [25].

Our results should be interpreted with caution to the extent that the small sample size leads to a model with precision limitations in the effect measurement. However, the big percentages of success with increased numbers of repetitions allowed us to think there would be similar results with bigger sample sizes. The number of models was chosen based on practical issues and the ACEP recommendations to assess the quality of the ultrasound images, even without being validated. In consequence, future research must include an extensive group of individuals, local models, and operators.

Accordingly, the scope of the results is in some way limited to our own background. As far as we know, this is the first study in Colombia designed for building a learning curve for this technique, and controlled by the operators' adaptation. Moreover, in so far as the agreement between residents and the expert regarding the perception of the best ultrasound window was partially assessed, finding a measure of collapsibility or vena cava diameter may require a similar number of repetitions. In this regard, Fields et al. suggested at least 15 repetitions in order novice operators to obtain a reliable measure of IVC diameter through the subxiphoid ultrasound window. This result was not generated from a curve, but based on the assumption that an additional five repetitions above the baseline of 10 repetitions increases the degree of congruence between the residents and the experts [26].

Finally, although these results correspond to the practical verification of the average time used to improve the technique of IVC ultrasound window in the Colombian context, they set a precedent for the evaluation of this type of diagnostic procedures in the local and regional community. Lastly, methodology used makes it easy to extrapolate the evaluation process carried out here to other areas of medical education assessment, particularly with regard to obtaining other, more complex, good quality ultrasound windows.

### Authors' contributions

MGB conceived the study; had primary responsibility for design, overall planning, and interpretation; and drafted the manuscript. JCO participated in the conception and design. JMM participated in the design, data analysis, and manuscript drafting. AMB participated in study design and manuscript drafting. YFB participated in study design and manuscript drafting. All authors read and approved the final manuscript.

### Author details

[1] Emergency Medicine Specialist, Universidad del Rosario, Bogotá, Colombia. [2] Epidemiology, Biostatistics and Public Health Research Group, EPIBIOS_UR, Escuela de Medicina y Ciencias de la Salud (EMCS), Universidad del Rosario, Bogotá, Colombia. [3] Chief of the Department of Emergency Medicine and Director of the Simulation Center, Escuela de Medicina y Ciencias de la Salud (EMCS), Universidad del Rosario, Bogotá, Colombia.

### Acknowledgements

The authors thank the residents of the EM program at the Universidad del Rosario for their participation. We also thank Universidad del Rosario for the use of the Simulation Laboratory facilities and equipment.

### References

1. American College of Emergency Physicians (ACEP) (2008) Emergency ultrasound Guidelines. Am Coll Emerg Physicians 53:1–38
2. Sippel S, Muruganandan K, Levine A, Shah S (2011) Review article: use of ultrasound in the developing world. Int J Emerg Med 4:72. doi:10.1186/1865-1380-4-72
3. Beaulieu Y, Marik PE (2005) Bedside ultrasonography in the ICU. Chest 128:1766–1781
4. Perera P, Mailhot T (2012) The RUSH exam 2012: rapid ultrasound in shock in the evaluation of the critically Ill patient. Ultrasound Clin 7:255–278. doi:10.1016/j.cult.2011.12.010
5. Weekes AJ, Quirke DP (2011) Emergency echocardiography. Emerg Med Clin North Am 29:759–787. doi:10.1016/j.emc.2011.08.002
6. Lanctôt J-F, Valois M, Beaulieu Y (2011) EGLS: echo-guided life support. Crit Ultrasound J 3:123–129. doi:10.1007/s13089-011-0083-2
7. Rudski LG, Lai WW, Afilalo J et al (2010) Guidelines for the echocardiographic assessment of the right heart in adults: a report from the Ameri-

can Society of Echocardiography endorsed by the European Association of Echocardiography, a registered branch of the European Society of Cardiology, and t. J Am Soc Echocardiogr 23:685–688. doi:10.1016/j.echo.2010.05.010

8. Via G, Hussain A, Wells M et al (2014) International evidence-based recommendations for focused cardiac ultrasound. J Am Soc Echocardiogr 27:1–683. doi:10.1016/j.echo.2014.05.001
9. Henwood PC, Beversluis D, Genthon A et al (2014) Characterizing the limited use of point-of-care ultrasound in Colombian emergency medicine residencies. Int J Emerg Med 7:7
10. Enomoto TM, Harder L (2010) Dynamic indices of preload. Crit Care Clin 26:307–321. doi:10.1016/j.ccc.2009.12.004
11. American College of Emergency Physicians (2009) Emergency ultrasound guidelines. Ann Emerg Med 53:550–570
12. Mandeville JC, Colebourn CL (2012) Can transthoracic echocardiography be used to predict fluid responsiveness in the critically ill patient? A systematic review. Crit Care Res Pract 2012:513480. doi:10.1155/2012/513480
13. Ma OJ, Gaddis G, Norvell JG, Subramanian S (2008) How fast is the focused assessment with sonography for trauma examination learning curve? Emerg Med Australas 20:32–37. doi:10.1111/j.1742-6723.2007.01039.x
14. SonoSite Edge C60x Transducer. http://www.umiultrasound.com/ultrasound-transducers/sonosite/edge/c60-transducer. Accessed 11 May 2015
15. Parker R, Browne W (2014) The place of experimental design and statistics. ILAR J 55:477–485
16. Kleinbaum D, Klein M (2010) Interaction Assessment Stage. In: Gail M, Krickeberg K, Samet JM, Tsiatis A (eds) Logist regres a self-learning Text, 3rd edn. Springer, New York, pp 207–210
17. American College of Emergency Physicians (ACEP) (2011) Emergency Ultrasound Standard Reporting Guidelines. http://www.acep.org/workarea/DownloadAsset.aspx?id=82679. Accessed 3 May 2015
18. Fieller E, Hartley H, Pearson E (1957) Tests for rank correlation coefficients. Biometrika 44:470–481
19. Zunzunegui M, García De Yébenes M, Forster M et al (2004) Aplicaciones de los modelos multinivel al análisis de medidas repetidas en estudios longitudinales. Rev Esp Salud Publica 78:177–188
20. Aparicio A, Morera M (2007) La conveniencia del análisis multinivel para la investigación en salud. Población y Salud en Mesoamérica. doi:10.15517/psm.v4i2.4556
21. StataCorp. 2015. Stata Statistical Software: Release 14. College Station, TX: StataCorp LP
22. Gaspari J, Dickman E, Blehar D (2009) Learning curve of bedside ultrasound of the gallbladder. J Emerg Med 37:51–56
23. Hertzberg B, Kliewer M, Bowie J et al (2000) Physician training requirements in sonography: how many cases are needed for competence? Am J Roentgenol 174:1221–1227
24. Jang TB, Ruggeri W (2010) Learning curve of emergency physicians using emergency bedside sonography for symptomatic first-trimester pregnancy. J Ultrasound Med 29:1423–1428
25. Jang T, Aubin C, Naunheim R (2004) Minimum training for right upper quadrant ultrasonography. Am J Emerg Med 22:439–443
26. Fields J, Lee P, Jenq K et al (2011) The interrater reliability of inferior vena cava ultrasound by bedside clinician sonographers in emergency department patients. Acad Emerg Med 18:98–101

2

# A unique method for estimating the reliability learning curve of optic nerve sheath diameter ultrasound measurement

Frederick A. Zeiler[1], Markus T. Ziesmann[1], Patrick Goeres[2], Bertram Unger[3], Jason Park[1], Dimitrios Karakitsos[4], Michael Blaivas[5], Ashley Vergis[1] and Lawrence M. Gillman[1*]

**Abstract**

**Background:** Optic nerve sheath diameter (ONSD) measurement using ultrasound has been proposed as a rapid, non-invasive, point of care technique to estimate intra-cranial pressure (ICP). Ultrasonic measurement of the optic nerve sheath can be quite challenging and there is limited literature surrounding learning curves for this technique. We attempted to develop a method to estimate the reliability learning curve for ONSD measurement utilizing a unique definition of reliability: a plateau in within-subject variability with unchanged between-subject variability.

**Methods:** As part of a previously published study, a single operator measured the ONSD in 120 healthy volunteers over a 6-month period. Utilizing the assumption that the four measurements made on each subject during this study should be equal, the relationship of within-subject variance was described using a quadratic-plateau model as assessed by segmental polynomial (knot) regression.

**Results:** Segmental polynomial (knot) regression revealed a plateau in within-subject variance after the 21st subject. However, there was no difference in overall mean values [3.69 vs 3.68 mm ($p = 0.884$)] or between-subject variance [14.49 vs 11.92 ($p = 0.54$)] above or below this cutoff.

**Conclusions:** This study suggests a significant finite learning curve associated with ONSD measurements. It also offers a unique method of calculating the learning curve associated with ONSD measurement.

**Keywords:** Point of Care ultrasound, Optic nerve sheath diameter, Ultrasound, Intracranial pressure, Education, Learning curve

## Background

In head injured patients, elevated intra-cranial pressure (ICP) is associated with worse outcomes [1]. One of the fundamental tenants of management involves identifying those with elevated ICP and intervening to lessen and control this pressure [2]. Optic nerve sheath diameter (ONSD) measurement using ultrasound has been proposed as a rapid, non-invasive, point of care technique to estimate ICP [3]. This has been suggested as a screening tool for, or even an alternative to, invasive ICP measurement. Traditionally ICP is measured via a surgically inserted, intracranial (subdural, intra-parenchymal or intra-ventricular) pressure monitor. While this is a fairly common procedure it carries a finite but not insignificant rate of complications (most notably intracranial hemorrhage and infection) [4] and is for the most part limited to centres with neurosurgical capabilities. Given the growing use of ultrasound in the emergency department, critical care units and even in the field, point-of-care estimation of ICP using ultrasound is appealing as it can be performed in a wide variety of locations, is easily repeatable and does not require transport of the patient or large diagnostic equipment (such as CT scanners). Its utility has been substantiated by a number of small studies in diverse populations including traumatic brain

*Correspondence: gillmanlm@yahoo.ca
[1] Departments of Surgery, University of Manitoba, 409 Tache Avenue, Winnipeg, MB R2H 2A6, Canada
Full list of author information is available at the end of the article

injury, mass lesion, infection and post transplant reperfusion injury [5–9].

The technique, however, can be quite challenging. It requires the measurement of an often moving, sub-centimeter structure, estimated to the nearest 0.1 of a millimeter, stretching both the limits of the operator and the resolution of the ultrasound unit. Significant inter-rater variance early in the learning curve is a potential concern that could affect the utility of this approach in more novice users. The literature surrounding learning curves for point of care ultrasound in general is limited [10] and even more so for the specific technique of ONSD measurement [11]. Here we attempt to employ a unique statistical method for estimating the potential learning curve for ONSD measurement.

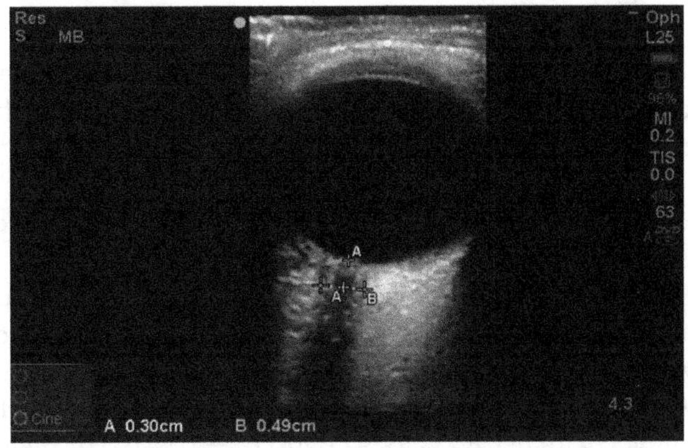


**Fig. 1** Sample image of ultrasonic ONSD measurement (measurement "*B*"), measured 3 mm behind the optic nerve head (measurement "*A*")

## Methods

### Ultrasound technique

As part of a previously published study [12] a single trained operator (LG) measured the ONSD in 120 healthy volunteers over a 6-month period. This operator was trained in this technique during a World Interactive Network Focused On Critical Ultrasound (WINFOCUS) ultrasound course and has a number of previous publications in this area [12–14]. All subjects signed a consent form approved by the University of Manitoba Health Research Ethics Board (H2013:199).

Subjects were placed in the supine position and images were obtained through a closed eyelid. A 13–6 MHz linear array ultrasound transducer (L25x transducer with a Sonosite M-Turbo Ultrasound Machine, SonoSite Inc, Bothell, WA) was used with the ophthalmic preset thus minimizing the power and acoustic output of the ultrasound system. The probe was placed gently on the upper eyelid. The ONSD was measured in a direction perpendicular to the axis of the nerve, in each eye, in the horizontal and sagittal plane, 3 mm behind the optic nerve head (Fig. 1), for a total of four measurements per subject.

### Method for assessing the learning curve

For the sake of the learning curve analysis it was assumed that the four measurements (left, right, horizontal, sagittal) in each patient should be identical and any differences in these values are the result of measurement error.

The relationship of within-subject variance was described using a quadratic–plateau model as assessed by segmental polynomial regression [15] to determine how many subject measurements were needed before the operator achieved a stable within-subject variance. Segmental polynomial regression, or knot regression, allows the opportunity to fit multiple regression lines to different portions of a dataset, which then join at a "knot" value which represents the intersection of these two regression lines (in this case the plateau of the learning curve). In this specific variant of segmental polynomial regression, the quadratic-plateau model, a quadratic curve is fit to the early data and a flat line (plateau) to the later data. This model is able to predict the exact point of plateau in the learning curve as it describes how many subjects were needed before the ultrasonographer achieved a stable within-subject variance.

### Assessing data before and after the "knot"

To ensure there was no inherent differences in the data other than the plateau of within-subject variance before and after the "knot" variable as described above, the means of the early (subjects before the "knot" or plateau) versus late (subjects after the "knot") measurements were compared using Welch Two Sample *t* tests. As well, the homogeneity of the between-subject variance was examined for early versus late measurements utilizing Levene's test for homogeneity of variance.

Analysis was completed using both the Statistical Analysis Software version 9.3 (SAS Institute, Cary, NC) and R Statistical Library (R Core Team, 2013).

## Results

Subjects included 65 males and 55 females. Mean age was 29.3 (range 18–65). Overall mean ONSD measurement was 3.68 (95 % CI 2.85–4.40) [12]. Segmental polynomial (knot) regression revealed a plateau in within-subject variance, var($I$), at subject index ($I$) 21 (Fig. 1). Below the knot (Subject 21), the best-fit equation is:

$$\text{var}(I) = 19.73 - 1.614I + 0.03843I^2$$

Above the knot, the best-fit equation is simply the plateau value:

$$\mathrm{var}(I) = 2.78$$

Based on the segmental polynomial regression and the plateau of within-subject variance at subject 21 we utilized this as the cut-off for defining early (subjects before the "knot" or plateau) vs late (subjects after the "knot") measurements. The mean measurements for each subject were compared between the early and late groups using Welch Two Sample $t$ tests (Table 1) with no difference seen. In addition, utilizing Levene's test for homogeneity, the between-subject variance was compared in these two groups revealing no difference between early and late groups [14.49 (early) vs 11.92 (late) ($p = 0.54$)]. For males and females, respectively, it was 12.64 (early) vs 9.48 (late) ($p = 0.33$) and 12.50 (early) vs 11.71 (late) ($p = 0.95$).

## Discussion

Determining the learning curve associated with point of care ultrasound has been investigated in multiple studies across a number of techniques. The most commonly studied technique is the focused assessment with sonography in trauma (FAST) exam [10]. Estimates for the learning curve associated with this technique have been extremely variable, however, and range from 10 [16, 17] to 200 studies [18] and even up to 500 scans [19]. The heterogeneity in these results likely results from the fact that there is no clear, accepted definition of what is an acceptable performance. The majority of these studies utilized clinical endpoints (correct identification of free fluid) to define the learning curve with varying thresholds of acceptable results [10, 16–18, 20–23], while only a single study utilized an assessment of image quality and technique [24].

To our knowledge, only a single study to date has commented on the learning curve associated with ONSD measurement. In their 2007 study, Tayal et al. [11] concluded that this technique can be learned relatively quickly with a learning curve of between 10 and 25 scans depending on previous ultrasound experience. However, the origin of these estimates is not clearly discussed within the manuscript and in discussion with the senior author of this paper, these figures were estimated based on qualitative observation and not based on objective measures (personal communication).

**Table 1 Welch two sample *t* test comparing mean of early versus late mean ONSD measurements using subject 21 as a cutoff**

| | Early ONSD mean (mm) | Late ONSD mean (mm) | *p* value |
|---|---|---|---|
| Overall | 3.69 | 3.68 | 0.884 |
| Males | 3.88 | 3.78 | 0.454 |
| Females | 3.52 | 3.55 | 0.869 |

As in other forms of point of care sonography, one of the challenges associated with determining a learning curve involves the definition of acceptable performance. This is even more so an issue for ONSD measurement as it requires a quantitative assessment of a specific structure that is inherently difficult to measure making comparison to a control or reference value challenging. For example, in comparison with the work done in FAST one could use clinical outcomes and prediction of elevated ICP as a surrogate of competency but this does not determine if the numeric measurement of ONSD is accurate. Alternatively, one could use an assessment tool of ONSD image quality and generation but currently as apposed to FAST [25], no such validated tool exists. One could use comparison of results to another imaging technique (MRI or CT scan). While this has been used to assess the utility of ultrasound ONSD measurement [6] to date this has not been used to assess learning curves. One could also compare to the results of an expert but again this requires the definition of an expert. Finally, one could use a model with known ONSD measurements as was recently developed by our group [13, 14]. While measurements in the model tend to be easier than real life and may underestimate the learning curve-crisper borders to the simulated optic nerve sheath, and no eye movement to contend with-of the options available, it certainly seems the most feasible and reproducible and an area requiring further study.

One important dimension in proficiency with this skill is the ability to making reliable measurements. In this study, we utilized a unique definition of reliability. First, by assuming the presence of an internal control between each measurement in each eye and assuming any error/variance between these measurements is due measurement error. There are a number of recent ultrasound studies that give credence to this assumption by suggesting there may be no difference between right and left ONSD measurements [26–28]. In addition, since the variance did indeed plateau over time it does lend some credibility to the technique (Fig. 2). In addition, the use of the quadratic plateau polynomial regression model is unique to this study but presents a seemingly reliable way to determine the learning curve. This model allows a quadratic regression curve to be fit to the early data and a flat line (plateau) to the later data thus allowing the model to predict the exact point of plateau in the learning curve as it describes how many subjects were needed before the sonographer achieved a stable within-subject variance. Given four measurements per subject and a plateau at subject 21, this suggests that the error may plateau after approximately 80 individual measurements of ONSD.

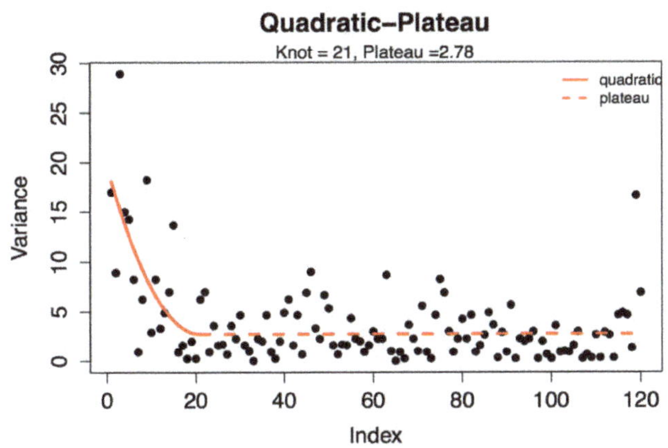


**Fig. 2** Segmental polynomial (knot) regression of within-subject variance showing a plateau (knot) at subject 21

Due to the difference in variance in early versus late subjects we questioned the validity of the measurements in the initial 21 subjects in our previous publication. However, despite the increased variability, since our original data was reported using the mean of four measurements any random measurement error should cancel out. By defining the early group as all subjects measured up to subject 21 and the late group as subjects 22–120 we compared both the mean measurements and the between-subject variance between these two groups. Neither of these revealed a difference confirming that despite the increased within-subject variance in the first 21 subjects, the overall mean and between subject variance was equal between these groups meaning the first 21 measurements were still valid.

### Study limitations

There are a number of significant limitations to this study performed in healthy volunteers. First, as mentioned earlier, when calculating the learning curve it is assumed that the actual ONSD measurement should be identical in each subject in both the right and left eye. However, even if these measurements are not identical [and our results would substantiate this since there still is some within-subject variability remaining even after the plateau (Fig. 2)] the plateau in this variability may still represent a useful definition of reliability. This is an area that requires further confirmation. Second, we have used a single operator to minimize inter-observer bias and hence to test the new statistical method for the estimation of the learning curve in a rather small group of healthy volunteers. This operator was not blinded to the measurements but the calculation of learning curve was a post hoc analysis and not the initial intention of the original study. Further studies are clearly required including in larger number of subjects and with more observers to confirm the current results. Finally, the operator in this study was in fact not a novice but his previous experience with this technique, although considerable, was on a more sporadic basis prior to this study. This does not lessen the finding of the learning curve but does suggest that the learning curve may be significantly longer than we have estimated in the case of true novices. In addition, it may also suggest a significant decay of skills if the technique is not practiced regularly and could suggest the need for retraining after a prolonged period of inactivity or regular maintenance of skills through simulation. The aforementioned concepts will be a focus of a future study.

## Conclusions

Despite the obvious limitations, this study offers a unique method of calculating the learning curve associated with ONSD utilizing a new definition of reliability by looking at within-subject variability and a unique statistical model to calculate the plateau in this variability.

#### Abbreviations

ONSD: optic nerve sheath diameter; FAST: focused assessment with sonography in trauma; ICP: intra-cranial pressure.

#### Authors' contributions

All authors were involved in study design, data analysis and manuscript composition. LG and PG were involved in data collection. All authors read and approved the final manuscript.

#### Author details

[1] Departments of Surgery, University of Manitoba, 409 Tache Avenue, Winnipeg, MB R2H 2A6, Canada. [2] Undergraduate Medical Education, University of Manitoba, Winnipeg, MB, Canada. [3] Medical Education, University of Manitoba, Winnipeg, MB, Canada. [4] Departments of Internal Medicine, University of South Carolina, School of Medicine, Columbia, SC, USA. [5] Departments of Internal Medicine and Emergency Medicine, University of South Carolina, School of Medicine, Columbia, SC, USA.

#### References

1. Jones PA, Andrews PJ, Midgley S et al (1994) Measuring the burden of secondary insults in head-injured patients during intensive care. J Neurosurg Anesthesiol 6:4–14
2. Brain Trauma Foundation, American Association of Neurological Surgeons, Congress of Neurological Surgeons (2007) Guidelines for the management of severe traumatic brain injury. J Neurotrauma 24(Suppl 1):S1–106. doi:10.1089/neu.2007.9999
3. Gangemi M, Cennamo G, Maiuri F, D'Andrea F (1987) Echographic measurement of the optic nerve in patients with intracranial hypertension. Neurochirurgia 30:53–55. doi:10.1055/s-2008-1053656
4. Guyot LL, Dowling C, Diaz FG, Michael DB (1998) Cerebral monitoring devices: analysis of complications. Acta Neurochir Suppl 71:47–49
5. Geeraerts T, Launey Y, Martin L et al (2007) Ultrasonography of the optic nerve sheath may be useful for detecting raised intracranial pressure after severe brain injury. Intensive Care Med 33:1704–1711. doi:10.1007/s00134-007-0797-6
6. Geeraerts T, Newcombe VFJ, Coles JP et al (2008) Use of T2-weighted magnetic resonance imaging of the optic nerve sheath to detect raised intracranial pressure. Crit Care 12:R114. doi:10.1186/cc7006
7. Moretti R, Pizzi B (2011) Ultrasonography of the optic nerve in neurocritically ill patients. Acta Anaesthesiol Scand 55:644–652. doi:10.1111/j.1399-6576.2011.02432.x

8. Dubourg J, Javouhey E, Geeraerts T et al (2011) Ultrasonography of optic nerve sheath diameter for detection of raised intracranial pressure: a systematic review and meta-analysis. Intensive Care Med 37:1059–1068. doi:10.1007/s00134-011-2224-2
9. Seo H, Kim Y-K, Shin WJ, Hwang GS (2013) Ultrasonographic optic nerve sheath diameter is correlated with arterial carbon dioxide concentration during reperfusion in liver transplant recipients. Transplant Proc 45:2272–2276. doi:10.1016/j.transproceed.2012.12.032
10. Thomas B, Falcone RE, Vasquez D et al (1997) Ultrasound evaluation of blunt abdominal trauma: program implementation, initial experience, and learning curve. J Trauma Inj Infect Crit Care 42:384–388 **(discussion 388–90)**
11. Tayal VS, Neulander M, Norton HJ et al (2007) Emergency department sonographic measurement of optic nerve sheath diameter to detect findings of increased intracranial pressure in adult head injury patients. Ann Emerg Med 49:508–514. doi:10.1016/j.annemergmed.2006.06.040
12. Goeres P, Zeiler FA, Unger B et al (2015) Ultrasound assessment of optic nerve sheath diameter in healthy volunteers. J Crit Care 31:168–171. doi:10.1016/j.jcrc.2015.10.009
13. Zeiler FA, Unger B, Kramer AH et al (2013) A unique model for ultrasound assessment of optic nerve sheath diameter. Can J Neurol Sci 40:225–229
14. Zeiler FA, Unger B, Zhu Q et al (2014) A unique model for ONSD Part II: inter/intra-operator variability. Can J Neurol Sci 41:430–435
15. SAS Institute Inc. (2008) NLIN Procedure. SAS/STAT 9.2 user's guide. SAS Institute Inc., Cary
16. Smith RS, Kern SJ, Fry WR, Helmer SD (1998) Institutional learning curve of surgeon-performed trauma ultrasound. Arch Surg 133:530–535 **(discussion 535–6)**
17. Shackford SR, Rogers FB, Osler TM et al (1999) Focused abdominal sonogram for trauma: the learning curve of nonradiologist clinicians in detecting hemoperitoneum. J Trauma Inj Infect Crit Care 46:553–562 **(discussion 562–4)**
18. Scalea TM, Rodriguez A, Chiu WC et al (1999) Focused assessment with sonography for trauma (FAST): results from an international consensus conference. J Trauma 46:466–472
19. American Institute of Ultrasound in Medicine (2014) Training guidelines for physicians who evaluate and interpret diagnostic abdominal/general ultrasound examinations. http://www.aium.org/resources/viewStatement.aspx?id=47. Accessed 3 Nov 2015
20. Rozycki GS (1998) Surgeon-performed ultrasound: its use in clinical practice. Ann Surg 228:16–28
21. Frezza EEE, Solis RLR, Silich RJR et al (1999) Competency-based instruction to improve the surgical resident technique and accuracy of the trauma ultrasound. Am Surg 65:884–888
22. McCarter FD, Luchette FA, Molloy M et al (2000) Institutional and individual learning curves for focused abdominal ultrasound for trauma: cumulative sum analysis. Ann Surg 231:689–700
23. Gracias VH, Frankel HL, Gupta R et al (2001) Defining the learning curve for the focused abdominal sonogram for trauma (FAST) examination: implications for credentialing. Am Surg 67:364–368
24. Jang T, Kryder G, Sineff S et al (2012) The technical errors of physicians learning to perform focused assessment with sonography in trauma. Acad Emerg Med 19:98–101. doi:10.1111/j.1553-2712.2011.01242.x
25. Ziesmann MT, Park J, Unger BJ et al (2015) Validation of the quality of ultrasound imaging and competence (QUICk) score as an objective assessment tool for the FAST examination. J Trauma Acute Care Surg 78:1008–1013. doi:10.1097/TA.0000000000000639
26. Asghar A, Hashmi M, Hussain A (2015) Optic nerve sheath diameter evaluated by transorbital sonography in healthy volunteers from Pakistan. Anaesth Pain Intensive Care 19:282–286
27. Lovrencic-Huzjan A, Simicevic DS, Popovic IM, Puretic MB, Cvetkovic VV, Gopcevic A et al (2012) Ultrasonography of the optic nerve sheath in brain death. Perspect Med 1:414–416
28. Chen H, Ding G-S, Zhao Y-C, Yu R-G, Zhou J-X (2015) Ultrasound measurement of optic nerve diameter and optic nerve sheath diameter in healthy Chinese adults. BMC Neurol 15:106

# 3

# Diagnostic accuracy of lung ultrasonography combined with procalcitonin for the diagnosis of pneumonia

Peiman Nazerian[1*], Gabriele Cerini[1], Simone Vanni[1], Chiara Gigli[1], Maurizio Zanobetti[1], Maurizio Bartolucci[2], Stefano Grifoni[1] and Giovanni Volpicelli[3]

**Abstract**

**Background:** The diagnostic value of lung ultrasonography (LUS) and procalcitonin (PCT) in the diagnosis of lung infections is known. No studies evaluated the combination of LUS and PCT for the diagnosis of pneumonia in the emergency department (ED). We evaluated the diagnostic accuracy of the combination of LUS and PCT in the diagnosis of pneumonia.

**Methods:** Patients with respiratory symptoms of unexplained origin who underwent a chest CT in ED were included in the study if PCT assay was available. LUS was performed before CT and was targeted to the detection of lung consolidations with the morphologic features of pneumonia. A PCT assay was performed at presentation, and cut-off of 0.25 and of 0.5 ng/ml were used to rule-out and rule-in pneumonia. The final diagnosis of pneumonia was established by independent clinicians, on the basis of clinical chart review including CT results.

**Results:** We enrolled 128 patients and pneumonia was the final diagnosis in 61 (47.7%). In 38 patients (29.7%) LUS and PCT were negative (PCT < 0.25 ng/ml). The overall accuracy, sensitivity and negative predictive value of LUS/PCT were 88.8, 96.7 and 94.7% respectively. Sensitivity of the LUS/PCT test was significantly superior to LUS alone (85.2%) and PCT alone (73.8%) ($p < 0.05$ for both). Specificity and positive predictive value of the combination of positivity of LUS/PCT (PCT > 0.5 ng/ml) were 94% and 83.3% respectively. Specificity of LUS/PCT was not significantly different to LUS alone (88.1%) ($p = 0.125$).

**Conclusions:** The sensitivity of the combination of LUS with PCT for the diagnosis of pneumonia was significantly superior when compared with the sensitivity of LUS and PCT alone.

**Keywords:** Biomarkers, Diagnosis, Pneumonia, Ultrasound, Procalcitonin

## Background

Pneumonia is an infection that involves alveoli, distal airways, and interstitium leading to lung inflammatory consolidations and is one of the major infection-related cause of death in developed countries [1, 2].

The mainstay of the diagnosis is based on symptoms and signs consistent with acute infection of the lower respiratory tract associated with the visualization of at least one pulmonary consolidation at chest imaging. For the purpose of imaging the consolidation, chest computed tomography (CT) is the diagnostic gold standard. Unfortunately CT can't be used routinely because of high cost, radiation exposure and scarce availability in low resources settings [3]. Thus, in clinical practice, chest radiography (CXR) represents the standard of care and is mostly used to diagnose pneumonia. However, in patients evaluated in the emergency department (ED), CXR showed a poor sensitivity (43.5%) when compared to CT [4]. Therefore, reliance on CXR to diagnose pneumonia may lead to significant rates of misdiagnosis.

*Correspondence: pnazerian@hotmail.com
[1] Department of Emergency Medicine, Careggi University Hospital, Largo Brambilla 3, 50134 Florence, Italy
Full list of author information is available at the end of the article

Lung ultrasonography (LUS) is an emerging bedside diagnostic tool with a sensitivity of 94% and a specificity of 96% for the diagnosis of pneumonia according to a recent metanalysis [5]. Procalcitonin (PCT) expression in parenchymal tissue is induced by bacterial infection and its concentrations have been successfully used to diagnose and guide antibiotic therapy in lower respiratory tract infections [6, 7].

No previous studies have evaluated the accuracy of a combination of LUS and PCT for the diagnosis of pneumonia in the ED. Thus, the aim of our study was to assess the diagnostic accuracy of the combination of LUS with PCT when the final diagnosis was supported by a chest CT imaging.

## Methods

### Study subjects and design

This is a prospective accuracy study, in which patients enrolled in a registry from December 2011 to August 2012 were included if PCT level at admission was available [8]. Patients were recruited in the ED with an annual census of 130,000 visits. The study was approved by the local institutional review board. Written informed consent was obtained for inclusion in the study.

Consecutive patients aged >18 years with at least one unexplained respiratory complaint among dyspnea, chest pain, cough or hemoptysis with or without fever, for which the attending emergency physician ordered a chest CT were considered in the study. PCT was ordered by the attending emergency physician, independent from the study protocol, when a infective cause was suspected.

### Methods

Lung ultrasonography was performed before and within 3 h from chest CT by one of eight sonographer investigators who participated to the study. The investigators were four internal and emergency medicine staff physicians with at least 5 years experience on point-of-care emergency ultrasonography and four resident physicians (two in Internal Medicine and two in Emergency Medicine) with at least 6 months training in emergency ultrasound. The investigators were aware of the presenting symptoms and the evident physical signs, but were blinded to all the other general clinical information including any radiologic finding and laboratory results. The following multi-probe machines were used: MyLab30 Gold (Esaote, Genova, Italy) and HD7 (Philips, Amsterdam, Holland). LUS was performed by using a 4–8 MHz linear probe or a 3.5–5 MHz curved array probe. The lung was examined by longitudinal and oblique scans on anterior, lateral and posterior chest. The patient was preferably examined in the sitting position. When this latter position could not be maintained, due to critical clinical conditions or poor compliance, the examination was performed in the supine or semi-recumbent position. The posterior areas were scanned in the sitting position or, when not feasible, by turning the patient in the lateral decubitus on both sides. The LUS examination was targeted to the detection of typical subpleural lung consolidations with tissue-like or anechoic pattern and blurred, irregular margins with associated focal B-lines [9]. The consolidations due to infection usually show dynamic air bronchograms (branching echogenic structures with centrifuge movement with breathing) or multiple hyperechogenic lentil-sized spots, due to air trapped in the small airways. LUS was considered positive when at least one consolidation showing the above-described features was detected. Pleural effusion could be associated with consolidation and has been interpreted as an auxiliary sign, but its detection was not considered individually as sign of suspected pneumonia.

Chest radiography was performed using a Practix 300 Bucky diagnostic equipment (Philips Medical Systems, Hamburg, Germany) by posterior-anterior and lateral views in the upright patients and anterior-posterior view in the supine patients, following standardized hospital diagnostic protocol. The film was digitally reviewed by an expert radiologist blinded to the results of LUS and CT. The radiologist had the possibility to review also previous CXR, when available, as part of standard clinical care. The radiologist was asked to detect and locate the opacities that might correlate with the diagnosis of pneumonia. CXR was considered positive when at least one typical consolidation was visualized.

Procalcitonin, requested by the treating physician at ED presentation for clinical reason, was measured using an automated Enzyme-Linked Fluorescent Assay (ELFA): VIDAS® B.R.A.H.M.S PCT™ (Vidas, BioMerieux). Samples were processed by personnel blinded from any patient data. We considered two PCT cut-off of 0.25 and 0.5 ng/ml based on previous studies [6, 7, 10–12]. These studies suggested that a PCT level <0.25 ng/ml can be used to rule out bacterial pneumonia in patients with suspected respiratory tract infections and a PCT level >0.5 ng/ml is considered to rule in bacterial pneumonia and to support antibiotic therapy. Patients that didn't consent or didn't undergo LUS within the time limit were excluded from the study. Patients in which PCT was not requested in ED were also excluded.

Chest CT was performed by one Somatom Definition AS128 (Siemens, Erlangen, Germany), only for clinical purposes independent from the study protocol. An expert radiologist, other than the attending radiologist and blinded to LUS and CXR results, reviewed the studies investigating one or more consolidations related to pneumonia, defined as homogeneous increase in pulmonary parenchymal attenuation obscuring the margins of vessels and airway walls, with or without air bronchograms [13].

The final diagnoses of pneumonia were determined by two expert internal medicine physicians, blinded to CXR, LUS and PCT results, who independently reviewed all available clinical data including CT data and medical records for hospitalized patients. In case of discordance, a third senior physician adjudicated the diagnosis.

### Statistical analysis

The sample size was calculated considering a prevalence of pneumonia of 50% among suspected patients in ED and a sensitivity of LUS for the diagnosis of pneumonia when chest CT was used as gold standard of 80% [8]. Wanting to prove that PCT increased the sensitivity of 10% and considering a type I error of 5% and a power (1-ß) of 80%, it was estimated that this would require approximately 120 patients.

Data points are expressed as mean $\pm$ standard deviation (SD). The unpaired Student's $t$ test was used to compare normally distributed data. Fisher's exact test was used for the comparison of non-continuous variables expressed as proportions. $p < 0.05$ indicates statistical significance. All $p$ values are two sided. The diagnostic performance of LUS, CXR and PCT and the combination of LUS and CXR with PCT was assessed by calculating sensitivity, specificity, positive predictive value, negative predictive value and likelihood ratios. The extended McNemar and the McNemar tests were used to evaluate if there was a significant difference in the accuracy, sensitivities and specificities of LUS, CXR, PCT and the combination of imaging tests with PCT [14]. Receiver operating characteristic (ROC) curves were constructed to assess the sensitivity and specificity of white blood cells count (WBC), PCT and multivariable models to compare the ability of LUS and CXR combined with PCT to predict pneumonia. Calculations were performed by using SPSS statistical package (version 17.0; IBM).

## Results

### Baseline characteristics

A total of 308 patients with respiratory complains underwent chest CT in the ED during the study period. Four patients did not consent to participate. In 19 patients LUS was not performed before chest CT or within the time limit. In 157 patients PCT was not requested by the attending emergency physician at presentation in the ED. Thus, 128 patients were included in the final analysis (Fig. 1). These patients had a mean age of 70.7 $\pm$ 15.8 years (range 23–100) and 64 (50%) were female. Pneumonia was the final diagnosis in 61 patients (47.7%). The patients' characteristics according to the presence or absence of pneumonia are shown in Table 1. Alternative diagnoses in patients without pneumonia are reported in Table 2.

### Main results

Lung ultrasonography was feasible in all patients, but in 11 cases (8.2%), included in the study, pulmonary examination was limited only to the anterior-lateral areas mainly due to uncooperative patients. LUS was positive for at least one consolidation in 60 patients (46.9%). Fifty-two (86.7%) out of 60 patients with positive LUS had a final diagnosis of pneumonia (Fig. 1). LUS was false positive in eight cases (6.2%) and false negative in nine patients (7%). In three out of nine (33%) false negative cases pulmonary examination was limited only to the anterior-lateral areas. The sensitivity and the specificity of LUS were 85.2% (95% CI 73.8–93%) and 88.1% (95% CI 77.8–94.7%) respectively.

Procalcitonin median in patients with and without pneumonia were 0.3 and 0.1 ng/ml respectively ($p = 0.05$). The sensitivity and the specificity of PCT $\geq$ 0.25 ng/ml were 73.8% (95% CI 61–84.2%) and 47.8% (95% CI 35.4–60.3%) respectively, whereas the sensitivity and the specificity of $PCT > 0.5$ ng/ml were 42.6% (95% CI 30–55.9%) and 67.2% (95% CI 54.6–78.1%) respectively.

Chest radiography was performed with the patient in the up-right position in 29 (23%) cases. Thirty-seven out of 45 patients (82.2%) with positive CXR had a final diagnosis of pneumonia. CXR showed false positive examination in 8 (6.2%) patients and false negative examination in 24 (18.7%) patients. The sensitivity and the specificity of CXR were 60.7% (95% CI 47.3–72.9%) and 88.1% (95% CI 77.8–94.7%) respectively.

In 38 cases (29.7%) we observed the combination of negative LUS and negative PCT (<0.25 ng/ml). A false negative combination of LUS/PCT test was observed in 2 cases (1.6%). In one of these two patients the final diagnosis was infective endocarditis and heart failure associated to pneumonia. The other patient had a final diagnosis of pneumonia complicated by heart failure and non-ST elevated myocardial infarction. The derived sensitivity of negative LUS/PCT test was 96.7% (95% CI 88.6–99.5%) with a significant superiority to LUS alone and PCT alone ($p < 0.05$ for both). Negative predictive value (NPV) and negative likelihood ratio (LR) were 94.7% (95% CI 88.2–99.2%) and 0.06 (95% CI 0.02–0.24) respectively. In 24 patients (18.8%) we observed the combination of positive LUS and positive PCT (>0.5 ng/ml). Out of these, four were false positive (3.1%). The derived specificity, positive predictive value (PPV) and positive LR were 94% (95% CI 85.4–98.3%), 83.3% (95% CI 62.6–95.2%) and 5.49 (95% CI 1.99–15.17) respectively. Specificity of the LUS/PCT

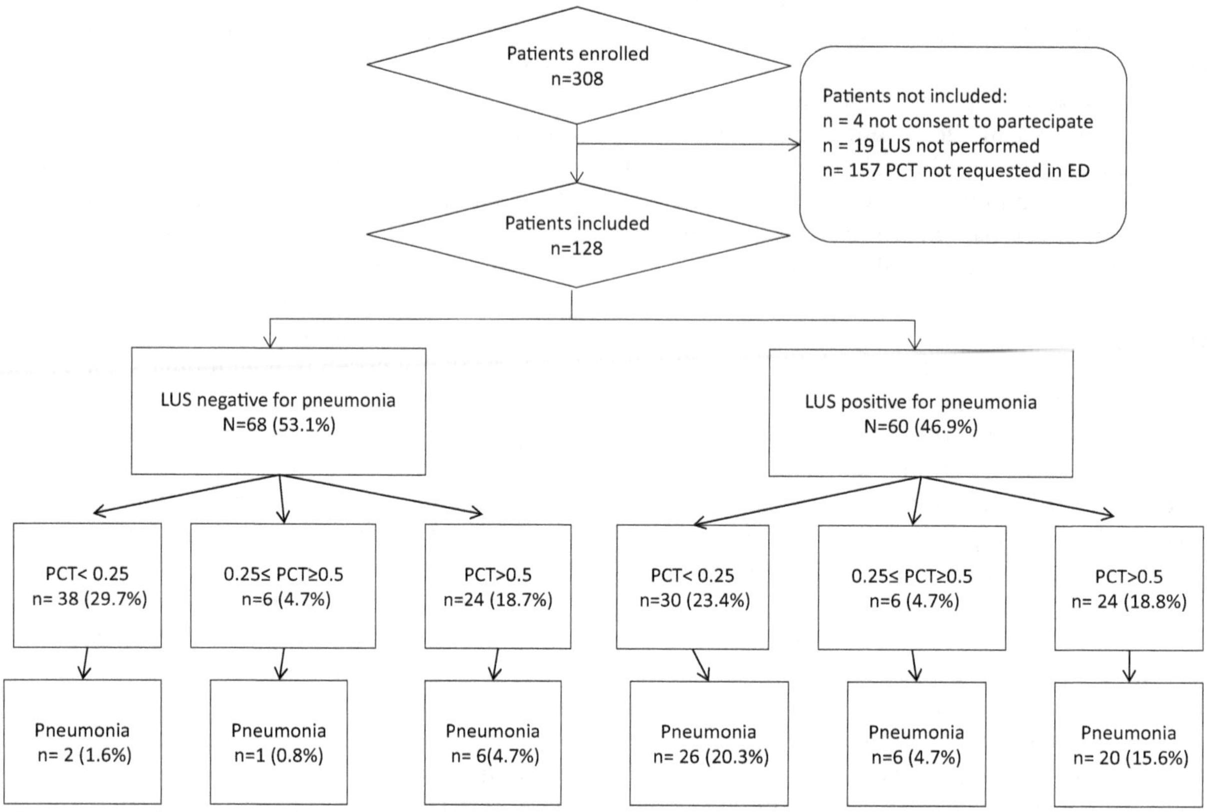


**Fig. 1** Characteristics of patients according to the presence or absence of pneumonia. *LUS* lung ultrasonography; *PCT* procalcitonin

**Table 1 Characteristics of the study population according to final diagnosis**

| | Pneumonia ($n = 61$) | No pneumonia ($n = 67$) | $p$ value |
|---|---|---|---|
| Mean age ± SD, y | 69.8 ± 18.8 | 71.6 ± 12.6 | 0.51 |
| Women | 25 (41%) | 39 (58.2) | 0.076 |
| *Medical history of lung disease* | | | |
| Chronic obstructive pulmonary disease | 7 (11.5) | 10 (14.9) | 0.611 |
| Lung cancer | 2 (3.3) | 5 (7.5) | 0.444 |
| Heart failure | 11 (18) | 14 (20.9) | 0.824 |
| Previous pulmonary embolism | 1 (1.6) | 3 (4.5) | 0.621 |
| *Signs and symptoms at presentation* | | | |
| Dyspnea | 44 (72.1) | 49 (73.1) | 1 |
| Cough | 26 (42.6) | 12 (31.6) | 0.003 |
| Pleuritic chest pain | 8 (13.1) | 8 (11.9) | 1 |
| Shock/hypotension | 17 (27.9) | 13 (19.4) | 0.3 |
| SBP ± SD, mmHg | 121.7 ± 30.5 | 124.9 ± 37.3 | 0.6 |
| Heart rate >100 bpm | 42 (68.9) | 30 (44.8) | 0.008 |
| Respiratory rate/min | 26.1 ± 8.2 | 23.3 ± 6.8 | 0.2 |
| $PaO_2/FiO_2$ ± SD | 292.6 ± 83.9 | 309.5 ± 94 | 0.29 |
| Temperature >37.8 °C | 31 (50.8) | 22 (32.8) | 0.049 |
| White blood cells count/$mm^3$ | 12,494 ± 10,130.3 | 11,906 ± 6657 | 0.7 |
| *Mechanical invasive ventilation* | 4 (6.6) | 6 (9) | 0.747 |

Data are given as no. (%) or mean ± standard deviation (SD)

*SD* standard deviation; *SBP* systolic blood pressure; *$PaO_2$* arterial oxygen pressure express in mmHg; *$FiO_2$* fraction of inspired oxygen; *bpm* beats/min; *ED* emergency department

**Table 2 Final diagnosis in the study patients**

| Diagnosis | No (%) |
|---|---|
| Pneumonia | 61 (47.7) |
| Pulmonary embolism | 21 (16.4) |
| Heart failure | 9 (7) |
| Pleural effusion | 8 (6.3) |
| Sepsis with no pulmonary involvement | 8 (6.2) |
| Chronic obstructive pulmonary disease | 4 (3.1) |
| Acute coronary syndrome | 3 (2.3) |
| Tachyarrhythmia | 1 (0.8) |
| Respiratory failure in pulmonary malignancy | 1 (0.8) |
| Pericardial effusion/pericarditis | 1 (0.8) |
| Miscellaneous | 11 (8.6) |

Data are given as no. (%) unless otherwise indicated

test was not significantly different when compared to LUS alone ($p = 0.125$).

In 46 patients (35.9%), CXR was negative for pneumonia and PCT was <0.25 ng/ml. False negative cases where 12 (9.4%). The derived sensitivity, NPV and negative LR were 80.3% (95% CI 68.1–89.4%), 73.9% (95% CI 58.9–85.7%) and 0.39 (95% CI 0.22–0.68) respectively. In 16 patients (12.5%) CXR was positive for pneumonia and PCT was >0.5 ng/ml (16, 12.5%), with one false positive case (0.8%). The derived specificity, PPV and positive LR were 98.5% (95% CI 91.9–99.7%), 93.7% (95% CI 69.7–98.9%) and 16.48 (95% CI 2.24–121.05%) respectively.

The sensitivity of negative LUS/PCT (<0.25 ng/ml) was significantly higher than negative CXR/PCT (96.7 vs 80.3%, $p < 0.05$), whereas the specificity of positive LUS/PCT (>0.5 ng/ml) was not significantly different to positive CXR/PCT (94 vs 98.5%, $p = 0.68$). Overall test characteristics of LUS, CXR and PCT and of LUS and CXR combined with PCT are reported in Tables 3 and 4.

According to ROC curve, the diagnostic accuracy of LUS associated with PCT (88.8% $\pm$ 3.1) was higher than the total count of white blood cells (WBC) (49.1% $\pm$ 5.2), PCT alone (60.7% $\pm$ 5) and CXR associated with PCT (77.4% $\pm$ 4.2) (Fig. 2).

## Discussion

To our knowledge, this is the first study evaluating the diagnostic performance of LUS combined with PCT for the diagnosis of pneumonia in the ED. Research on the diagnosis of pneumonia is usually hampered by difficulties in obtaining a systematic comparison with CT scan. The lack of a gold standard that supports the visual diagnosis of pneumonia, may lower the significance of many studies. One strength of our study is that the final diagnosis of pneumonia in all patients is supported by a post hoc review of the clinical chart, and based on the detection of typical consolidations at chest CT read by an expert radiologist. In many previous studies LUS showed to be an accurate bedside tool for the diagnosis of pneumonia [8, 15–17]. In our study LUS alone ruled in pneumonia with a good positive likelihood ratio and ruled out this condition with a moderate negative likelihood ratio. The superiority of LUS over CXR is reported in literature [9]. In our study, despite the two methods showed similar specificities, the sensitivity of LUS was superior to CXR. We have to consider that in 8% of patients, pulmonary ultrasound examination was limited only to the anterior-lateral areas and that 33% of all false negative cases belong to this group. In these patients, most dependent pulmonary areas were not scanned and consolidations were not detected and this was the cause of a reduction in overall sensitivity of LUS for the diagnosis of pneumonia.

Procalcitonin is an emerging biomarker, whose practical application is increasingly common, not only in the diagnosis and follow-up of sepsis but also in pneumonia [18]. A PCT value below the threshold level makes unlikely a severe pneumonia with bacteraemia and is used to withhold antibiotic therapy [19–21]. Müller et al. analysed data from two randomized prospective studies with a total of 545 patients with suspected infection of the lower respiratory tract. In their post-hoc analysis, they found that the diagnostic accuracy to predict radiographically suspected community acquired pneumonia was significantly higher for PCT (87%) than for WBC (64%) [22]. In our study, the diagnostic accuracy of PCT, although inferior to the performance obtained by Müller et al., was still higher than WBC (49%).

**Table 3 Diagnostic performance of lung ultrasonography, chest radiograph and procalcitonin for the diagnosis of pneumonia**

| | Sens % (95% CI) | Spec % (95% CI) | PPV % (95% CI) | NPV % (95% CI) | +LR % (95% CI) | −LR (95% CI) |
|---|---|---|---|---|---|---|
| LUS | 85.2 (73.8–93) | 88 (77.8–94.7) | 86.7 (75.4–94) | 86.8 (76.3–93.7) | 7.14 (3.70–13.79) | 0.17 (0.09–0.31) |
| CXR | 60.7 (47.3–72.9) | 88.1 (77.8–94.7) | 82.2 (67.9–92) | 71.1 (60.1–80.5) | 5.08 (2.57–10.04) | 0.45 (0.32–0.62) |
| PCT $\geq$ 0.25 | 73.8 (61–84.2) | 47.8 (35.4–60.3) | 56.2 (44.7–67.3) | 66.7 (51.6–79.6) | 1.41 (1.07–1.86) | 0.55 (0.34–0.90) |

*Sens* sensitivity; *Spec* specificity; *PPV* positive predictive value; *NPV* negative predictive value; *+LR* positive likelihood ratio; *−LR* negative likelihood Ratio; *95% CI* 95% confidence interval; *CXR* chest X-ray; *LUS* lung ultrasonography; *PCT* procalcitonin value express in ng/ml

**Table 4 Diagnostic performance of lung ultrasonography and chest radiograph combined with procalcitonin for the diagnosis of pneumonia**

| | Sens % (95% CI) | Spec % (95% CI) | PPV % (95% CI) | NPV % (95% CI) | +LR (95% CI) | −LR (95% CI) |
|---|---|---|---|---|---|---|
| Positive LUS or PCT ≥0.25 | 96.7 (88.6–99.5) | 53.7 (41.1–66) | 65.6 (54.8–75.3) | 94.7 (82.2–99.2) | 2.09 (1.61–2.72) | 0.06 (0.02–0.24) |
| Positive LUS and PCT >0.5 | 32.8 (21.3–46) | 94 (85.4–98.3) | 83.3 (62.6–95.1) | 60.6 (50.5–70) | 5.49 (1.99–15.17) | 0.71 (0.59–0.86) |
| Positive CXR or PCT ≥0.25 | 80.3 (68.1–89.4) | 50.7 (38.2–63.2) | 59.8 (48.3–70.4) | 73.9 (58.9–85.7) | 1.63 (1.2–2.1) | 0.39 (0.22–0.68) |
| Positive CXR and PCT >0.5 | 24.6 (14.5–37.3) | 98.5 (91.9–99.7) | 93.7 (69.7–98.9) | 58.9 (49.2–68.1) | 16.48 (2.24–121.05) | 0.77 (0.66–0.89) |

*Sens* sensitivity; *Spec* specificity; *PPV* positive predictive value; *NPV* negative predictive value; *+LR* positive likelihood ratio; *−LR* negative likelihood Ratio; *95% CI* 95% confidence interval; *CXR* chest X-ray; *LUS* lung ultrasonography; *PCT* procalcitonin value express in ng/ml; or means that at least one test was positive; and means that both tests were positive

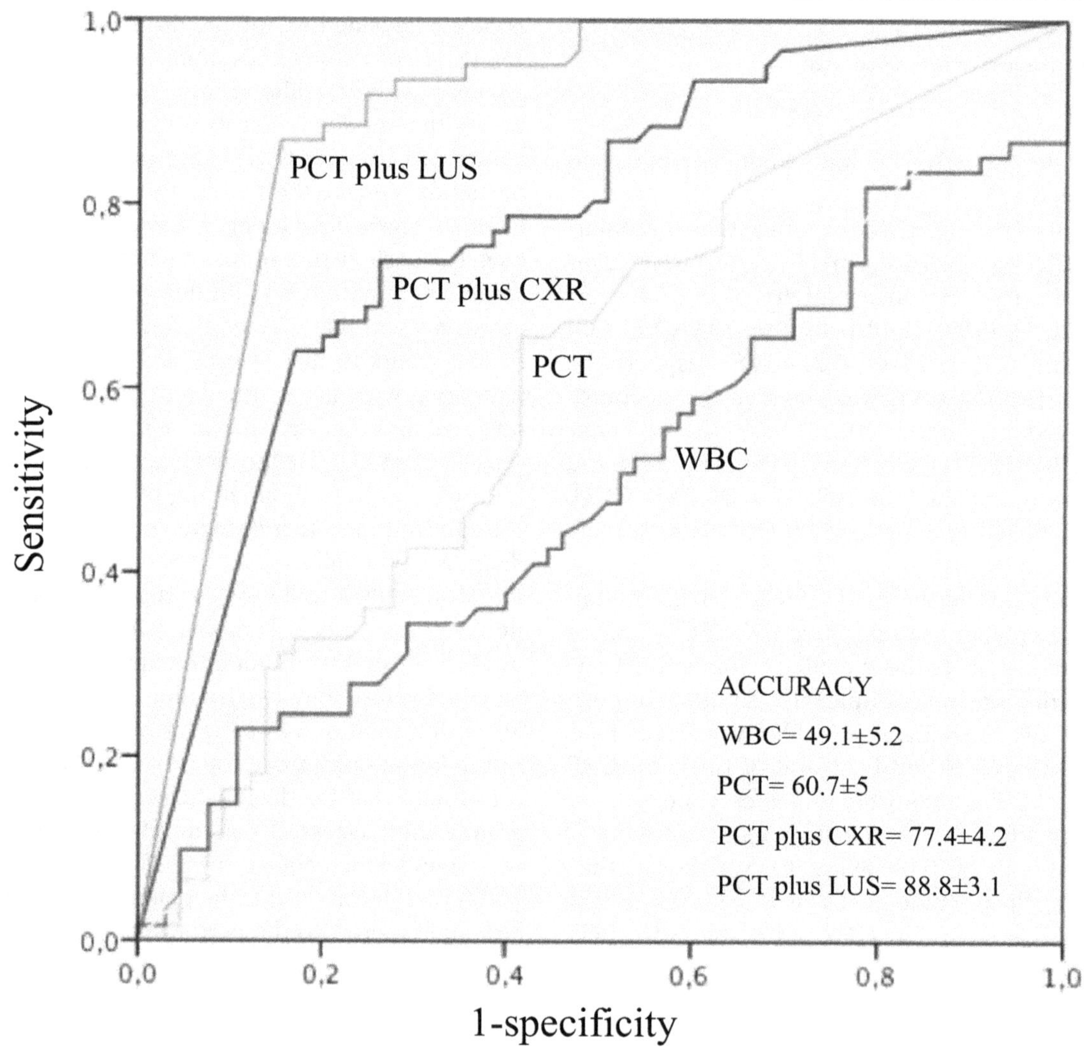


**Fig. 2** ROC curve of WBC, PCT, LUS and CXR and their combination. *WBC* white blood cells; *PCT* procalcitonin; *LUS* lung ultrasonography; *CXR* chest X-ray

The lower accuracy of PCT found in our study compared with the study by Müller may be due to a different selection of patients and to the different gold standard used for the diagnosis of pneumonia.

Despite its known role in the confirmation of bacteraemia in sepsis, in our study PCT alone was not sufficiently accurate in the diagnosis of pneumonia. This can be explained considering that while the final diagnosis of pneumonia was only confirmed in presence of typical clinical signs with at least one typical consolidation detected at chest CT, we cannot confirm that in our patients the radiologic consolidations were always due to a bacterial infection with bacteraemia. The majority of patients with a final diagnosis of pneumonia were in a stable condition and showed an isolated pulmonary infection not necessarily associated with bacteraemia. It is well known that in cases of localized organ infections, PCT is usually lower as compared to septicaemia with positive blood cultures [23].

No previous studies evaluated the association of LUS and PCT for the bedside diagnosis of pneumonia in the ED. However, a recent study by Zagli et al. performed on critically ill patients in the intensive care unit, evaluated a new score, CEPPIS (chest echography and procalcitonin pulmonary infection score), based on a combination of PCT and LUS for the diagnosis of ventilator associated pneumonia (VAP) [24]. The new proposed score differed from the traditional clinical pulmonary infection score (CPSI) basically in two items: WBC was replaced by PCT and CXR by LUS. The study showed that sensitivity of CEPPIS (80.5%) was superior then CPSI (39.8%) for the diagnosis of VAP, while specificity was similar (85.2 vs 83.3%). There are many methodological differences between the study of Zagli et al. and our study, but both showed that the sensitivity of LUS/PCT is superior to other diagnostic approach based on CXR in the diagnosis of pneumonia.

In our study the association of a negative LUS examination with a PCT level <0.25 ng/ml significantly improved sensitivity of LUS for the diagnosis of pneumonia, reducing the occurrence of false negative diagnoses and decreasing the negative LR. We can argue that the clinician, in approximately one-third of "difficult" diagnosis in patients with unexplained respiratory symptoms, may rule-out pneumonia with a sufficient level of certainty by combining LUS and PCT. On the other hand, our study showed that when LUS visualizes a consolidation with the typical ultrasonography features, the specificity and positive predictive value for the diagnosis of pneumonia is not significantly influenced by the addiction of PCT.

Lung ultrasonography is a powerful, cheap, easy to perform, and safe tool for the diagnosis of many pulmonary conditions at bedside and its use is exponentially increasing among specialists and general practitioners in and out of hospitals. Moreover, the diagnostic accuracy of LUS for pneumonia is at least as good as CXR in different settings and patients. Considering that a point-of care PCT measurement will become available for clinical practice [10], the results of this preliminary study opens new perspectives for improving the diagnostic approach to pneumonia at the bedside, by combining LUS and PCT in the general population. Further studies could also evaluate the usefulness of this combined diagnostic strategy in some subgroup of patients where CXR is less accurate or contraindicated such as bedridden patients in particular patients in invasive and not invasive ventilation, immunocompromised patients and pregnant women. Furthermore, using multiple biomarkers combined with LUS could further increase diagnostic accuracy of physicians and be useful to triage patients at the bedside in many different clinical scenarios[25].

#### Study limitations

A questionable characteristic of our protocol is that patients were not enrolled on the basis of a direct suspicion for pneumonia. We concentrated our study on patients with respiratory complains, who demanded CT scan for ambiguous diagnosis. In case of suspected uncomplicated lung infection, where the diagnosis is mainly based on clinical findings and CXR, it is unusual to undergo CT scans. Thus, our specific patient population does not allow generalization of our results. However, a systematic application of CT studies in all suspected low respiratory tract infection is not feasible because it does not represent a standard of care, and it is not ethical for its radiation burden and not sustainable for high cost. Another limitation of our study, is that the final diagnosis of pneumonia was based on the detection of a consolidation at chest CT, while the possibility of interstitial pneumonia was not considered. We have also to consider that it is not known if the consolidation identified at chest CT was due to bacterial, viral or other germ infection. Regarding the comparison between LUS and CXR, a consideration should be done on the criteria of enrolment. In fact, the patients enrolled in the study underwent chest CT once the physician was aware of CXR results, and this could have selected a population with not diagnostic CXR. Thus, this criteria probably affected the low sensitivity of CXR. However, in the real practice, the role of LUS is often to confirm negative chest films in patients with high suspicion of pneumonia. Thus, the difference in sensitivity between the two methodologies is still confirmed. Indeed, the fact that in our study the majority of CXR were not performed in the upright position, may have influenced more significantly the comparison between the two methods. The anterior-posterior radiographic view is undoubtedly less accurate for the study of the lungs. However, the evaluation of suboptimal chest films is largely representative of the real daily practice and the main cause of inconclusive CXR studies. Finally, the lack of systematic and consecutive PCT assays in the population studied may have biased our results. Indeed, a PCT assay was only based on the personal judgement of the attending physician facing challenging diagnostic situations and was independent from the study protocol. However, these situations are exactly those deserving more accurate and sometimes alternative diagnostic tools, that is the possible future role of a combined LUS/PCT protocol.

## Conclusions

The combination of LUS and PCT showed a high sensitivity for the diagnosis of pneumonia in patients presenting with respiratory complaints of uncertain origin that underwent chest CT and the sensitivity of this combination was significantly higher when compared with the sensitivity of LUS alone and PCT alone.

### Authors' contributions

PN, SV, GV conceived and design the study, CG, MB, GC acquired data; PN, SV conducted statistical analysis; PN, SV, GC, MZ, GV analyzed and interpreted the data and wrote the article; all the authors participated in manuscript review and revision and provided final approval of the version to be published. PN had full access to all the data in the study and takes responsibility for the integrity of the data and the accuracy of the data analysis, including and especially any adverse effects. PN assumes full responsibility for the integrity of the submission as a whole, from inception to published article. PN takes responsibility for the paper as a whole. All the authors have participated in the preparation of the final manuscript. All authors read and approved the final manuscript.

### Author details

[1] Department of Emergency Medicine, Careggi University Hospital, Largo Brambilla 3, 50134 Florence, Italy. [2] Radiology Department, Careggi University Hospital, Florence, Italy. [3] Department of Emergency Medicine, San Luigi Gonzaga University Hospital, Turin, Italy.

### Acknowledgements

The work was conducted at Careggi University Hospital, Firenze, Italy.

### References

1. Mortensen EM, Coley CM, Singer DE, Marrie TJ, Obrosky DS, Kapoor WN, Fine MJ (2002) Causes of death for patients with community-acquired pneumonia: results from the Pneumonia Patient Outcomes Research Team cohort study. Arch Intern Med 162:1059–1064
2. Niederman MS, Mandell LA, Anzueto A, Bass JB, Broughton WA, Campbell GD et al (2001) Guidelines for the management of adults with community-acquired pneumonia. Diagnosis, assessment of severity, antimicrobial therapy, and prevention. Am J Respir Crit Care Med 163:1730–1754
3. Brenner DJ, Hall EJ (2007) Computed tomography an increasing source of radiation exposure. N Engl J Med 357:2277–2284
4. Self WH, Courtney DM, McNaughton CD, Wunderink RG, Kline JA (2013) High discordance of chest x-ray and computed tomography for detection of pulmonary opacities in ED patients: implications for diagnosing pneumonia. Am J Emerg Med 31:401–405
5. Chavez MA, Shams N, Ellington LE, Naithani N, Gilman RH, Steinhoff MC et al (2014) Lung ultrasound for the diagnosis of pneumonia in adults: a systematic review and meta-analysis. Respir Res 23(15):50
6. Christ-Crain M, Jaccard-Stolz D, Bingisser R, Gencay MM, Huber PR, Tamm M, Muller B (2004) Effect of procalcitonin-guided treatment on antibiotic use and outcome in lower respiratory tract infections: cluster-randomised, single-blinded intervention trial. Lancet 363:600–607
7. Schuetz P, Christ-Crain M, Wolbers M, Schild U, Thomann R, Falconnier C et al (2009) Effect of procalcitonin based guidelines compared to standard guidelines on antibiotic use in lower respiratory tract infections: the randomized-controlled multicenter ProHOSP Trial. JAMA 302:1059–1066
8. Nazerian P, Volpicelli G, Vanni S, Gigli C, Betti L, Bartolucci M et al (2015) Accuracy of lung ultrasound for the diagnosis of consolidations when com- pared to chest computed tomography. Am J Emerg Med 33:620–625
9. Volpicelli G, Elbarbary M, Blaivas M, Lichtenstein DA, Mathis G, Kirkpatrick AW et al (2012) International evidence-based recommendations for point-of-care lung ultrasound. Intensive Care Med 38:577–591
10. Briel M, Schuetz P, Mueller B, Young J, Schild U, Nusbaumer C et al (2008) Procalcitonin- guided antibiotic use vs a standard approach for acute respiratory tract infections in primary care. Arch Intern Med 168:2000–2007
11. Christ-Crain M, Stolz D, Bingisser R et al (2006) Procalcitonin guidance of antibiotic therapy in community acquired pneumonia: a randomized trial. Am J Respir Crit Care Med 174(1):84–93
12. Stolz D, Christ-Crain M, Bingisser R et al (2007) Antibiotic treatment of exacerbations of COPD. Chest 131(1):9–19
13. Hansell DM, Bankier AA, MacMahon H, McLoud TC, Muller NL, Remy J (2008) Fleischner society: glossary of terms for thoracic imaging. Radiology 246:697–722
14. Hawass NE (1997) Comparing the sensitivities and specificities of two diagnostic procedures performed on the same group of patients. Br J Radiol 70:360–366
15. Cortellaro F, Colombo S, Coen D, Duca PG (2012) Lung ultrasound is an accurate diagnostic tool for the diagnosis of pneumonia in the emergency department. Emer Med J 29:19–23
16. Reissig A, Copetti R, Mathis G, Mempel C, Schuler A, Zechner P et al (2012) Lung ultrasound in the diagnosis and follow-up of community-acquired pneumonia: a prospective, multicenter, diagnostic accuracy study. Chest 142:965–972
17. Shah VP, Tunik MG, Tsung JW (2013) Prospective evaluation of point-of-care ultrasonography for the diagnosis of pneumonia in children and young adults. JAMA Pediatr 167:119–125
18. Christ-Crain M, Opal SM (2010) Clinical review: the role of biomarkers in the diagnosis and management of community-acquired pneumonia. Crit Care. doi:10.1186/cc8155
19. Simon L, Gauvin F, Amre DK, Saint-Louis P, Lacroix J (2004) Serum procalcitonin and C-reactive protein levels as markers of bacterial infection: a systematic review and meta-analysis. Clin Infect Dis 39:206–217
20. Schuetz P, Chiappa V, Briel M, Greenwald JL (2011) Procalcitonin algorithms for antibiotic therapy decisions: a systematic review of randomized controlled trials and recommendations for clinical algorithms. Arch Intern Med 171:1322–1331
21. Schuetz P, Müller B, Christ-Crain M, Stolz D, Tamm M, Bouadma L et al (2012) Procalcitonin to initiate or discontinue antibiotics in acute respiratory tract infections. Cochrane Database Syst Rev 9:CD007498
22. Müller B, Harbarth S, Stolz D, Bingisser R, Mueller C, Leuppi J et al (2007) Diagnostic and prognostic accuracy of clinical and laboratory parameters in community-acquired pneumonia. BMC Infec Dis 7:10
23. Soderquist B, Jones I, Fredlund H, Vikerfors T (1998) Bacterial or crystal-associated arthritis? Discriminating ability of serum inflammatory markers. Scand J Infect Dis 30:591–596
24. Zagli G, Cozzolino M, Terreni A, Biagioli T, Caldini AL, Peris A (2014) Diagnosis of ventilator-associated pneumonia: a pilot, exploratory analysis of a new score based on procalcitonin and chest echography. Chest 146:1578–1585
25. Schuetz P, Hausfater P, Amin D, Amin A, Haubitz S, Faessler L, Kutz A, Conca A, Reutlinger B, Canavaggio P, Sauvin G, Bernard M, Huber A, Mueller B (2015) Biomarkers from distinct biological pathways improve early risk stratification in medical emergency patients: the multinational, prospective, observational TRIAGE study. TRIAGE Study group. Crit Care 19:377

4

# Lung ultrasound in internal medicine

Chiara Mozzini*, Anna Maria Fratta Pasini, Ulisse Garbin and Luciano Cominacini

**Abstract**

**Background:** Lung ultrasound (LUS) represents an emerging technique for bedside chest imaging in different clinical settings. A standardized approach allows the diagnosis, the quantification, and the follow-up of different conditions for which acute respiratory failure is the main clinical presentation. The aim of this study was to test what skill targets could be achieved in LUS, with a short-training course offered to 19 Medical Doctors attending the certification board school in Internal Medicine at the University of Verona, Italy.

**Methods:** The training course (theoretical and practical) consisted of 9 h subdivided in 4 days. Each trainee examined three healthy volunteers during the first day that was also the day of the theoretical lessons. Moreover, they examined nine patients per day (a total of 27 patients). Trainees were tested in the recognition of the basic signs in LUS, the managing of the Bedside Lung Ultrasound Evaluation (the BLUE protocol), and the recognition of the broad clinical scenarios recognized by the LUS. Kappa statistic was used to calculate the inter-observer agreement (trainees/tutor).

**Results:** Twenty-seven patients were examined by the 19 trainees (ten trainees had previous limited experience in general ultrasound). The agreement among the trainees and the tutor in the recognition of the LUS basic signs and in the recognition of the BLUE protocol profiles ranged from "fair" to "excellent". In particular, the agreement among the trainees and the tutor in the final LUS diagnosis was "excellent" for the recognition of the interstitial syndrome and the pleural effusion, "substantial" for the recognition of the normal lung, and "moderate" for the recognition of consolidation and pneumothorax. LUS outcome gave useful information and drove change in therapy in 16 patients. It affected immediate management in nine patients. The concordance between the previous X chest ray and LUS was observed in 21 patients.

**Conclusions:** A short training in LUS provided good proficiency in the recognition only of the main signs of the BLUE protocol, but allowed a correct LUS diagnosis in the Internal Medicine most frequent clinical settings of acute respiratory failure. This study supports incorporating LUS into Internal Medicine fellowship training programs.

**Keywords:** Lung ultrasound (LUS), Internal Medicine, Training, Clinical practice

## Background

The evaluation of the lungs has been considered an "off-limits" area for ultrasound for many years, considering the air as the main obstacle. Nevertheless, in the last years, lung ultrasound (LUS) has emerged in different clinical settings, such as in emergency and critical care medicine [1–3], but also in cardiology [4] and in Internal Medicine [5]. LUS represents an adjunct to the physical examination to recognize specific ultrasonic signs that represent a narrow list of potential diagnoses in specific clinical settings [6–8]. A standardized approach allows the diagnosis, the quantification, and the follow-up of different conditions for which acute respiratory failure is the main clinical presentation. In particular, the main fields of LUS applications are: the pneumothorax (PNX), the interstitial syndrome, the lung consolidation, and the pleural effusion [6–8]. Recently, the World interactive network focused on critical ultrasound (WINFOCUS) has proposed a document [9] reporting evidence-based recommendations on the clinical use of LUS. LUS uses

*Correspondence: chiaramozzini@libero.it
Department of Medicine, Section of Internal Medicine, University of Verona, Piazzale L.A. Scuro, 10, 37134 Verona, Italy

the basic technology (only 2D and M-mode are required and every probe can be appropriate), it is free of ionizing radiations, and it is not invasive, repeatable and effective. It does not require transfer of patients [10]. Nevertheless, it is largely operator dependent, and a scientific assessment of the learning curve remains to be assessed [11]. The main limitation of LUS is that it does not rule out any pulmonary abnormality that does not reach the pleura [10].

The primary aim of this study was to test what skill targets could be achieved in LUS. A relatively short-training course was offered to already certified Medical Doctors attending the certification board school in Internal Medicine. Part of this aim was established more precise rules in training courses based on the previous expert consensus recommendations [9]. The desired level of competence consisted in acquiring technical skills and interpretative skills. The essence of LUS is mainly a dichotomous interpretation of the findings. The diagnostic approach is qualitative or semi-quantitative. The objectives were: the recognition of the basic signs in LUS, the managing of the bedside lung ultrasound evaluation (the BLUE protocol) [12, 13], and the recognition of the broad clinical scenarios recognized by LUS [8]. The second aim of this study was to depict the clinical utility of LUS in an Internal Medicine department. The goal was to show the usefulness of LUS in the management of the most common causes of acute respiratory failure in this department.

## Methods

### Participants

The study setting was the Internal Medicine department of the University Hospital of Verona, Italy, already certified as a first level ultrasound centre by the Società Italiana di Medicina Interna (SIMI). Nineteen Medical Doctors attending the certification board school in Internal Medicine at the University of Verona accepted to follow a short-training course in LUS. The training course consisted of a total of 9 h of theoretical and practical lessons over a period of 4 days. The tutor was a general ultrasound certified Internal Medicine specialist with the formal competency from the Società Italiana di Ultrasonologia in Medicina e Biologia (SIUMB). A subgroup of the trainees had previous limited theoretical and practical experience in general ultrasound (basic principles of ultrasound and basic knowledge of the devices) and in focused cardiac ultrasound (no competence certification, nor daily practice of ultrasound).

### Ethics statement

The study was conducted in accordance with the ethical standards laid down in the Helsinki Declaration of 1975 and its late amendments. The participants provided written consent prior to starting the study (for collecting and publishing data). The procedure did not require a particular approval by the local Ethical Committee.

### Description of the training and evaluation program

First, the tutor did theoretical lessons of 2 h and 20 min which included these precise lectures: introduction, contents, advantages, and disadvantages of LUS (5 min); brief theoretical summary of the basic principles of ultrasound and of the characteristics of the device used (EnVisor C HD, Philips, equipped with linear, convex, and sector transducers) (5 min); the international evidence-based recommendations for point of care lung ultrasound [9] (15 min); and the flow chart of different diagnoses according to the BLUE protocol [12, 13] (15 min). Particular attention was paid to the patient's position and to the correct scanning technique, as previously recommended [6, 7, 9]: the eight-zone examination modality (15 min); the twenty-eight scanning site scheme (10 min); and the possibility of a more rapid two-region scan as an option for the critically ill patients (5 min). Photos and video clips were used to demonstrate the LUS signs and patterns. The signs of the BLUE protocol [12, 13] were explained (30 min): bat sign; lung sliding; seashore sign (in M-mode); A lines (normal lung tissue yields, lung sliding, and horizontal repetition artifacts arising from the pleural line); quad sign; sinusoid sign; fractal sign; tissue-like sign; stratosphere sign; lung point (M-mode); lung pulse; and dynamic air bronchogram, and B lines (artifacts that correlate with interstitial edema, and, if three or more between two ribs, are called lung rockets). Then, the profiles of the BLUE protocol derived from the association of the signs were explained, and the BLUE protocol "decision tree" [12, 13] was analysed (10 min): A profile; A' profile; B profile; B' profile; C profile; and A/B profile. Then, according to the international recommendations [9], the main clinical scenarios were discussed (30 min): normal lungs; PNX; interstitial syndrome; and lung consolidation. Then, in the first session for each group, the training course was performed with healthy volunteers, tested as "without any lung abnormalities" by the trainer (three examinations for each trainees). In the other sessions, patients enrolled from the same Internal Medicine department were studied. Didactic material for the theoretical lectures was provided (bibliographic indexes, online material) to invite the trainees to study also on their own. During the practical sessions, each theoretical point was discussed in depth, with the aim of refreshing and fixing the main concepts. The desired level of competence consisted in acquiring technical skills (the recognition of the LUS signs and the different patterns) and in making the correct focused diagnosis. The time allotted for each examination and diagnosis making was a maximum of 3 min, according to the BLUE protocol. The trainees were blinded to the LUS examination report previously made by the tutor. The sector probe was the first choice of use, but the convex and the linear ones were also available. No specific attendance certification was issued.

The inter-observer agreement was assessed with kappa statistics based on Cohen and Fleiss' works [14, 15]. The strength of agreement of kappa coefficients was guided by the boundaries suggested by Landis and Koch [16].

## Results

The study was conducted in Spring and Autumn 2014. Nineteen certified Medical Doctors attending the certification board school in Internal Medicine accepted to participate on the training program. The trainees were subdivided into four groups of five or four students for each one. The training course (theoretical and practical) consisted of 9 h subdivided in 4 days (3 h on the first day and 2 h on the following days). Each trainee examined three healthy volunteers during the first day that was also the day of the theoretical lessons. Moreover, they examined nine patients per day (a total of twenty-seven patients were examined) blinded to each other as regarding the final diagnosis. The patients were not selected on the basis of the difficulty in acoustic windows images acquisition or on the basis of the diagnosis difficulty. They were selected on the basis of their actual needs.

The average time to acquire and interpret LUS was tested only when patients were examined, while free time was allowed for healthy volunteer's examination. Baseline demographics of the patients and the indications to perform LUS examination are reported in Table 1.

**Table 1 Baseline characteristics of the examined patients and indications requested by physicians to perform the examination**

| Characteristics/indications | $N = 27$ patients |
|---|---|
| Median age (years) | 71 ± 5 |
| Male/female | 15/12 |
| Obese: BMI (kg/m$^2$) ≥30 | 5 |
| Day of the examination from the admission day | 2 ± 1 |
| Acute respiratory failure as indication | 12 |
| Short time follow-up in already diagnosed pathology as indication | 10 |
| Guide for thoracentesis/exclusion of PNX after thoracentesis | 3 |
| Exclusion of PNX after central venous catheter placement | 2 |
| X chest ray at the admission (in the Emergency Medicine department) | 24 |

*BMI* body mass index

The agreement ($k$) and the strength of agreement between the trainees and the tutor in the recognition of the LUS basic signs, in the recognition of the profiles of the BLUE protocol, and in the final LUS diagnosis are displayed in Tables 2, 3, and 4.

The agreement among the trainees and the tutor in the recognition of the LUS basic signs and in the recognition of the BLUE protocol profiles ranged from "fair" to "excellent". In particular, the agreement among the trainees and the tutor in the final LUS diagnosis was "excellent" for the recognition of the interstitial syndrome and the pleural effusion, "substantial" for the recognition of the normal lung, and "moderate" for the recognition of consolidation and pneumothorax.

Table 5 shows the LUS outcome for the examined patients (the results were reported on the basis of the findings of the formal examination performed by the tutor). LUS outcome gave useful information and drove change in therapy in 16 patients. It affected immediate management in nine patients. The concordance between previous X chest ray and LUS was observed in 21 patients.

Changing in therapy or management included: diuretic therapy dosage improvement or lowering, antimicrobial therapy insertion, rapid fluid administration, thoracic surgeon consultation, thoracentesis execution, thoracic computed tomography examination, patient's discharge from the Internal Medicine department, and their admission to the Intensive Care Unit.

Table 6 depicts the final discharge diagnosis (with respect to lung findings) cited in the discharge report from the department. For some patients, the coexistence of two or more pathologies was reported. Heart failure, pneumonia, and pleural effusion were the most common final discharging diagnosis.

## Discussion

This study has been designed to assess the feasibility and the clinical utility of a short-training course in LUS for Internal Medicine certification board school attending Medical Doctors. The primary aim was to collect experience that could promote the assessment of systematic standards in training courses. Nowadays, the absence of appropriate and validated teaching models and programs is a great obstacle in this area. The training course has been precisely structured, starting with lectures (photos and video clips) and then hands-on training. The model to start with normal volunteers seems to be a convenient and effective method to teach the key elements of images acquisition, ability in probe manipulation, and spatial orientation. The beginning was the exploration of the normal lung. The sonographic technique was conducted based only on the current international evidence-based

**Table 2 Agreement between the trainees and the tutor in the recognition of the LUS basic signs**

| LUS basic signs (recognition of) | Students without any previous experience in ultrasound ($n = 9$) | | | Students with previous limited experience in Cardiac ultrasound ($n = 10$) | | |
|---|---|---|---|---|---|---|
| | *k* | 95 % CI | Agreement strength | *k* | 95 % CI | Agreement strength |
| The bat sign | 0.30 | 0.28–0.33 | Fair | 0.28 | 0.26–0.31 | Fair |
| The lung sliding | 0.71 | 0.65–0.79 | Substantial | 0.77 | 0.73–0.80 | Substantial |
| The seashore sign (M-mode) | 0.45 | 0.41–0.49 | Moderate | 0.70[a] | 0.68–0.72 | Substantial |
| The A lines | 0.90 | 0.81–1.00 | Excellent | 0.91 | 0.81–1.00 | Excellent |
| The quad sign | 0.33 | 0.29–0.40 | Fair | 0.28 | 0.25–030 | Fair |
| The sinusoid sign | 0.44 | 0.41–0.46 | Moderate | 0.44 | 0.41–0.46 | Moderate |
| The fractal sign | 0.30 | 0.27–0.32 | Fair | 0.35 | 0.28–0.40 | Fair |
| The tissue-like sign | 0.80 | 0.78–0.82 | Substantial | 0.80 | 0.79–0.81 | Substantial |
| The B lines recognition | 0.90 | 0.88–0.92 | Excellent | 0.90 | 0.86–0.94 | Excellent |
| The B lines quantification | 0.70 | 0.67–0.73 | Substantial | 0.72 | 0.70–0.74 | Substantial |
| The lung rockets | 0.50 | 0.48–0.52 | Moderate | 0.52 | 0.51–0.53 | Moderate |
| The stratosphere sign (M-mode) | 0.80 | 0.78–0.82 | Substantial | 0.84[a] | 0.82–0.84 | Excellent |
| The lung point | 0.80 | 0.78–0.82 | Substantial | 0.79 | 0.78–0.80 | Substantial |
| The lung pulse | 0.80 | 0.80–0.80 | Substantial | 0.78 | 0.77–0.79 | Substantial |
| The dynamic air bronchogram | 0.78 | 0.77–0.79 | Substantial | 0.76 | 0.73–0.79 | Substantial |

*CI* confidence intervals

[a] Significantly different between the two groups

**Table 3 Agreement between the trainees and the tutor in recognition of the BLUE protocol profiles**

| The profiles of the BLUE protocol (recognition of) | Students without any previous experience in ultrasound ($n = 9$) | | | Students with previous limited experience in cardiac ultrasound ($n = 10$) | | |
|---|---|---|---|---|---|---|
| | *k* | 95 % CI | Agreement strength | *k* | 95 % CI | Agreement strength |
| The A profile | 0.77 | 0.73–0.80 | Substantial | 0.71 | 0.61–0.80 | Substantial |
| The A' profile | 0.76 | 0.75–0.77 | Substantial | 0.76 | 0.74–0.78 | Substantial |
| The B profile | 0.77 | 0.76–0.78 | Substantial | 0.75 | 0.74–0.76 | Substantial |
| The B' profile | 0.72 | 0.70–0.72 | Substantial | 0.72 | 0.66–0.78 | Substantial |
| The C profile | 0.32 | 0.30–035 | Fair | 0.35 | 0.29–0.41 | Fair |
| The A/B profile | 0.50 | 0.48–0.52 | Moderate | 0.51 | 0.49–0.53 | Moderate |

*CI* confidence intervals

**Table 4 Agreement between the trainees and the tutor in the final LUS diagnosis**

| Final LUS diagnosis | Students without any previous experience in ultrasound ($n = 9$) | | | Students with previous limited experience in cardiac ultrasound ($n = 10$) | | |
|---|---|---|---|---|---|---|
| | *k* | 95 % CI | Agreement strength | *k* | 95 % CI | Agreement strength |
| The normal lung | 0.65 | 0.61–0.69 | Substantial | 0.66 | 0.61–0.72 | Substantial |
| The pneumothorax | 0.46 | 0.45–0.47 | Moderate | 0.48 | 0.46–0.50 | Moderate |
| The interstitial syndrome | 0.82 | 0.81–0.83 | Excellent | 0.84 | 0.82–0.86 | Excellent |
| The consolidation | 0.45 | 0.44–0.46 | Moderate | 0.48 | 0.47–0.49 | Moderate |
| The pleural effusion with the correct recognition of its nature (transudates/exudates) | 0.82 | 0.81–0.83 | Excellent | 0.83 | 0.82–0.84 | Excellent |

*CI* confidence intervals

**Table 5 LUS outcome for the examined patients**

| LUS outcome | N = 27 patients |
|---|---|
| Affected immediate management | 9 |
| Gave useful information and drove change in therapy | 16 |
| No useful information nor change in therapy | 2 |
| Concordance between previous X chest ray and LUS | 21 |
| X chest ray examination or thoracic computed tomography need to confirm the management | 4 |

*LUS* lung ultrasound

**Table 6 Summary of the final discharging diagnosis (for some patients two or more diagnosis were reported)**

| Discharging diagnosis cited in the final report | N = 27 patients |
|---|---|
| Heart failure | 22 |
| Pneumonia | 12 |
| Pleural effusion | 10 |
| PNX | 2 |
| Pulmonary fibrosis | 1 |
| ARDS | 1 |

*ARDS* acute respiratory distress syndrome, *PNX* pneumothorax

recommendations [9], focusing in particular on the BLUE protocol [12, 13]. This choice was to standardize knowledge and skills. The results of the present study suggest an acceptable ability level in performing LUS and in allocating the patients in one of its principal clinical scenarios. However, some tasks were more difficult to acquire and interpret. In general, there was not a significant difference in performing LUS on the basis of previous knowledge and practice in cardiac ultrasound, except for obese patients (data not analysed). The same results for the detection of those signs for which M-mode evaluation is required. The lack of substantial difference could be due to the fact that the trainees with previous knowledge in focused cardiac ultrasound had limited experience and practice. Therefore, these data confirm that LUS is relatively easy to perform even in non-ultrasound-experienced physicians [11, 17]. Regarding the average time to acquire and interpret the LUS, the results of this training course substantially agree with the time allotted by the BLUE protocol (maximum 3 min) [12, 13]. The adherence to the BLUE protocol was mandatory for the trainer, with the aim of standardizing the procedure. More time was required (and consented) by the trainers during the management of the healthy volunteers. Regarding the training period, previous experiences [11] have shown that a 1 day course could be sufficient to acquire theoretical and practical skills in LUS. More work has to be done to standardize these training courses. The precise time to devote and the examination number to be done to have the ability to perform a useful LUS has to be identified.

Although the study was principally assessed to evaluate a model of LUS training, some remarks could be made about the indications to perform LUS. They reflect the most common indications in an Internal Medicine department. In particular, heart failure is one of the most common admission diagnoses. In this context, the main sign that has to be considered is the presence of B lines. They surely represent an easy to acquire and highly reproducible sign, but their limitation is the low specificity [18]. B lines due to cardiogenic pulmonary edema are usually diffusing or recovering symmetrically. In fact, their regular distribution allows to differentiate cardiogenic pulmonary edema from ARDS and from pulmonary fibrosis [2]. This last is also characterized by irregularities of the pleural line and sub-pleural small consolidations. The B lines have to be used both as diagnostic modality and in monitoring heart failure therapy [18]. The clearance of the B lines represents a direct sign of effective treatment in heart failure and, as we have demonstrated, a careful assessment and quantification of them is useful also in the follow-up. It has been shown [4, 18] that ultrasound accuracy has even higher sensitivity than chest X ray in the detection of the early signs of interstitial thickening due to the pulmonary congestion. Sonographic B-lines' assessment is surely of particular interest in LUS. A recent study [19] has evaluated the agreement among trained and novice Medical Doctors in an Emergency department. Authors tried to determine which thoracic zones could represent the highest level of inter-observer reliability for B-lines' assessment. They found that agreement was best in the anterior/superior thoracic zones, and it was highest at extreme high or low numbers of B lines. This study has to be mentioned, because training assessment in B-lines' recognition is a promising area of investigation, relatively simple but mandatory. Moreover, the precise thoracic zone definition is a more detailed information. It is not present in our study. This fact could be a limitation of our current training program.

In addition, pneumonia represents a very common diagnosis in the Internal Medicine department, associated with increasing morbidity and mortality, hospitalization rate, and health costs [20]. Pneumonia LUS pattern is constituted by consolidations and dynamic air bronchograms. These signs could be frequently associated with pleural effusion or interstitial syndrome images [21]. It is well established that computed tomography represents the gold standard and that chest X ray remains the daily reference for lung imaging in the diagnosis of pneumonia [21]. However, recent studies have confirmed excellent sensitivity and specificity of LUS, with percentages comparable with chest X ray [18, 21, 22] (the main limitation is that LUS may only detect lesions reaching the pleura). Nevertheless, it is to mention that these comparable results could be obtained only with experienced LUS operators. Therefore, in this context, the importance of precise training courses and a common level of proficiency are mandatory. As described in "Results", LUS gave useful information and drove change in therapy in the majority of the analysed cases. It affected immediate management in a consistent number of cases. This point underlines its importance. The LUS operator was not blinded to the patients' clinical situation (while the Radiologist usually does not see the patients but only an information summary about them). This modality underlines the usefulness of this imaging examination. It could be performed at the bedside by the physician who is looking after the patient and who is better able to place any LUS finding in a more appropriate context with other clinical problems.

Nevertheless, this study has several limitations. The results do not address what level of experience is needed to maintain the skills. They inform only about the initial training assessment required. Second, the post-course performance of the trainees was tested just shortly after the completion of the program. This is an important point to be considered in each area of ultrasound. Trainees' skills decrease as a function of time, particularly when ultrasound techniques are not conducted regularly and further supervised teaching is not available. Moreover, this is an Internal Medicine department experience. No patients directly derived from the emergency setting were tested. According to the admission characteristics in the Internal Medicine department, the evaluation of a sufficient number of PNX, ARDS, and artificial ventilation patients was not possible. In fact, the study reflects the real need of this department, focusing on interstitial syndrome, pleural effusion, and consolidation (both as acute and as follow-up indication for LUS). In particular, the ability to rule out the PNX was critical after procedures, such as the insertion of central venous catheter but mostly after the thoracentesis. This procedure is not so unusual for the Internal Medicine department. LUS should be mandatory both as procedure guide and as procedure monitoring to reduce the iatrogenic complications [23, 24].

## Conclusions

This study supports incorporating LUS into Internal Medicine fellowship training programs. It should facilitate the design of future training courses. The maximum effectiveness of the method is obtained through a clinically driven, focused and methodologically learned assessment. As mentioned by Lichtenstein, who significantly improved the expansion of LUS explaining his "ten good reasons to practice ultrasound in critical care" [25], it is hopeful that these good reasons could reach also the Internal Medicine care. This contributes to a widespread and routine use of LUS in this department with rigorous and scientific training courses protocols.

**Abbreviations**

ARDS: acute respiratory distress syndrome; BLUE: bedside lung ultrasound evaluation; BMI: body mass index; LUS: lung ultrasound; PNX: pneumothorax; SIMI: Società Italiana di Medicina Interna; SIUMB: Società Italiana di Ultrasonologia in Medicina e Biologia; WINFOCUS: World interactive network focused on critical ultrasound.

**Authors' contributions**

CM designed and performed the study and wrote the manuscript, AFP and UG analysed the data, and LC designed and organized the study. All authors read and approved the final manuscript.

**Acknowledgements**

None.

**References**

1. Bouhemad B, Zhang M, Lu Q, Rouby JJ (2007) Clinical review: bedside lung ultrasound in critical care practice. Crit Care 11(1):205–213
2. Via G, Storti E, Gulati G, Neri L, Mojoli F, Braschi A (2012) Lung ultrasound in the ICU: from diagnostic instrument to respiratory monitoring tool. Minerva Anestesiol 78:1282–1296
3. Reissig A, Copetti R, Kroegel C (2011) Current role of emergency ultrasound of the chest. Crit Care Med 39(4):839–845
4. Gargani L (2011) Lung ultrasound: a new tool for the cardiologist. Cardiovasc Ultrasound 9:6–12
5. Filopei J, Siedenburg H, Rattner P, Fukaya E, Kory P (2014) Impact of pocket ultrasound use by internal medicine house staff in the diagnosis of dyspnoea. J Hosp Med 9(9):594–597
6. Lichtenstein D (2014) Lung ultrasound in the critically ill. Curr Opin Crit Care 20:315–322
7. Lichtenstein D (2014) Lung ultrasound in the critically ill. Ann Intensiv Care 4:1–12
8. Volpicelli G (2013) Lund sonography. J Ultrasound Med 32:165–171
9. Volpicelli G, International Liaison Committee on Lung Ultrasound (ILC-LUS) for the International Consensus Conference on Lung Ultrasound (ICC-LUS) (2012) International evidence-based recommendation for point of care lung ultrasound. Intensive Care Med 38:577–591
10. Gargani L, Volpicelli G (2014) How I do it: lung ultrasound. Cardiovasc Ultrasound 12:25–35
11. Breitkreutz R, Dutinè M, Scheiermann P, Hempel D, Kujumdshiev S, Ackermann H (2013) Thorax, trachea, and lung ultrasonography in emergency and critical care medicine: assessment of an objective structured training concept. Emerg Med Int. doi:10.1155/2013/312758
12. Lichtenstein D, Meziere GA (2008) Relevance of lung ultrasound in the diagnosis of acute respiratory failure. The BLUE protocol. Chest 134:117–125
13. Lichtenstein D (2009) Lung ultrasound in acute respiratory failure: an introduction to the BLUE protocol. Minerva Anestesiol 75:313–317
14. Cohen J (1960) A coefficient of agreement for nominal scales. Educ Psychol Meas 20:37–46
15. Fleiss J (1971) Measuring nominal scale agreement among many raters. Pyschol Bull 76(5):378–382
16. Landis JR, Koch GG (1977) Measurement of observer agreement for categorical data. Biometrics 33:159–174
17. Martindale JL, Noble VE, Liteplo A (2013) Diagnosing pulmonary edema: lung ultrasound versus chest radiography. Eur J Emerg Med 20(5):356–360

18. Ang SH, Andrus P (2012) Lung ultrasound in the management of acute decompensated heart failure. Curr Cardiol Rev 8:123–136
19. Gullett J, Donnelly JP, Sinert R, Hosek B, Fuller D, Hill H, Feldman I, Galetto G, Auster M, Hoffmann B (2015) Interobserver agreement in the evaluation of B-lines using bedside ultrasound. J Crit Care 30(6):1395–1399
20. Welte T, Torres A, Nathwani D (2012) Clinical and economic burden of community-acquired pneumonia among adults in Europe. Thorax 67:71–79
21. Reissig A, Copetti R, Mathis G, Mempel C, Schuler A, Zechner P (2012) Lung ultrasound in the diagnosis and follow up of community-acquired pneumonia. A prospective, multicentre, diagnostic accuracy study. Chest 142(4):965–972
22. Lichtenstein D, Goldstein I, Mourgeon E, Cluzel P, Grenier P, Rouby JJ (2004) Comparative diagnostic performances of auscultation, chest radiography and lung ultrasonography in acute respiratory distress syndrome. Anesthesiology 100:9–15
23. Mercaldi CJ, Lanes SF (2013) Ultrasound guidance decreases complications and improves the cost of care among patients undergoing thoracentesis and paracentesis. Chest 143(2):532–538
24. Perazzo A, Gatto P, Barlascini C, Ferrari Bravo M, Nicolini A (2013) Can ultrasound guidance reduce the risk of pneumothorax following thoracentesis? J Bras Pneumol 40(1):6–12
25. Lichtenstein D, van Hooland S, Malbrain M (2014) Ten good reasons to practice ultrasound in critical care. Anaesthesiol Intensiv Ther 6(5):323–335

# 5

# Current status of emergency department attending physician ultrasound credentialing and quality assurance in the United States

Devjani Das[1*], Monica Kapoor[1], Cara Brown[1], Afoma Ndubuisi[1] and Sanjey Gupta[2]

**Abstract**

**Background:** The use of emergency ultrasonography (EUS) has gained much popularity in the past few decades, and is now a mainstay of diagnostic decision-making. This expanded use is now highlighting the substantial issue of individual hospitals in credentialing its emergency medicine attending physicians in EUS in the United States. This issue is also of importance as more hospitals are now requesting reimbursements for emergency ultrasounds. The objective of this study is to gain an understanding of how many emergency departments are currently credentialing its attending staff in EUS, what the internal structure and staffing are of these emergency departments, and how they are currently performing quality assurance of the ultrasounds performed.

**Methods:** This was a cross-sectional, web-based survey sent to 160 ACGME-accredited EM residency programs from July 2013 to November 2013. The survey consisted of 23 questions regarding: (1) number of emergency medicine attendings on staff, (2) presence of an EUS fellowship, (3) quality assurance (QA) process, and (4) current US credentialing process.

**Results:** There was a 50 % response rate. Fifty percent of the total respondents ($n = 40$) had an EUS fellowship program. Of the sites with an EUS fellowship, 36 had EUS fellowship-trained attendings. Of the sites without an EUS fellowship, 19 had EUS fellowship-trained faculty, $p \leq 0.0001$. Sites with an EUS fellowship had a greater percentage of staff credentialed to perform EUS as compared to sites with no EUS fellowship, $p = 0.0161$. All sites with an EUS fellowship had EUS-credentialed attendings. In sites with an EUS fellowship, 35 conducted a formal QA of ED performed EUS scans versus 22 at sites without an EUS fellowship, $p = 0.003$.

**Conclusions:** The survey results support hiring emergency attendings that have completed postgraduate training in emergency ultrasonography to aid in credentialing staff. This also seems to be helpful in completing a timelier QA of all ED ultrasounds.

**Keywords:** Emergency ultrasonography, Education, Survey, Credentialing, Quality assurance

## Background

The use of emergency ultrasonography (EUS) has gained much popularity, since it was first introduced in the 1980s and is now a mainstay of diagnostic decision-making in the emergency department [1]. In 2011, the Accreditation Council for General Medical Education (ACGME) Residency Review Committee (RRC) adopted an outcomes-based approach to residency accreditation in the United States. As part of this endeavor, EUS was deemed as one of the essential components in Patient Care, which is one of six core competencies for emergency medicine residency training. Since adoption of this mandate, every emergency medicine (EM) residency program must teach

*Correspondence: devdas2@gmail.com
[1] Department of Emergency Medicine, Northwell Health-Staten Island University Hospital, 475 Seaview Ave, Staten Island, NY 10305, USA
Full list of author information is available at the end of the article

and assess ultrasound competency as part of its education [2]. As a result of this directive, improvements in US technology and research into new potential applications for US, the use of EUS has increased in the emergency department (ED). This expanded use is now highlighting the substantial issue of individual hospitals in credentialing its emergency medicine attending physicians in EUS in the United States. This issue is also of importance as an increasing number of hospitals is now requesting reimbursement for emergency ultrasounds.

Numerous organizations within EM have proposed guidelines on how to train physicians in EUS applications. Foremost among these are the 2008 American College of Emergency Physicians (ACEP) guidelines that recommend 150 ultrasound examinations in six specific applications [3]. However, several studies have shown that though there is an increase in EP training in EUS, there remains a wide variation in the type and extent of teaching in individual academic training programs [4, 5]. This variability in teaching and education presents a challenging situation for EDs to credential attending physicians in the use of EUS.

An extensive review of the current literature has shown that no standardized method of ED attending credentialing in EUS exists in the United States. Furthermore, credentialing is primarily an individual hospital function. This lack of a universal credentialing process in EUS may lead to a discrepancy in the delineation of privileges for a physician from hospital to hospital, i.e., a physician credentialed in performing ultrasound in one hospital may not be credentialed to do so in another hospital [6]. The objective of this study is to gain an understanding of how many emergency departments are currently credentialing its attending staff in EUS, what the internal structure and staffing are of these emergency departments, and how they are currently performing quality assurance of the ultrasounds performed.

## Methods

### Study design

This was a cross-sectional, web-based survey that was sent to 160 ACGME-accredited EM residency programs from July 2013 to November 2013. This was the total number of ACGME-accredited EM residency programs in existence during this time frame. A cover letter explaining the research study was initially sent to all EM residency program directors who were identified through the SAEM Residency Directory website. If deemed appropriate, the residency directors were instructed to share the survey with the US credentialing authority in their emergency department to acquire more accurate answers. A reminder email was sent 1 month after the initial survey request and again 2 months later to hospitals that had not completed the survey. The survey consisted of 23 questions created by the study authors regarding: (1) number of emergency attendings on staff, (2) presence or absence of an EUS fellowship, (3) quality assurance (QA) process, and (4) current EUS credentialing process (Figs. 1, 2). The survey required about 5–10 min to complete and included multiple choice and free text answers.

The survey was initially tested on a focus group consisting of three EUS program directors at various academic institutions. Questions were adjusted as suggested by the focus group for wording clarification purposes. Each academic institution that was sent a survey was provided with a unique numerical identifier after responses were obtained. All answers to the survey were de-identified and confidential prior to statistical analysis. This survey study was approved by the Institutional Review Board and was granted a waiver of signed consent at the authors' home institution.

### Data analysis

The survey was distributed and results directly extracted from the online survey tool Surveymonkey©. Categorical data were analyzed utilizing descriptive statistics. The differences between groups were analyzed with the Chi-square analysis. Multivariate analysis was performed with a logistical regression model. Ordinal data were analyzed with a Mann–Whitney test and Spearman correlation.

## Results

There was a 50 % response rate to the survey study for a total of 80 respondents out of 160 programs (Table 1). All responses were from academic institutions in either a community ($n = 22$) or academic setting ($n = 58$). Of all respondents, 68.75 % ($n = 55$) had US-trained faculty on site. Fifty percent of total respondents ($n = 40$) had an EUS fellowship program. Of the sites with an EUS fellowship, 36 had EUS fellowship-trained attendings. Of the sites without an EUS fellowship, 19 had EUS fellowship-trained faculty, $p \leq 0.0001$. Sites with an EUS fellowship had a greater percentage of staff credentialed to perform EUS as compared to sites with no EUS fellowship, $p = 0.0161$.

### Ultrasound credentialing

Ultrasound credentialing was done by a variety of methods at different sites. All sites with an EUS fellowship had EUS-credentialed attendings. The designated EUS director usually performed the process of credentialing at these sites. At sites without an EUS fellowship, 7 had no credentialing for emergency attendings to perform EUS in the emergency department, $p = 0.025$ (Table 2).

1. What position do you hold at your institution?
   a. Ultrasound Director
   b. Residency Director
   c. Department Director
   d. Other, please specify ______________________
2. How would you describe your institution?
   a. Academic
   b. Community
   c. Rural
   d. Urban
   e. Suburban
   f. Mixture
3. What is the annual volume of your Emergency Department?
   a. <50,000 patient visits per year
   b. 50,000 – 90,0000 patient visits per year
   c. >90,0000 patient visits per year
4. What is the format of your residency program?
   a. PGY I-III
   b. PGY I-IV
   c. PGY II-IV
5. Do you have any ultrasound-fellowship trained emergency physicians on staff?
   a. Yes
   b. No
6. How many emergency medicine attendings are on staff? _______________
7. Are all of your emergency medicine attendings board-certified in emergency medicine?
   a. Yes
   b. No
8. If not, how many are not board-certified in emergency medicine? ____________
9. Do you have a portable ultrasound machine in your Emergency Department?
   a. Yes
   b. No
10. If so, how often is the ultrasound machine available for use by your emergency medicine attending staff in your department?
    a. All of the time
    b. Some of the time
    c. Very rarely
11. Roughly how many ultrasounds do your emergency medicine attending staff order through your radiology department **yearly**?
    a. <100
    b. 100-500
    c. >500
12. What type of ultrasounds does your attending staff mostly order through the Radiology Department? (Circle all that apply)
    a. DVT
    b. AAA
    c. FAST
    d. Torsion (ovarian and/or testicular)
    e. Transabdominal/transvaginal pregnancy
    f. Gallbladder
    g. Cardiac
    h. Renal
    i. Musculoskeletal (including abscess, cellulitis or foreign body)
    j. Lung
    k. Ocular

**Fig. 1** Survey questionnaire

13. How often is the Radiology Department available to perform the ultrasounds ordered by your attending staff?
    a. <12 hours per day
    b. 12-24 hours
    c. 24 hours a day
14. On average, how many **TOTAL** ultrasounds does your emergency medicine attending staff perform yearly on their own?
    a. <50
    b. 50-100
    c. >100
15. What percentage of your emergency medicine staff is credentialed to perform bedside ultrasound?
    a. 0-25%
    b. 25-50%
    c. 50-75%
    d. 75-100%
16. Who credentials your attending staff to perform emergency ultrasound?
    a. Department Director
    b. Ultrasound Director
    c. Hospital credentialing board
    d. We don't credential our staff in ultrasound
    e. Other, please specify ______________________
17. If you are credentialing your staff to perform emergency ultrasound, what are some of the barriers you have come across in doing so?
18. What procedure do you use to credential your staff to perform emergency ultrasounds?
19. Is there a formal quality assurance (QA) process for ultrasounds performed by your emergency medicine attending staff?
    a. Yes
    b. No
20. If so, what kind of QA process do you use?
    a. US scans reviewed weekly
    b. US scans reviewed monthly
    c. US scans reviewed yearly
    d. US scans are not reviewed
    e. Other, please specify ______________________
21. If a QA process exists, who performs the QA?
    a. US director
    b. Radiology department
    c. Other, please specify ______________________
22. Do you currently submit ultrasounds performed by your emergency medicine attending staff for reimbursement?
    a. Yes
    b. No
23. If not, are there plans to do so in the future?
    a. Yes
    b. No

**Fig. 2** Survey questionnaire

## Quality assurance

In sites with an EUS fellowship, 35 conducted a formal QA of ED performed EUS scans versus 22 at sites without an EUS fellowship, $p = 0.003$. At hospital sites with an EUS fellowship that conducted formal QA, 100 % (35) had the QA process performed by the EUS director. In the non-EUS fellowship sites, 18 had the QA performed by the EUS director, $p = 0.019$. At non-EUS fellowship sites without an EUS director who are conducting QA, 4 utilized the following for QA: (1) assigned faculty member, (2) program director/director of pediatric ED, (3) hospital EUS credentialing committee, or (4) radiology department. At hospitals with an EUS fellowship that conducted a formal QA, 29 conducted QA weekly or less, 5 conducted QA bi-weekly-to-monthly, and 1 conducted QA in another format. At non-EUS fellowship

**Table 1 Demographics of study population**

| Respondents | N (percentage) |
|---|---|
| Respondent demographics | |
| Number of respondents | 80 |
| Position in the institution | |
| Ultrasound director | 23 (28.75) |
| Residency director | 42 (52.5) |
| Department director | 1 (1.25) |
| Other faculty | 16 (20) |
| Institution description | |
| Academic | 58 (72.5) |
| Community | 22 (27.5) |
| Annual departmental volume (k visits) | |
| <50 | 6 (7.5) |
| 50–90 | 35 (43.75) |
| >90 | 40 (50) |
| Residency program format | |
| PGY 1–3 | 53 (66.25) |
| PGY 1–4 | 26 (32.5) |
| EM/IM or EM/FM | 1 (1.25) |
| Ultrasound demographics | |
| Does the site have portable ultrasound in the ED? | |
| Yes | 80 (100) |
| No | 0 (0) |
| Does the site have an ultrasound fellowship? | |
| Yes | 40 (50) |
| No | 40 (50) |
| Does the site have ultrasound trained faculty? | |
| Yes | 55 (68.75) |
| No | 25 (31.25) |

**Table 2 Credentialing and quality assurance responses**

| Respondents | N (percentage) |
|---|---|
| Percentage of ED attendings credentialed for EUS | |
| 0–25 % | 15 (18.75) |
| 25–50 % | 22 (27.5) |
| 50–75 % | 12 (15) |
| 75–100 % | 31 (38.75) |
| Who credentials the staff to perform EUS? | |
| Department director | 16 (20) |
| Ultrasound director | 50 (62.5) |
| Hospital credentialing board | 32 (40) |
| Do not credential | 7 (8.75) |
| Other | 1 (1.25) |
| Is there a formal QA process for EP performed US? | |
| Yes | 57 (71.25) |
| No | 23 (28.75) |
| If a QA process exists, who performs the QA? | |
| Ultrasound director | 56 (98.25) |
| Radiology department | 1 (1.75) |
| N/A | 23 |

sites, 5 conducted QA weekly or less, 13 conducted QA bi-weekly-to-monthly, 4 performed QA in another format (including rolling, yearly, or quarterly), $p < 0.001$. (Table 2).

## Discussion

The response rate to this survey study was on par with other studies conducted on similar topics. What differentiates this data set from other studies was that 50 % of total respondents were affiliated with sites supporting EUS fellowship programs, while 50 % were not. This allowed for a greater understanding of the difference in the credentialing and QA process at hospital sites with and without an EUS fellowship.

The survey results support that there is a great deal of variation in the number of EUS-credentialed staff and method for credentialing emergency attendings in EUS. This variability seemed to depend largely on the presence or absence of an EUS fellowship program at the institution. Having an EUS fellowship and a dedicated EUS director seems to be associated with wider credentialing of attending staff. This is likely due to having a greater number of faculty members to provide the additional training required to credential staff. However, this does not necessarily apply to institutions that have EUS fellowship-trained faculty, but no EUS fellowship on site. In addition, institutions without an EUS fellowship and without an EUS director are largely not credentialing their faculty to perform ultrasounds.

Similarly, there is variability in the QA process at hospital sites with and without an EUS fellowship program. Based on the results of the survey, hospital sites with an EUS fellowship are more likely to perform a formal QA process. Overwhelmingly, the majority of the hospitals manage their QA process within the ED. However, at hospital sites without an EUS fellowship program, there was greater variability in the method by which the QA process is currently being performed. Of hospital sites with a formal QA process, ultrasounds are likely to be reviewed on a weekly basis. However, if no EUS fellowship program is present, there is a greater likelihood that the QA process is not being conducted on a weekly basis. However, studies have shown that a weekly QA process is the optimal method to provide feedback, performance improvement, and assurance that ultrasounds are being performed and interpreted correctly [7].

In contrast to other medical specialties that utilize ultrasound, the examinations performed by emergency physicians are highly focused, limited, and goal-directed

[8]. As Jang, et al. put forth in his recent article regarding competency-based mandate in EUS, to be considered competent in EUS, physicians must have (1) an understanding of the disease process and indications for the diagnostic modality, (2) technical skills to acquire appropriate and interpretable images, (3) the ability to reliably interpret sonograms, and (4) management skills to apply the findings in light of their patient's clinical presentation [8]. The American Board of Emergency Medicine (ABEM) has been seeking to gain approval amongst its members to offer physician certification in clinical ultrasonography through the American Board of Medical Specialties (ABMS). ABEM envisions that once this is approved, physicians who do not achieve certification in clinical ultrasonography might eventually have a more difficult time practicing or billing for ultrasonography in some institutions. However, the process by which this may occur will require rigorous review through ABMS and may not occur for several years. As this move by ABEM highlights, it is becoming increasingly apparent that EUS is a vital skill in the ED management of patients. Currently, there exist evidence-based recommendations and expert consensus recommendations for specific applications for EUS, including for point-of-care lung and cardiac ultrasound [9, 10]. There have also been well-researched and comprehensive proposed guidelines/curriculum for teaching EUS and providing a foundational knowledge of point-of-care ultrasonography. However, these guidelines have not been prospectively validated [11]. Therefore, training and assessment of ultrasound education among different residency programs vary greatly [12]. What this study poses is the understanding that having an EUS fellowship, or at least staff that have completed an EUS fellowship, is associated with increased training of attendings in emergency ultrasonography.

Another key factor that was highlighted in this study was the variability in which hospitals are currently performing their QA process. As hospitals are moving forward with more widespread use of EUS, many hospitals are already, or are soon planning, to request reimbursement for ultrasounds performed in the ED. Each US that is performed, used to make clinical decisions and are subsequently submitted for reimbursement require appropriate documentation regarding the indication for the examinations, written interpretation of the examinations, description of the organs or structures studied, who performed the examinations, and documentation of the scope of the study [13]. For patient safety purposes, it is, therefore, imperative that all of these studies be reviewed for QA on a timely basis. Having an EUS fellowship is likely conducive to having additional staff to review all of these ultrasounds and to ensure that the QA process is more streamlined.

### Limitations

There are inherent limitations to any study based on survey results. This survey was subject to selection bias in that hospital sites that regularly utilize EUS are more likely to respond to the questionnaire. However, our response rate allowed for a unique data subset to analyze given that exactly 50 % had an EUS fellowship program versus 50 % that did not.

This study was also limited because hospital sites were chosen exclusively for having an ACGME-accredited EM residency program. This was done so that a greater understanding of the credentialing and QA process could be made at sites that are likely to be invested in having a robust EUS education program. However, results may be quite different if applied to hospital sites without an EM residency program and may not be generalizable to non-academic institutions.

## Conclusions

The spectrum of growth of EUS in daily practice within EDs nationwide is evident over the past several decades. This was exemplified by the RRC, which has made US education one subcomponent of its six emergency medicine core competencies. It is clear, therefore, that all hospitals, especially those with an ACGME-accredited residency program, will need to ensure that its staff is well versed in their US knowledge and technical skills. Credentialing their emergency attendings in EUS is a hospital-specific issue, but is a complex one when considering the extensive requirements that all physicians must meet to be considered competent in emergency ultrasonography. Our survey results seem to support hiring staff that has completed extra training in emergency ultrasonography to aid in credentialing other staff in EUS. This also seems to be helpful in completing a more timely QA process of all ultrasounds performed in the ED. In the future, we hope to look into what methods hospitals are currently using to credential their staff in EUS and which of these methods appear to be most effective.

#### Abbreviations

EUS: emergency ultrasonography; ACGME: Accreditation Council for General Medical Education; RRC: Residency Review Committee; EM: emergency medicine; ED: emergency department; ACEP: American College of Emergency Physicians.

#### Authors' contributions

DD contributed to the development of the concept of the research, research design, data acquisition, and development of manuscript. MK contributed to the development of the concept of the research and research design. CB contributed to the development of the concept of the research and research design. AN contributed to the development of the concept of the research, research design, and data acquisition. SG contributed to the development of the concept of the research, research design, statistical analysis, and development of manuscript. All authors read and approved the final manuscript.

### Authors' information

DD is the Associate Director of Emergency Ultrasound and Co-Fellowship Director in the Department of Emergency Medicine at Northwell Health-Staten Island University Hospital. She is currently involved in the development of the quality assurance process and credentialing of attending physicians in emergency ultrasound in her department.

MK is the Director of Emergency Ultrasound and Co-Fellowship Director in the Department of Emergency Medicine at Northwell Health-Staten Island University Hospital. She is currently involved in the development of the quality assurance process and credentialing of attending physicians in emergency ultrasound in her department.

CB is a member of the Emergency Ultrasound Division in the Department of Emergency Medicine at Northwell Health-Staten Island University Hospital. She is currently involved in the development of the quality assurance process and credentialing of attending physicians in emergency ultrasound in her department.

AN is an attending in the Department of Emergency Medicine at Northwell Health-Staten Island University Hospital.

SG is the Director of the Emergency Department at Northwell Health-Franklin Hospital.

### Author details

[1] Department of Emergency Medicine, Northwell Health-Staten Island University Hospital, 475 Seaview Ave, Staten Island, NY 10305, USA. [2] Department of Emergency Medicine, Northwell Health-Franklin Hospital, 900 Franklin Ave, Valley Stream, NY 11580, USA.

### References

1. Moore CL, Molina AA, Lin H (2006) Ultrasonography in Community Emergency Departments in the United States; access to ultrasonography performed by consultants and status of emergency physician-performed ultrasonography. Ann Emerg Med 47(2):147–153
2. Jang TB, Coates WC, Liu YT (2012) The competency-based mandate for emergency bedside sonography training and a tale of two residency programs. J Ultrasound Med 31:515–521
3. American College of Emergency Physicians (ACEP) (2008) "Policy statement: emergency ultrasound guidelines."
4. Moore CL, Gregg S, Lambert M (2004) Performance, training, quality assurance, and reimbursement of emergency physician-performed ultrasonography at academic medical centers. J Ultrasound Med 23:459–466
5. Ahern M, Mallin MP, Weitzel S et al (2010) Variability in ultrasound education among emergency medicine residencies. West J Emerg Med 11(4):314–318
6. Lanoix R (1997) Credentialing issues in emergency ultrasonography. Emerg Med Clinics of North America 15(4):913–920
7. Budhram G, Elia T, Rathlev N (2013) Implementation of a successful incentive-based ultrasound credentialing program for emergency physicians. W J Emer Med 14(6):602–608
8. Jang TB, Coates WC, Liu YT (2012) The competency-based mandate for emergency bedside sonography training and a tale of two residency programs. J Ultrasound Med 31:515–521
9. Via G, Hussain A, Wells M et al (2014) International evidence-based recommendations for focused cardiac ultrasound. J Am Soc Echocardiogr 27(7):683
10. Volpicelli G, Elbarbary M, Blaivas M et al (2012) International evidence-based recommendations for point-of-care lung ultrasound. Intensive Care Med 38(4):577–591
11. Atkinson P, Bowra J, Lambert M et al (2015) International federation for emergency medicine point of care ultrasound curriculum. CJEM 17(2):161–170
12. Cohen JS, Teach SJ, Chapman J (2012) Bedside ultrasound education in pediatric emergency medicine fellowship programs in the United States. Pediatr Emerg Care 28(9):845–850
13. Cardenas E (2004) Emergency medicine ultrasound policies and reimbursement guidelines. Emerg Med Clinics of N Am 22(3):829–838

# 6

# The Sierra Leone Ultrasound Rainbow4Africa Project (SLURP): an observational study of ultrasound effectiveness in developing countries

Alessandro Lamorte[1*], Enrico Boero[2], Paola Crida[3], Abdul R. Conteh[4], Marco Foletti[5] and Paolo Narcisi[5]

**Abstract**

**Background:** Diagnostic tools available in low-income countries are often really basic even if patients can be as sick as those of the richer countries. Point-of-care ultrasound could be a solution for this problem. We studied the impact of ultrasound at the Holy Spirit Hospital, Makeni, Sierra Leone.

**Methods:** This is a prospective, observational study on outpatients presenting at the HSH. We enrolled continually for 1 month 105 patients asked for ultrasound examination by the caring physician that had to indicate the differential diagnosis hypothesized, the confidence degree about these on a 5-point Likert scale, and the therapy before and after the US. The primary outcome was to measure the difference in the number of differential diagnoses. Secondary outcomes were the rate of new diagnoses, the confidence changes of the visiting physician, and the changes in prescribed therapy or management. Categorical variables were compared using the Chi-square test, and continuous ones using two-tailed Student's test and Likert with the Wilcoxon rank-sum test.

**Results:** 194 differential diagnoses were formulated, with a mean of 1.85 (DS 0.87) diagnoses per patient. 89 (46%) were excluded on the basis of US, reducing the mean of differential diagnosis per patient to 1, 0 ($p < 0.001$). US also introduced 53 new diagnoses in 42 patients (mean 1.26; SD 0.54), raising the final differential diagnosis from 105 to 158 (+50.5%) that is 1.51 (DS 0.79) per patient. There is a statistically significant reduction (18.6%) in diagnoses per patient after having performed the ultrasound ($p < 0.001$). The certainty level increased (Wilcoxon rank-sum test: $p < 0.001$). We did not reach the statistical significance studying the changes in therapy and management because the subgroups for analysis were too small. Nonetheless, we saw interesting changes in drug prescription and referral rate before and after the US.

**Conclusion:** Ultrasound is feasible in low-income countries; with it diagnostic hypotheses were reduced and new unexpected diagnoses were introduced. Further studies are needed to explore other strong outcomes like mortality, length of stay in hospital, and money saved with the use of ultrasound in developing countries.

**Keywords:** Point-of-care ultrasound, Low-income countries, Developing Countries, Rural context, Emergency medicine, Diagnostic, Clinical decision making, Abdominal ultrasound

*Correspondence: alessandro.lamorte86@gmail.com
[1] Emergency Department, San Luigi Gonzaga Hospital, Regione Gonzole 10 Orbassano, 10043 Turin, Italy
Full list of author information is available at the end of the article

## Background

The struggle to diagnose and treat diseases is usually one of the hardest. But it can be worse in a low-resource country where Diagnostic tools available are really basic especially for doctors used to the western standards of technology. Especially if we consider that the low-income countries patients can be as sick as those of the richer countries.

Sierra Leone has been dramatically influenced by a decade of civil war that affected over two million people. The country is among the last countries in the Human Development Index and has a mortality rate of 36.8% in adults. The main pathologies present in the country are malaria, tuberculosis, and HIV. Access to health services is difficult and very often patients must pay for these services and travel for long distances on foot, or face new charges for transport. So much of the population turns to traditional healers, which in many areas of the country are the only chance of cure.

Ultrasonography and specifically point-of-care ultrasound (POCUS) could be a solution for this lack of diagnostic possibilities because of some intrinsic features of the technology. Ultrasonography (US) is cheap, dynamic, repeatable, bedside (if the machine can be moved or has a battery), and can answer any questions the physician could have. To date, ultrasonography was used almost in every condition, from war to the Amazon jungle to Tibet [1, 2], from space to Everest [3, 4], and has shown to fit in all of these conditions.

We planned to study the impact of the ultrasound performed by a specifically trained nurse at the Holy Spirit Hospital, Makeni, Sierra Leone. Our primary outcome was to measure the difference in the number of differential diagnosis before and after US. Secondary outcomes were the rate of introduction of new unexpected diagnoses after the US exam; the confidence changes of the visiting physician in diagnoses hypothesized before and after the US; and the last point was to evaluate changes in prescribed therapy or inpatient management (surgical referral, medical only therapy).

## Methods

### Study design and sample selection

This is a prospective, observational study on outpatients presenting at the Holy Spirit Hospital of Makeni in Bombali district, Sierra Leone. Patients were continuously enrolled from April 28, 2014 to May 21, 2014 from the outpatient department (OPD) where four physicians examined them and indicated the need for an ultrasound exam. All patients requiring an ultrasound examination, as directed by the physician on duty, were eligible for enrollment. Exclusion criteria were age <18, refusal to participate by the patient. Each enrolled patient was given an explanation of the nature and purpose of the study and a written information sheet before collecting the consent (Additional file 1). The ultrasound examination was always performed by a local skilled sonographer (ARC) under the supervision of a Rainbow 4 Africa sonographer (AL, EB) experienced in lung, abdomen, and heart ultrasound. All ultrasound examinations were carried out with a Toshiba Memio 20.

### Study protocol and data collection

Common demographic variables were collected. The visiting physician was asked to fill out the first page of the case report form (CRF, Additional file 2) indicating the main complaint(s) of the patient, the differential diagnoses hypothesized (choosing from a list of the most typical diagnoses based on data from the previous year of US exam by ARC), the confidence degree about these diagnoses on a 5-point Likert scale and which area of therapy would have fit the patient's problems (i.e., medical, surgical, or the need for a referral). The clinician was able to ask for several US scans: cardiac, chest (i.e., pulmonary), abdominal, ob-gyn, and soft tissue, or a combination of them, according to proposed differential diagnosis; this selection was recorded too. The US exam was then performed in the room next to the examination one by a nurse who was the only staff trained in point-of-care ultrasound available. The sonographer was aware of the main complaints and formulated differential diagnoses. He reported the findings on the standard form used in the hospital to give feedback to the caring physician. After receiving the report, the visiting physician was asked to fill in the second page of the CRF, indicating the new list of differential diagnosis for the patient, if any new diagnosis had come up (yes/no), the final degree of confidence using the same 5-point Likert scale and the final therapy. The full database is available in Additional file 3.

### Statistical analysis

Descriptive analysis was carried out using common measures of synthesis; values are expressed as mean ± standard deviation (SD). Categorical variables were compared using the Chi-square test; Likert scales were compared with the Wilcoxon rank-sum test. Continuous variables were compared using two-tailed Student's t test after determining homoscedasticity. Statistical significance was set at 5%.

## Results

From April 24 to May 24, 2014, 105 patients were enrolled from the OPD of the Holy Spirit Hospital. Among them, 69 patients were female (65.7%) and the majority of the enrolled patients (62.9%) were less than 35 years old (Table 1; Fig. 1). 105 ultrasound exams were requested by

**Table 1 Overall relative frequencies of age classes among entire population and prevalence of genders**

| | N (%) |
|---|---|
| Sex | |
| Male | 36 (34.29) |
| Female | 69 (65.71) |
| Overall | 105 (100) |
| Age | |
| 18–25 | 35 (33.33) |
| 26–35 | 31 (29.52) |
| 36–45 | 17 (16.19) |
| 46–55 | 12 (11.43) |
| 56–65 | 7 (6.67) |
| 66+ | 3 (2.86) |
| Overall | 105 (100) |

four different physicians, asking, respectively, for 62, 21, 20, and 2 exams. The physician who requested the higher number of exams was also the one who visited the majority of the patients.

### Ultrasound exam requests

The most requested ultrasound exam was the abdominal one (43), followed by transabdominal obstetric-gynecological (35), combined chest and abdominal (22), soft tissue (4), and cardiac exam (1). The stratification of the requested exam according to the treating physician's level of confidence prior to the exam itself highlighted how ultrasound scans limited to the abdomen only were requested when facing higher level of confidence, while combined chest and abdominal scans where requested in case of lower levels of confidence ($\chi^2 = 139.9$; 16 g.l.; $p < 0.001$; Table 2).

### Main complaints and differential diagnosis

The most frequent symptom was abdominal pain (60 cases, 63%) followed by obstetric-gynecological problems (i.e., menstrual irregularities, vaginal discharge, other obstetric problems: 21 cases, 20%). Most of the patients (78%) reported more than one complaint. Table 3 shows all the complaints that led the patients to the hospital.

Considering all the patients, the treating physicians *hypothesized* an amount of 24 possible pathologies in formulating the differential diagnoses before the US exam. The most frequent was genitourinary tract infection or adnexitis (34 cases), followed by peptic ulcer disease (27) and pregnancy (17). Such diagnoses remained the most represented even after the US examinations, though with a different frequency (Table 4).

In 41 cases, the number of differential diagnoses reduced after the US, in 51 it remained the same (being 34 of them cases in which the caring doctor hypothesized only one diagnosis), and only in 13 cases the number of differential diagnosis increased after the US (Table 5).

For the whole 105 patients, a total amount of 194 differential diagnoses were formulated, with a mean of 1.85 (DS 0.87) diagnoses per patient at the first medical contact, with a statistically significant reduction to 1.51 (DS 0.79) diagnoses per patient after having performed the ultrasound ($p < 0.001$). The total amount of differential diagnoses after the US was 158, showing a reduction of 18.6%. This is a gross computation that can be divided in more subtle phenomena.

1. Out of the total amount of 194 hypotheses, 89 (46%) were *excluded* on the basis of US, reducing the mean of clinically based differential diagnosis per patient to 1.0 ($p < 0.001$). On the other hand, US *introduced* 53 new diagnosis in 42 patients (mean 1.26; SD 0.54), raising the final figure of total differential diagnosis from 105 to 158 (+50.5%).
2. In 51 cases, the number of differential diagnosis *remained the same*, due to two different mechanisms. 32 of these patients had only 1 or 2 clinical hypothesized differential diagnosis (mean 1.22; SD 0.42), and neither rule-out nor introduction of new diagnosis was due to ultrasonography. The other 19 patients had a mean of 1, 15 new differential diagnosis introduced by ultrasonography and the same amount of

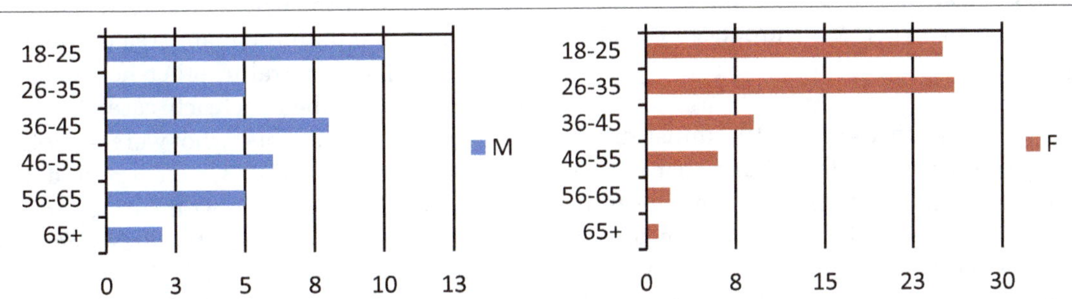


**Fig. 1** Relative frequencies of age classes among male (*left panel*) and female (*right panel*) population

**Table 2 Type of ultrasound exam requested according to the relative level of confidence of the attending physician**

| Type of ultrasound exam | Level of confidence before US | | | | | Totals |
|---|---|---|---|---|---|---|
| | 1 | 2 | 3 | 4 | 5 | N (%) |
| Cardiac | 1 | 0 | 0 | 0 | 0 | 1 (0.9) |
| Chest–abdomen | 0 | 12 | 9 | 0 | 1 | 22 (20.9) |
| Abdomen | 0 | 7 | 24 | 11 | 1 | 43 (40.9) |
| Ob/gyn | 0 | 10 | 5 | 19 | 1 | 35 (33.3) |
| Soft tissues | 0 | 3 | 1 | 0 | 0 | 4 (3.8) |
| Totals | 1 | 32 | 39 | 30 | 3 | 105 (100) |

**Table 3 Total amount of presenting symptoms in the sample and their distribution among male and female**

| Symptoms | Overall N (%) | Male | Female |
|---|---|---|---|
| Chest pain and burns | 22 (12) | 13 | 9 |
| Cough | 5 (3) | 5 | 0 |
| Dyspnea | 7 (4) | 6 | 1 |
| Palpitation | 5 (3) | 2 | 3 |
| Swelling of feet | 8 (4) | 4 | 4 |
| Abdominal pain | 64 (34) | 23 | 41 |
| Abdominal distension and discomfort | 11 (6) | 6 | 5 |
| Feeling of abdominal mass | 10 (5) | 5 | 5 |
| Swollen testes | 1 (1) | 1 | 0 |
| Difficulty in passing urine | 3 (2) | 1 | 2 |
| Obstetrics problems | 16 (9) | 0 | 16 |
| Menstrual problems | 20 (11) | 0 | 20 |
| Vaginal discharge | 15 (8) | 0 | 15 |
| Total | 187 (100) | 66 | 121 |

rule-outs. This second group of 19 patients presented to US exam with an amount of differential diagnosis before ultrasound that was significantly higher in comparison to the other 32 (p = 0.01).

3. 13 patients had their amount of differential diagnosis *increased* and it was always due to the introduction of new hypotheses by ultrasonography, with a mean of 1.6 for each patient; 5 of them also had 1 rule-out.
4. The amount of differential diagnosis *decreased* in 41 patients; they had an average of 1.51 rule-outs and 10 of them had a new hypothesis introduced by ultrasonography.

In summary, we found that 46% of 194 initial differential diagnoses were ruled out by US and that 33% of the final differential diagnoses considered were given by US. These percentages were calculated for each pathology (Table 4), showing that some pathologies had a high rate of exclusion (e.g., pneumonia/TB, splenomegaly, uterine myomatosis, ovarian cyst, cirrhosis, gastritis/PUD). Some other possible diagnoses were completely ruled out (i.e., appendicitis and nephrolithiasis). As mentioned, some diagnoses were added only after the US, like abdominal aortic dilation, pelvic mass, cholecystolithiasis, gynecomastia e pulmonary overload.

Finally, the number of differential diagnoses was not linked with the sex ($\chi^2 = 6.77$; 4 df; $p = 0.15$), or with the age of the patients ($\chi^2 = 21.35$; 20 df; $p = 0.37$).

New diagnoses were found in 42 patients, of whom 20 in male and 22 in female, even if our sample was composed by two-thirds of females. This means that the new diagnosis rate in males was two times higher than in female patients.

The thoracic-abdominal ultrasound gave the caring physician proportionally more new diagnoses than the abdominal and the cardiac alone ($\chi^2$ = 9,69; 3 df; p = 0.046).

### Physician level of confidence

The confidence level of the caring physicians before the US exam was distributed symmetrically around the modal value of 3. After the US, the distribution changed with a modal value of 5 asymmetrically distributed. The certainty level always increased (Wilcoxon rank-sum test: $p < 0.001$) except in 5 cases, in which it remained the same (Fig. 2).

### Therapy

The therapy proposed in every patient was recorded before and after the US, as described in Table 6.

We analyzed both the main area of therapy (i.e., medical, surgical, or referral to other hospital) and the drugs that were prescribed for each case. After the US exam among the 82 patients who were hypothesized to be treated only medically, 3 were referred (3, 6%) and 5 were treated also or only with surgery (6%). Conversely, surgical therapy remained the only one in 4 out of the 19 patients who would have had it (21%); 11 had a medical therapy and 4 a combined medical-surgical therapy.

**Table 4 Suspected diagnosis in the sample**

| Suspected diagnosis | Before-US N (%) | | After-US N (%) | | Ruled out N (%[a]) | | Added N (%[b]) | |
|---|---|---|---|---|---|---|---|---|
| Pneumonia/TB | 9 | (4.6) | 3 | (1.9) | 8 | (88.9) | 2 | (66.7) |
| Pleural effusion | 5 | (2.6) | 4 | (2.5) | 3 | (60.0) | 2 | (50.0) |
| Pulmonary overload | 0 | (0.0) | 3 | (1.9) | 0 | – | 3 | (100) |
| Cardiomyopathy | 12 | (6.2) | 6 | (3.8) | 7 | (58.3) | 1 | (16.7) |
| Aortic ectasia | 0 | (0.0) | 2 | (1.3) | 0 | – | 2 | (100) |
| Liver cirrhosis/schistosomiasis | 12 | (6.2) | 12 | (7.6) | 8 | (66.7) | 8 | (66.7) |
| Cholecystolithiasis | 0 | (0.0) | 1 | (0.6) | 0 | – | 1 | (100) |
| PUD | 27 | (13.9) | 24 | (15.2) | 6 | (22.2) | 3 | (12.5) |
| Gastritis/gerd | 10 | (5.2) | 7 | (4.4) | 5 | (50.0) | 2 | (28.6) |
| Gastroenteritis | 6 | (3.1) | 5 | (3.2) | 2 | (33.3) | 1 | (20.0) |
| Appendicitis | 2 | (1.0) | 0 | (0.0) | 2 | (100.0) | 0 | – |
| Acute/chronic nephritis | 7 | (3.6) | 5 | (3.2) | 3 | (42.9) | 1 | (20.0) |
| Nephrolithiasis/hydronephrosis | 2 | (1.0) | 1 | (0.6) | 2 | (100) | 1 | (100) |
| Abscess/mass | 11 | (5.7) | 16 | (10.1) | 4 | (36.4) | 9 | (56.3) |
| BPM | 0 | (0.0) | 1 | (0.6) | 0 | – | 1 | (100) |
| Pelvic muscle syndrome | 5 | (2.6) | 3 | (1.9) | 2 | (40.0) | 0 | (0.0) |
| Splenomegaly | 5 | (2.6) | 4 | (2.5) | 4 | (80.0) | 3 | (75.0) |
| Musculoskeletal pain | 2 | (1.0) | 4 | (2.5) | 1 | (50.0) | 3 | (75.0) |
| Gynaecomastia | 0 | (0.0) | 1 | (0.6) | 0 | – | 1 | (100) |
| Adnexitis/gut infection | 34 | (17.5) | 25 | (15.8) | 11 | (32.4) | 2 | (8.0) |
| Ovarian cyst | 16 | (8.2) | 8 | (5.1) | 11 | (68.8) | 3 | (37.5) |
| Uterus myomatosis | 7 | (3.6) | 2 | (1.3) | 6 | (85.7) | 1 | (50.0) |
| Miscarriage | 5 | (2.6) | 3 | (1.9) | 2 | (40.0) | 0 | (0.0) |
| Pregnancy | 17 | (8.8) | 18 | (11.4) | 2 | (11.8) | 3 | (16.7) |
| Total (%) | 194 | (100) | 158 | (100) | 89 | (45.9) | 53 | 33.5 |

First column: before ultrasound, based on clinical presentation. Second column: after the requested ultrasound scan and considering both the clinical and sonographical data. Third column: number of initial hypothesis excluded due to the ultrasound findings. Fourth column: number of final hypothesis added due to the ultrasound findings

[a] Percentage of ddx pre-US that has been excluded on US basis

[b] Percentage of ddx post-US that has been added on US basis

**Table 5 Variation of number of hypothesized differential diagnosis showed by coupling the figure before and after ultrasound scan (in the first coloumn the number of diagnosis before the US)**

| | 0 | 1 | 2 | 3 | 4 | Total |
|---|---|---|---|---|---|---|
| 1 | 2 | 34 | 6 | – | – | 42 |
| 2 | – | 22 | 15 | 3 | 3 | 43 |
| 3 | – | 4 | 8 | 2 | 1 | 15 |
| 4 | – | 1 | 3 | – | – | 4 |
| 5 | – | – | 1 | – | – | 1 |
| Total | 2 | 61 | 33 | 5 | 4 | 105 |

Finally, all of the 4 patients who were thought to need a combined therapy were addressed to a medical alone or a surgical therapy alone. Getting deep into the drug prescription changes after the US exam and clinical re-evaluation, we highlighted substantial differences in prescription for some classes of drugs.

- Antibiotics: we recorded a steep increase (+182%) in antibiotic prescription and antiparasitic drugs with the exception of metronidazole (−10%) and clarithromycin (−8%) in the eradicant therapy for H. pylori-related gastritis.

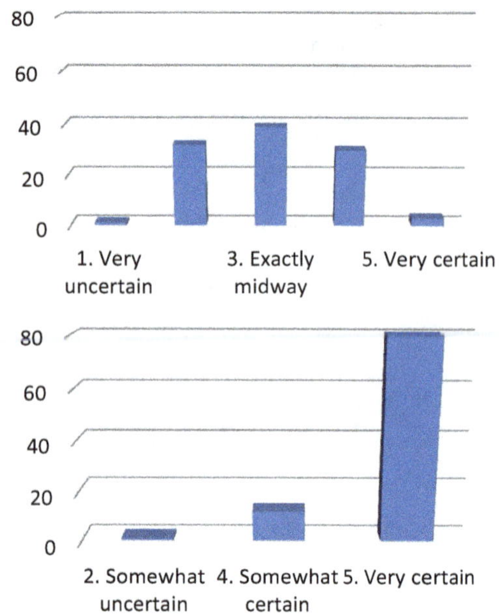


**Fig. 2** Distribution of level of confidence on the formulated differential diagnosis before the result of the ultrasound scan and after

**Table 6 Variation of the class of therapy (medical, surgical, or both) after the ultrasound results and variation of hypothesis**

| Kind of therapy (pre-US) | Medical (post-US) | Med and surg (post-US) | Referral (post-US) | Surgical (post-US) | Total (pre-US) |
|---|---|---|---|---|---|
| Medical | 74 | 3 | 3 | 2 | 82 |
| Medical and surgical | 3 | 0 | 0 | 1 | 4 |
| Surgical | 11 | 4 | 0 | 4 | 19 |
| Total (post-US) | 88 | 7 | 3 | 7 | 105 |

- PPI: we observed a 20% reduction in omeprazole prescription, according to a reduction in PUD or Gastro-Esophageal Reflux Disease (GERD) diagnosis of 17 out of the initial 37 (rule-out 45%), and then 11 (35% of final figure) were added after US.
- NSAIDs: we observed a 133% increase in NSAID prescription.
- Congestive heart failure drugs: we observed a moderate reduction (−21%) in furosemide and digoxin prescription related to the reduction in cardiomyopathy diagnosis made using US.

## Discussion

The construction of this study is based on ample literature that indicates how ultrasound can be considered the imaging technique of choice both in the ordinary European hospital environment and, thanks to its low cost and easy transportability, in low-resource contexts such as intra/extra-hospital emergencies or healthcare in developing countries. Another important reason is the consideration that the relationship between medicine and the population of developing countries is often influenced by cultural backgrounds rooted in distant traditions that clash with Western medicine's invasiveness. Ultrasound can therefore fill the role of a modern magic mirror that allows the doctor to "look inside" the patient without breaking through the "protective barrier" that surrounds the patient according to the animist culture. For this reason, it is often well accepted by people allowing for a great compliance between doctor and patient. Moreover, portability, costs, and steep learning curve on how to use the ultrasound machine make ultrasonography the most feasible imaging technique in this context.

As far as concern our results, abdominal pain was the most frequent symptom of presentation. In Sierra Leone, the only CT is a 3-hour drive from the HSH and the only imaging test locally available is plain X-ray, that is far less sensitive in the abdominal pain diagnostic pathway [5]. Taking this into account, US drastically improved the diagnostic possibility in our context. Moreover, the strongest barrier against the feasibility of US is not a big deal in Sierra Leone with only 3% of the population with a BMI >30 [6].

As mentioned in the results, most of the patients (78%) reported more than one complaint. In this situation, it is very likely to have a broad spectrum of differential diagnosis in which the US has been of paramount importance in leading to their reduction. In our primary outcome, it seems that with the US exam we obtained only a slight reduction in differential diagnoses from 1.8 diagnoses per patient to 1.5. Actually, we had a rule-out rate of 45% of pre-US diagnoses with 33% of new post-US diagnoses. This high turnover has led to the final result that can therefore be considered impressive. Moreover, the introduction of new potential and clinically unexpected diagnoses can be a valuable point since it can changes the management of the patient.

We noticed that the half of new unexpected diagnosis came in male patients, but male were only one-third of our sample. For this, the percentage of new unexpected diagnosis among men is nearly double than among women (56% for male, 32% for women, $\chi^2 = 5.5$; 1 df; $p < 0.02$). This could be quite surprising if we consider that one would expect to find with the US something unexpected in a female abdomen due to the greater amount of organs and therefore make the differential diagnosis of abdominal symptoms harder. Something was missing also in the possible explanation, given that abdominal presentation was fourfold in females rather than males. Analyzing our sample, we tried to find the confounding variable dividing abdominal or non-abdominal patients on the basis of the presenting symptom. Observing the odds ratio of new diagnosis, it came out that abdominal presentation did not conduce to greater number of diagnosis as being male did instead (OR 3.2; CI 1.04.9.81). This tells us that male presentation was probably a risk factor itself. The explanation could lay in two possible facts that we are not completely able to analyze: male patients came with worse clinical pictures in comparison with women or the visiting doctor formulated less diagnostic hypotheses when facing a man. This second explanation came out to be unlikely, since the average of differential diagnosis was not related to sex and average of new unexpected diagnosis was not correlated to the number of differential diagnosis.

The non-homogeneous distribution of new differential diagnosis prompted by the US thoraco-abdominal exam in comparison to sole abdominal or sole cardiac has to be related with the request of the complete abdominal-thoracic exam in the cases in which the physician was less sure of his diagnostic hypotheses.

Another strong point of US is the possibility to make some final diagnoses which would otherwise be impossible. For example, in two cases we have diagnosed an aortic dilation that has led to a follow-up for the patient. In the same way, we have diagnosed one case of nephrolithiasis (rare in African population) and one of cholecystolithiasis which could not have been recognized without the US.

Analyzing the differences in therapy before and after the US examination, we can underline some issues. As far as the therapeutic strategy is concerned, we can notice how 74% of unnecessary surgeries expected before the US have been avoided. On one hand, without US three cases would not have been referred in the right hospital and two patients would not have had the early surgery they needed. On the other hand, the changes in drugs prescription, the decrease in PPI, and eradication therapy can be explained with the PUD and gastritis diagnoses reduction. These diagnoses were typically general and not specific, made by the caring physician when there were no clear features of the abdominal pain referred by the patient. With the US exam, we increased the diagnostic performance of the caring physician on the abdominal pain, the most frequent main complaint. The most important variation between pre- and post-US therapy we observed was in NSAID prescription and was probably due to the after-US new diagnoses of painful abdominal masses, abscesses, and muscular pain. In the end, although the diagnosis of cardiomyopathy decreased after the US exam, the increase in spironolactone prescription can be explained with the increase in cirrhosis diagnosis.

This study presents some merits and limitations. Its one-hospital setting cannot be clearly representative of the whole population of all low-income countries; moreover, even in low-income countries there are differences in distribution of healthcare facilities and Sierra Leone itself represents one of most deprived countries. Despite an intuitive and consolidated idea of ultrasound utility in both high and low-income countries, the ability of the physician to give the right indication for US remains a big problem to deal with. Our hospital may have had physicians that are probably different in number, experience, and ability from the physicians of another service; specifically our visiting doctor were one young general practitioner from Pakistan, one older general practitioner from Nigeria, one surgeon, and one pediatrician. One big limit is due to the absence of a certain diagnosis to compare the variation in differential diagnosis to a standard reference. This problem is widespread and, in a certain sense, it will persist in those contexts in which diagnostic facilities, whether ultrasound or other, are unaffordable to people and services. Another limit is that, even with a good sample size, our 105 patients are not enough to make reliable deductions on the single pathologies encountered, since each pathology accounts for very few cases. We were not able to fulfill the typical features of point-of-care ultrasound [7] given that our examinations were not made directly by the caring physician. This was due to the lack of doctors trained in ultrasound at all. Actually, we decided to train a nurse in ultrasound for the low doctor/population ratio of Sierra Leone that amounted at 2.2 every 100,000 population [8]. For this reason, many medical competencies, that in Western countries are doctors' prerogative, in Sierra Leone can often be guaranteed by nurses, especially in rural zones. Finally, since US examination can be reassuring, the level of confidence of the visiting physician may have also risen because of this.

On the other hand, this study provide an example of well-integrated clinical and imaging diagnostic service, in which a point-of-care level of ultrasound facility was implemented by the collaboration between the visiting physician on duty and the sonographer, matching their ideas on the same patient in nearly real time. Both the reduction and emergence of new unexpected diagnoses are important parts of the diagnostic process and US showed to be a useful means to face this step. The confidence level of the caring physician is a point of great importance, since physician–patient relationship cannot relinquish a certain grade of confidence on the most probable diagnosis. In this context also blood tests are very expensive and limited in spectrum. Since US could aid to complete diagnostic needs, the introduction of widespread US could improve the diagnostic accuracy of local physician. The possibility to indicate an appropriate treatment instead of another, in particular a surgical one, is of paramount importance, from the point of view of safety, prognosis, and economic affordability. Finally, to our knowledge this is the first study exploring the gain in diagnostic accuracy after an ultrasound examination made by a specifically trained local nurse practitioner. In contexts with a severe lack of physician, like Sierra Leone, the results of our research highlight the usefulness of US training programs, which can be extended to all low-income countries.

Further studies are needed to explore other strong outcomes like mortality, length of stay in hospital, and money saved with the implementation of ultrasound services in low-income countries. Moreover, the Ebola epidemic brought many humanitarian resources to Sierra Leone, which could be useful to arrange a multicentric study, similar to this one, that can strengthen the results of this study.

## Conclusions

Ultrasound is feasible and practical because it is economic, repeatable, feasible, safe, portable, non-invasive, and actually well tolerated from a local anthropological point of view. It can work with electricity generators, using batteries and in difficult fields.

With ultrasound in a low-income country with a very low level of diagnostic and imaging facilities, clinical-based diagnostic hypotheses were strongly reduced and new unexpected imaging-based diagnostic hypotheses were introduced.

With the use of US, the level of confidence of the visiting physician on the final diagnosis of difficult patients rose.

The indication for a surgical treatment was reduced and global appropriateness augmented.

## Additional files

**Additional file 1.** Informed consent form.

**Additional file 2.** HSH ultrasound data sheet.

**Additional file 3.** Full database.

#### Abbreviations

HSH: Holy Spirit Hospital; HIV: human immunodeficiency virus; POCUS: point-of-care ultrasound; US: ultrasound; OPD: outpatient department; CRF: case report form; SD: standard deviation; PPI: proton pump inhibitor; PUD: peptic ulcer disease; GERD: gastro-esophageal reflux; NSAID: non-steroidal anti-inflammatory drugs; CT: computed tomography; BMI: body mass index.

#### Authors' contributions

AL and EB: Conception or design of the work, data collection, data analysis and interpretation, drafting the article, critical revision of the article, final approval of the version to be published. PC: Data collection, data analysis and interpretation, drafting the article, critical revision of the article, final approval of the version to be published. PN: Conception or design of the work, drafting the article, critical revision of the article, final approval of the version to be published. MF: Data analysis and interpretation, drafting the article, critical revision of the article, final approval of the version to be published. ARC: Data collection, critical revision of the article, final approval of the version to be published. All authors read and approved the final manuscript.

#### Author details

[1] Emergency Department, San Luigi Gonzaga Hospital, Regione Gonzole 10 Orbassano, 10043 Turin, Italy. [2] Department of Surgical Sciences, Turin University, Turin, Italy. [3] Turin University, Turin, Italy. [4] Holy Spirit Hospital, Makeni, Sierra Leone. [5] Rainbow for Africa NGO, Via Zuretti 29, Turin, TO, Italy.

#### Acknowledgements

The authors thank Fabrizio Bert MD (Department of Public Health and Pediatrics, University of Turin) for his help on data analysis and interpretation.

#### References

1. Blaivas M, Kuhn W, Reynolds B, Brannam L (2005) Change in differential diagnosis and patient management with the use of portable ultrasound in a remote setting. Wilderness Environ Med. 16:38–41
2. Giordani MT et al (2012) Ultrasound and infections on the Tibetan Plateau. J Ultrasound 15:83–92
3. Sargsyan AE et al (2005) FAST at MACH 20: clinical ultrasound aboard the International Space Station. J Trauma 58:35–39
4. Otto C et al (2009) Into thin air: extreme ultrasound on Mt Everest. Wilderness Environ Med. 20:283–289
5. Gans SL, Pols MA, Stoker J, Boermeester MA (2015) Guideline for the diagnostic pathway in patients with acute abdominal pain. Dig. Surg. 32:23–31
6. WHO: Prevalence obesity among adults. http://gamapserver.who.int/gho/interactive_charts/ncd/risk_factors/obesity/atlas.html. Accessed 20 Sep 2016
7. Moore CL, Copel JA (2011) Point-of-care ultrasonography. N Engl J Med 364:749–757
8. Physician density per 1000 population. http://apps.who.int/gho/data/node.main.A1444. Accessed 03 Oct 2016

# 7

# Systematic review and meta-analysis for the use of ultrasound versus radiology in diagnosing of pneumonia

Saeed Ali Alzahrani[1], Majid Abdulatief Al-Salamah[2], Wedad Hussain Al-Madani[3] and Mahmoud A. Elbarbary[4*]

**Abstract**

**Background:** Physicians are increasingly using point of care lung ultrasound (LUS) for diagnosing pneumonia, especially in critical situations as it represents relatively easy and immediately available tool. They also used it in many associated pathological conditions such as consolidation, pleural effusion, and interstitial syndrome with some reports of more accuracy than chest X-ray. This systematic review and meta-analysis are aimed to estimate the pooled diagnostic accuracy of ultrasound for the diagnosis of pneumonia versus the standard chest radiological imaging.

**Methods and main results:** A systematic literature search was conducted for all published studies comparing the diagnostic accuracy of LUS against a reference Chest radiological exam (C X-ray or Chest computed Tomography CT scan), combined with clinical criteria for pneumonia in all age groups. Eligible studies were required to have a Chest X-ray and/or CT scan at the time of clinical evaluation. The authors extracted qualitative and quantitative information from eligible studies, and calculated pooled sensitivity and specificity and pooled positive/negative likelihood ratios (LR). Twenty studies containing 2513 subjects were included in this meta-analysis. The pooled estimates for lung ultrasound in the diagnosis of pneumonia were, respectively, as follows: Overall pooled sensitivity and specificity for diagnosis of pneumonia by lung ultrasound were 0.85 (0.84–0.87) and 0.93 (0.92–0.95), respectively. Overall pooled positive and negative LRs were 11.05 (3.76–32.50) and 0.08 (0.04–0.15), pooled diagnostic Odds ratio was 173.64 (38.79–777.35), and area under the pooled ROC (AUC for SROC) was 0.978.

**Conclusion:** Point of care lung ultrasound is an accurate tool for the diagnosis of pneumonia. Considering being easy, readily availability, low cost, and free from radiological hazards, it can be considered as important diagnostic strategy in this condition.

**Keywords:** Systematic review, Ultrasound, Pneumonia, Point of care, lung, interstitial syndrome, and diagnosis

## Background

Acute pneumonia or acute respiratory tract infection is considered the most common cause of mortality in children around the globe [1]. In adult, pneumonia also is a serious disease with increased rate of mortality and hospitalization [2, 3]. The diagnosis of pneumonia can be difficult and challenging in the emergency setting or in critically ill patients [4]. Many of the commonly used radiological signs are non-specific [5]. In daily practice, pneumonia diagnosis is based on clinical presentation through patient history and physical exam, plus radiological imaging commonly chest X-ray (and infrequently CT scan) that may help confirm the diagnosis particularly with equivocal clinical status. Early diagnosing of pneumonia is very important to promptly starting the treatment; otherwise, it can be life-threatening or associated with high morbidity particularly in critically ill patients who need immediate decision.

There are many diagnostic approaches to diagnose and evaluate pneumonia and every tool has its own diagnostic accuracy.

*Correspondence: barbarym@ngha.med.sa; elbarbary.mahmoud@yahoo.com
[4] KSAUHS, Ministry of National Guard-Health Affairs, King Abdullah International Medical Research Center, Riyadh, Kingdom of Saudi Arabia
Full list of author information is available at the end of the article

Flexible bronchoscopy or endotracheal aspiration usually is reserved for intubated patients. Blood samples, urinary antigens, and expectorate collections are among routine examinations that are performed once pneumonia is suspected. Collected specimens are sent to microbiology laboratories [6] which may take several days to have conclusive results. Bronchoscope can give useful information; however, it has its own limitations and contraindications such as patients with severe hypoxemia, recent myocardial infarctions, or significant cardiac arrhythmia. Being relatively invasive technique, it is also not possible to perform bronchoscope in all patients but only in selected cases [7].

Another diagnostic tool is computed tomography, which is considered as the gold standard in lung imaging in general. This tool is particularly useful in lung masses or cavitary abnormality and any changes in lung parenchyma either acute or chronic such as the cases of pneumonia, interstitial lung disease, emphysema, and malignancy. The limitations are several but most important are radiation hazards, cost, and logistics that limit its routine use. A major limitation is difficulty in transporting patients with critical conditions to imaging section which precludes markedly unstable patients either respiratory or hemodynamically [8, 9].

Nevertheless, chest radiography remains an important imaging tool that been used for long and still helping in diagnosing many abnormalities in the chest. Chest X-ray is considered as the most common diagnostic tool that has been used traditionally in daily practice for diagnosis of pneumonia, especially in critical conditions [10]. Many limitations in using portable chest X-ray have been well described and noticed such as quality of an X-ray film in addition to the risk of repetitive radiation exposure [11]. Some reports claim that removal of chest radiography from daily practice may not affect intensive care unit mortality [12].

Relatively recently, lung ultrasound was promoted as a modality that can overcome many of the above-mentioned limitations of other tools in the diagnosis of pneumonia in multiple settings [13]. Through the last 2 decade, the ultrasound has shown that it could play a major role in medicine and common practice in assessing the lung [14]. Traditionally, the accessibility of the lung by ultrasound was considered poor due to the air barrier. However, this position has been dramatically changed with tremendous amount of literature supporting the use of LUS in multiple conditions [15–17]. This diagnostic tool can be used easily and immediately as a bedside tool which give it a huge advantage [18]. Lung ultrasound was reported with high accuracy in many pathological lung conditions such as consolidation, pleural effusion, and interstitial syndrome compared to bedside chest radiography [19].

The aim of our study is to conduct systematic review (SR) followed by meta-analysis for the diagnostic power of lung ultrasound versus chest radiological imaging for the diagnosis of pneumonia in both adult and pediatric population through estimation of the pooled diagnostic accuracy measures.

## Methods

A systematic search of electronic databases was conducted, including MEDLINE, EMBASE, and Cochrane databases from 1990 to 2016 to identify the relevant articles in the effectiveness of ultrasound in the diagnosis of pneumonia. Hand search was then conducted on references of relevant studies. The search strategy followed Cochrane guidelines with using the terms "Ultrasonography, ultrasound, sonography, ultrasonographies, sonogram"; "pneumonia, Bronchopneumonia, Pleuropneumonia, severe Acute Respiratory Syndrome, pulmonary inflammation, bronchiolitis"; and "sensitivity or specificity" with its MeSH terms. No restriction for language or type of patients was made at the time of the search. We included in this systematic review all studies evaluating diagnostic accuracy of lung ultrasound as index test against chest radiological imaging (CXR or CT) as reference standard. We included in this SR patients with respiratory disease and symptoms of acute respiratory failure. The evaluation of pneumonia is a combination of clinical data, laboratory results, and chest imaging. In addition, articles that evaluated any sign of respiratory disease, symptoms, or acute respiratory failure were included. We included all types of patients' pneumonia—both community- and hospital-acquired pneumonia—, children, adolescents, or adults. We have chosen to combine both adults and pediatric based on current literature suggesting that ultrasound findings in both are similar [17].

Two authors (SZ and WM) screened titles and abstracts for valid articles. Full-text articles were retrieved afterward. We developed an abstraction tables that includes year of publication, patients' baseline characteristics, and diagnostic study data (numbers of true positive, false positive, false negative, and true negative test results). Disagreement in study selection and abstraction was resolved by discussion with the third reviewer (ME).

Two reviewers (ME and SZ) independently used the QUADAS-2 instrument to assess the quality assessment of the included studies [20]. This tool consists of key domains covering patient selection, index test, reference standard, flow of patients through the study, and timing of the index test(s) and reference standard. Each domain was assessed in terms of the risk of bias and the concerns regarding applicability.

Risk of bias was judged as "Low," "High," or "Unclear." If all signaling questions for a domain are answered "Yes," then risk of bias can be judged "Low." If any signaling question is answered "No," this flags the potential for bias.

The meta-analysis was conducted using Meta-Disc 1.4 [21]. Random effect model was used in all analyses. The diagnostic accuracy measures used in the analysis were sensitivity, specificity, and likelihood ratio for positive and negative test (LR+ and LR−). Heterogeneity was assessed using the I-squared statistic and Q test.

## Results

We identified (431) studies that were relevant and fit our search strategy. After reviewing the articles and applying inclusion criteria and exclusion commentaries, we identified and enrolled 20 studies (see Fig. 1 flowchart). These 20 studies provided population of 2513 patients. The main reasons for exclusions were duplication of studies between the Pubmed and the Embase Databases and studies were not diagnostic.

Table 1 describes the basic characteristics of the 20 included studies. Among the included 20 studies, five of them are dealing with pediatrics patients [22–26]. Age of patients ranges from 1 month to 100 years. Some studies had comprehensive result of CT, clinical course, conventional tests, and follow-up outcomes as a diagnostic standard, which was considered clinical diagnosis. The quality of all studies was generally high, had low risk of bias, and satisfied the majority of the risk of bias criteria. Table 2 includes the chest imaging (reference standard) and other diagnostic criteria.

Overall pooled sensitivity and specificity for diagnosis of pneumonia by lung ultrasound were 0.85 (0.84–0.87) and 0.93 (0.92–0.95), respectively (Figs. 2, 3). Overall

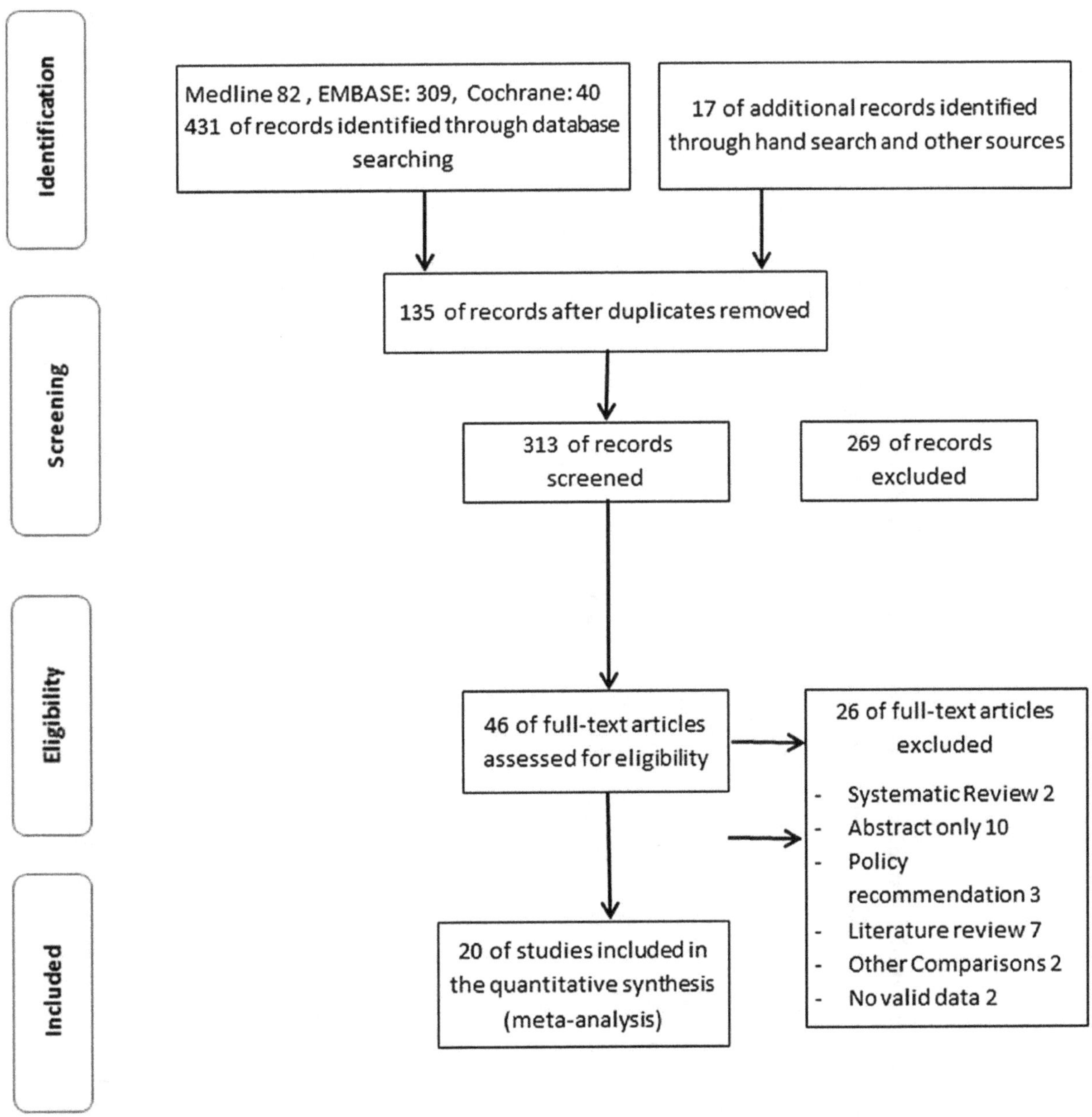


**Fig. 1** Flow chart for literature search process

**Table 1 Characteristics of studies and patients enrolled from studies retrieved for meta-analysis**

| Study | Year | Origin | Design | Sample size | Mean age (years) | M/F | True positive | False positive | False negative | True negative |
|---|---|---|---|---|---|---|---|---|---|---|
| Benci et al. [27] | 1996 | Italy | Prospective | 75 | 38.5 | 50/30 | 37 | 0 | 0 | 20 |
| Lichtenstein et al. [19] | 2004 | France | Prospective | 32 | 58 | Not mentioned | 111 | 0 | 8 | 265 |
| Lichtenstein et al. [28] | 2004 | France | Prospective | 117 | 53 | 37/23 | 59 | 1 | 6 | 51 |
| Lichtenstein et al. [29] | 2008 | France | Prospective | 260 | 68 | 140/120 | 74 | 10 | 9 | 167 |
| Parlamento et al. [30] | 2009 | Italy | Prospective | 49 | 60.9 | 31/81 | 31 | 0 | 1 | 17 |
| Cortellaro et al. [31] | 2010 | Italy | Prospective | 120 | 69 | 77/43 | 80 | 2 | 1 | 37 |
| Xirouchaki et al. [32] | 2011 | Greece | Prospective | 42 | 57.1 | 34/8 | 66 | 4 | 0 | 14 |
| Reissig et al. [33] | 2012 | Europe | Prospective | 356 | 63.8 | 228/134 | 211 | 3 | 15 | 127 |
| Testa et al. [34] | 2012 | Italy | Prospective | 67 | 55 | Not mentioned | 32 | 5 | 2 | 28 |
| Unluer et al. [24] | 2013 | China | Prospective | 72 | 66.3 | 35/37 | 27 | 7 | 1 | 37 |
| Luri [23] | 2009 | Italy | Prospective | 32 | 4.5 | 60 | 20 | 2 | 8 | 2 |
| Shah [35] | 2012 | US | Prospective | 200 | 3 | 112/88 | 31 | 18 | 146 | 5 |
| Hadeel and Dien [25] | 2013 | Egypt | Prospective | 75 | Neonates | Not mentioned | 64 | 4 | 7 | 0 |
| Copetti [36] | 2008 | Italy | Prospective | 144 | 77.6 | 72/72 | 60 | 0 | 0 | 19 |
| Caiulo VA [26] | 2013 | Italy | Prospective | 88 | 5.1 | 56/47 | 88 | 0 | 1 | 13 |
| Nafae [37] | 2013 | Egypt | Prospective | 100 | 50.6 | 56/44 | 61 | 1 | 1 | 17 |
| Liu [38] | 2014 | China | Prospective | 179 | 72 | 124/99 | 80 | 0 | 5 | 27 |
| Esposito [39] | 2014 | Italy | Prospective | 103 | 5.6 | 56/47 | 52 | 3 | 1 | 47 |
| Nazerian [40] | 2015 | Italy | Prospective | 285 | 71.14 | 133/152 | 72 | 9 | 15 | 189 |
| Bourcier [41] | 2014 | France | Prospective | 144 | 77.6 | 72/72 | 117 | 9 | 6 | 12 |

**Table 2 Chest imaging and diagnostic criteria of selected studies**

| Study | Imaging | Pneumonia diagnosis | Patient type | Inclusion criteria | Ultrasound operator | Diagnostic criteria | Blinding |
|---|---|---|---|---|---|---|---|
| Benci et al. [27] | CXR + Chest CT if CXR/LUS discordance | Clinical diagnosis or imaging | Hospitalized | Pneumonia symptoms | Experienced physicians | Consolidation | Yes |
| Lichtenstein et al. [19] | Chest CT | Imaging only | Critically ill | Acute respiratory distress syndrome | Experienced physicians | Consolidation | Yes |
| Lichtenstein et al. [28] | Chest CT | Imaging only | Critically ill | Chest pain or severe thoracic diseases | Two ED physician sonographers | Consolidation | Yes |
| Lichtenstein et al. [29] | CXR + Chest CT if possible | Clinical diagnosis or imaging | Critically ill | Acute respiratory failure | Experienced physicians | Alveolar and interstitial | Yes |
| Parlamento et al. [30] | CXR + Chest CT if CXR/LUS discordance | Imaging only | Presented to ED | CAP symptoms | Experienced physicians | Alveolar and interstitial | Yes |
| Cortellaro et al. [31] | CXR + Chest CT if possible | Clinical diagnosis or imaging | Presented to ED | CAP symptoms | Experienced physicians | Alveolar and interstitial | Yes |
| Xirouchaki et al. [32] | Chest CT scan | Imaging only | Critically ill | Mechanically ventilated patients scheduled for chest CT scan | Single physician (Expertise not mentioned) | Consolidation | Yes |
| Reissig et al. [33] | CXR + chest CT if CXR/LUS discordance | Clinical diagnosis or imaging | Presented to ED or hospitalized | CAP symptoms | Experienced physicians | Consolidation | Yes |
| Testa et al. [34] | CXR + chest CT if possible/indicated | Clinical diagnosis or imaging | Presented to ED | Suspected H1N1 infection | Experienced physicians | Alveolar and interstitial | Yes |
| Unluer et al. [24] | CXR + chest CT if possible/indicated | Imaging only | Presented to ED | CAP symptoms | Trained emergency physicians | Alveolar and interstitial | Yes |
| Nafae et al. [37] | Chest CT scan | Imaging only | Hospitalized | Pneumonia symptoms | Experienced physicians | Consolidation | No |
| Esposito et al. [39] | CR | Imaging only | Critically ill | CAP symptoms | Resident with limited experience | Alveolar and interstitial | Yes |
| Liu et al. [38] | CT scan | Imaging only | Presented to ED | CAP symptoms | Trained emergency physicians | Consolidation | Yes |
| Copetti et al. [36] | Electrocardiogram, Chest X-ray, and Color-Doppler echocardiography. | Imaging only | Critically ill | acute pulmonary edema | NA | Alveolar and interstitial | NA |
| Iuri [23] | Chest radiographs | Imaging only | admitted to the pediatric emergency ward | CAP symptoms | Two radiologists | Alveolar and interstitial | Yes |
| Shah [35] | Chest radiographs | Imaging only | patients had a routine clinical examination | Pneumonia symptoms | Trained physicians | Consolidation | Yes |
| Dien [25] | Chest radiographs | Imaging only | Critically ill | Pneumonia symptoms | One radiologist | Consolidation | NA |
| Caiulo [26] | Chest radiographs | Clinical diagnosis or imaging | Presented to ED | Pneumonia symptoms | One radiologist | Alveolar and interstitial | Yes |
| Nazerian [40] | Chest CT scan | Clinical diagnosis or imaging | Presented to ED | Any respiratory complaint | Trained emergency physicians | Consolidation | Yes |
| Bourcier [41] | Chest CT scan | Clinical diagnosis or imaging | Presented to ED | CAP pneumonia | Trained emergency physicians | Alveolar-interstitial syndrome | NA |

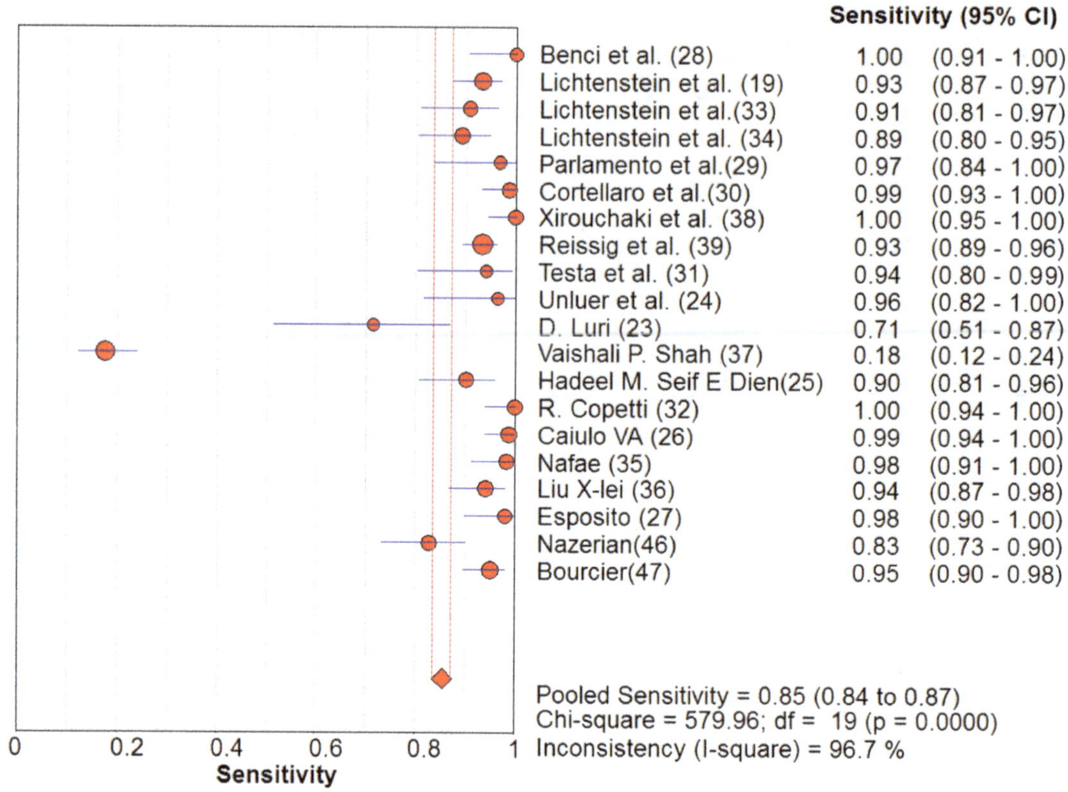


**Fig. 2** Pooled sensitivity of Ultrasound in ruling out pneumonia

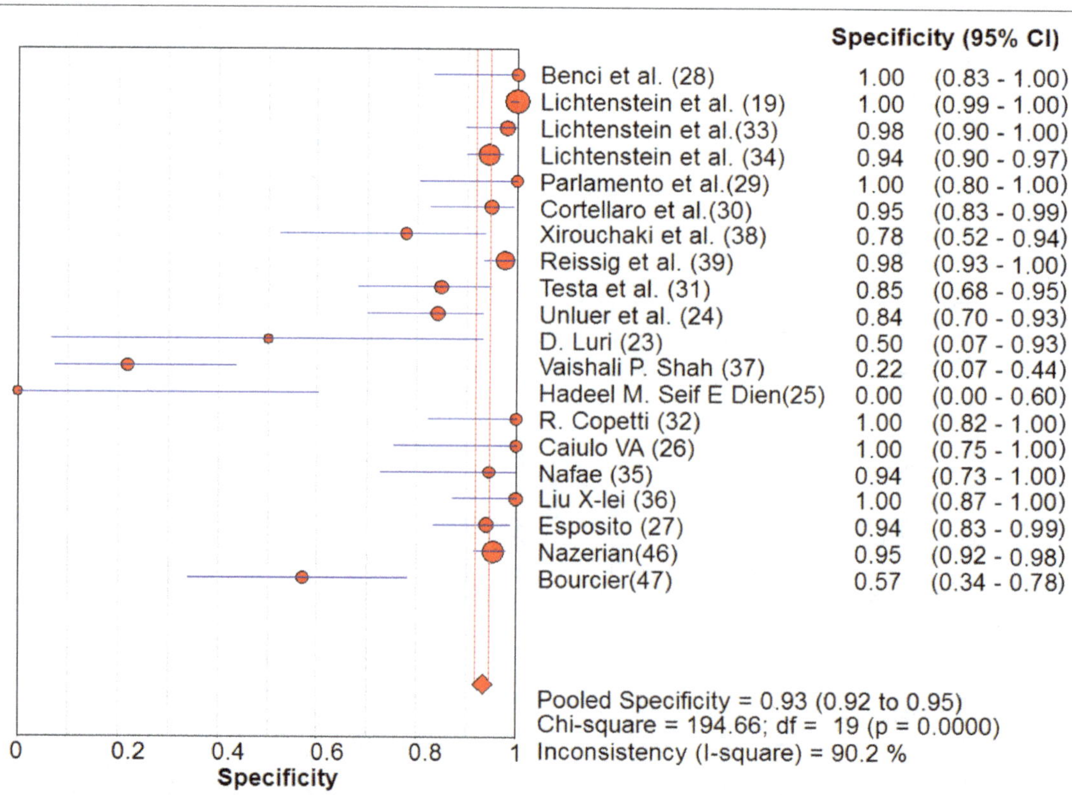


**Fig. 3** Pooled specificity of Ultrasound in ruling out pneumonia

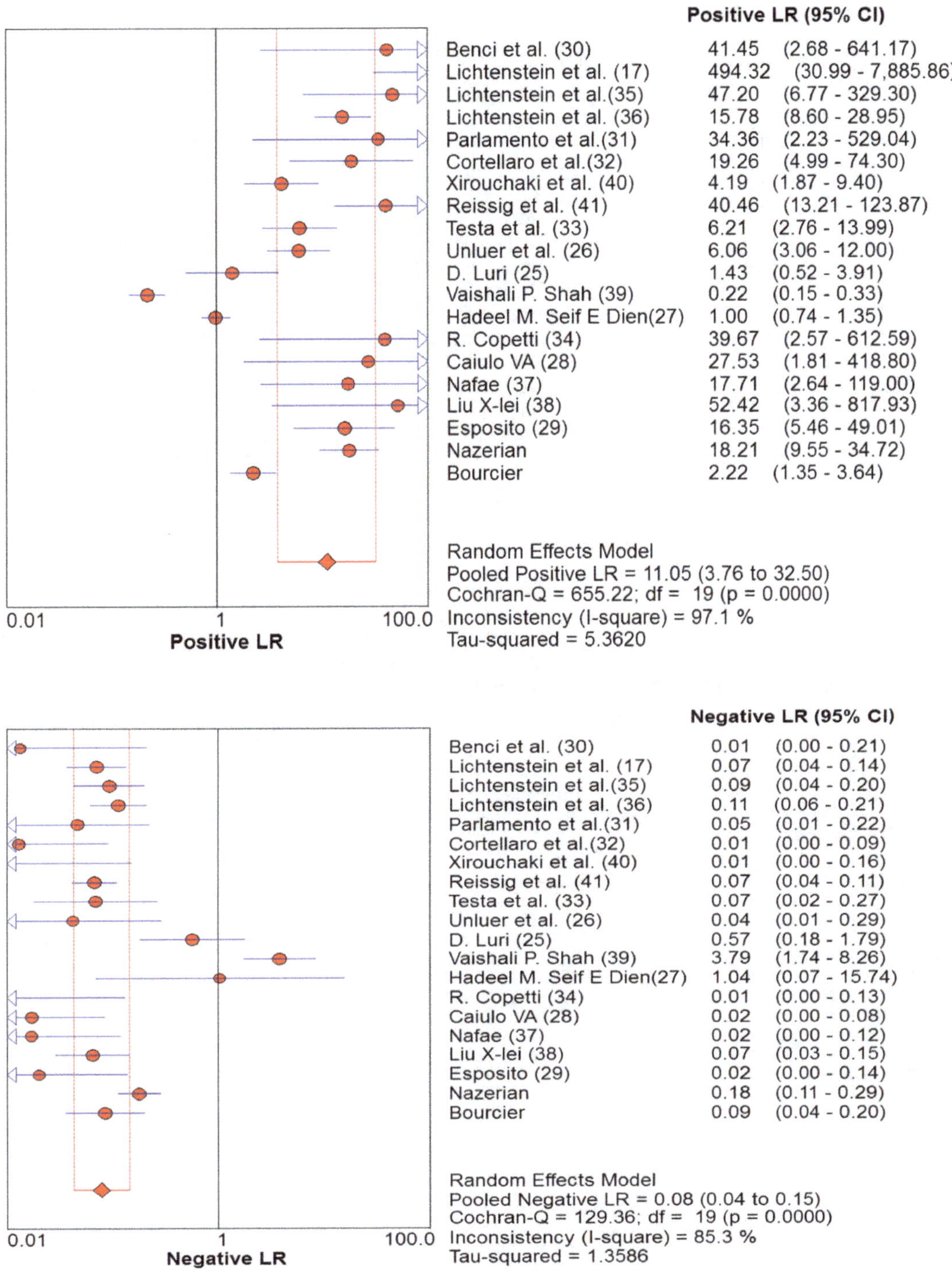


**Fig. 4** Pooled likelihood ratios of Ultrasound in diagnosing pneumonia

pooled positive and negative LRs (Fig. 4) were 11.05 (3.76–32.50) and 0.08 (0.04–0.15), pooled diagnostic Odds ratio (Fig. 5) was 173.64 (38.79–777.35), and area under the pooled ROC (AUC for SROC) was 0.978 (Fig. 6).

## Discussion

Pneumonia commonly leads to significant pulmonary consolidation that is demonstrated with a complete loss of aeration in the concerned lung region. On CXR, pulmonary consolidation is defined as a homogeneous

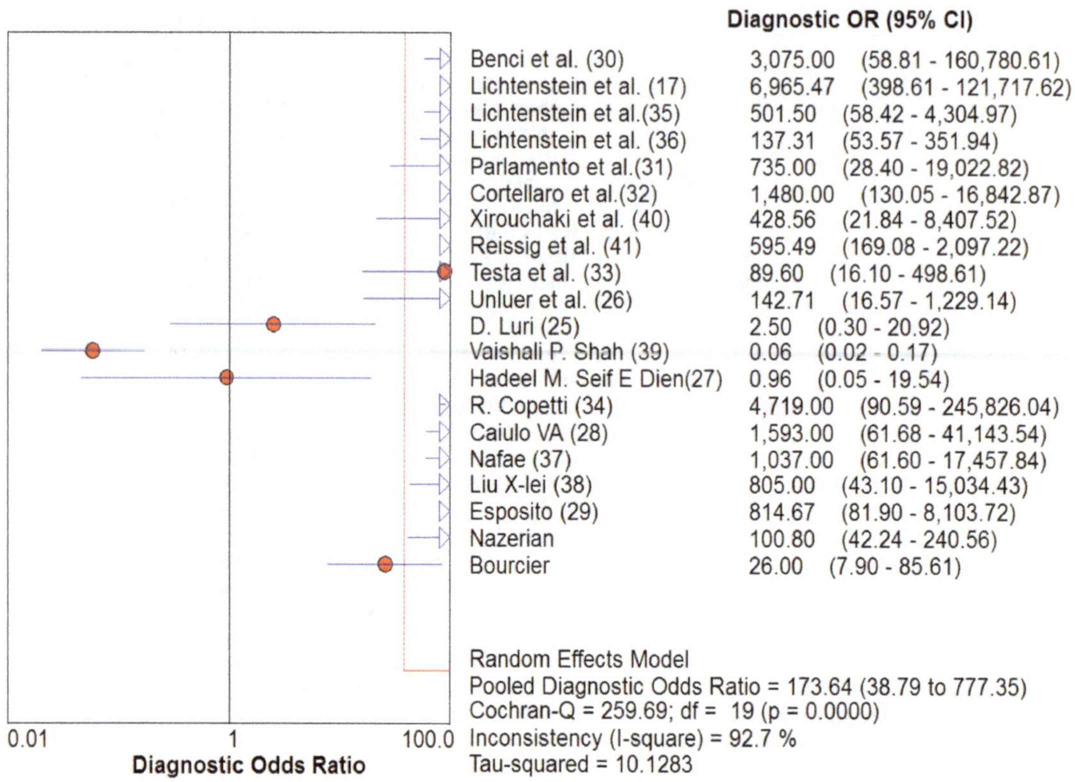


**Fig. 5** Pooled diagnostic Odds Ratio of Ultrasound in diagnosing pneumonia

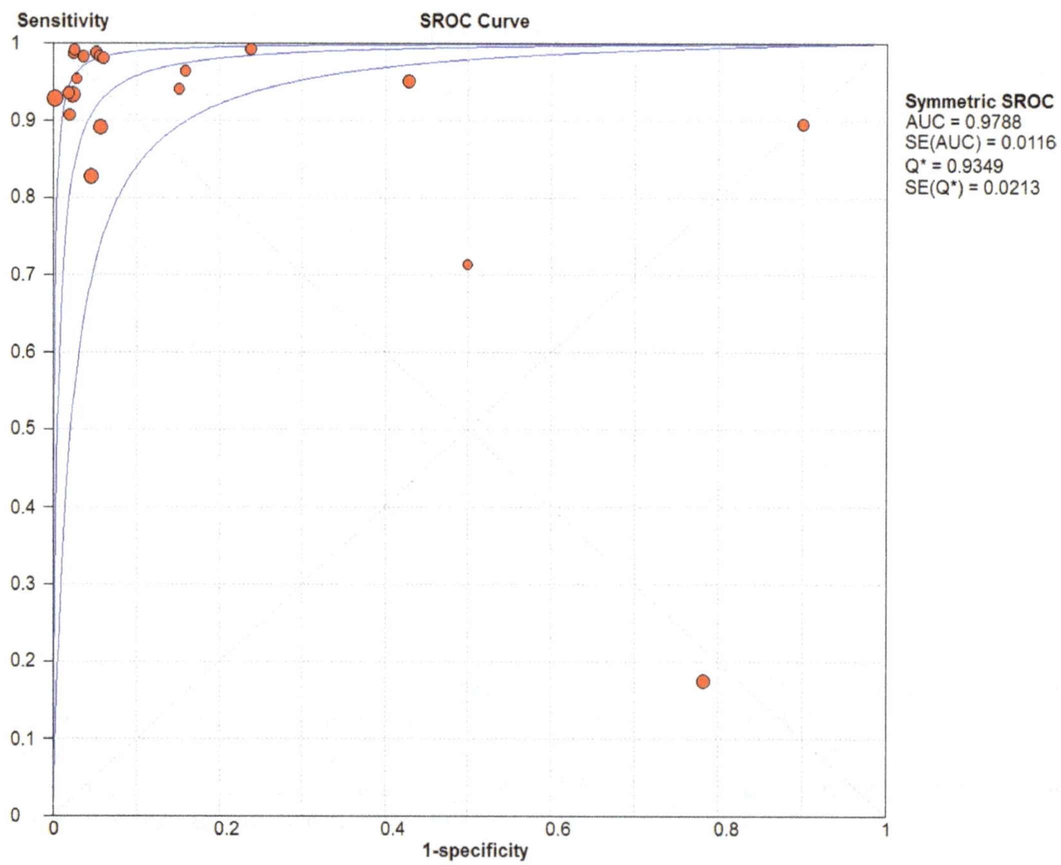


**Fig. 6** Pooled receiver operator characteristic curve of ultrasound in diagnosing pneumonia

opacity that may have effacement of blood vessel shadows and the presence of air bronchograms.

In lung ultrasound, the normal lung displays the "lung sliding" and A-lines. Lung sliding indicates sliding of the visceral pleura against the parietal pleura and A-lines are repetitive horizontal reverberation artifacts parallel to the pleural line generated by normally present subpleural air in the alveoli.

On ultrasound examination, consolidation is defined as tissue-like pattern reminiscent of the liver, sometimes called "hepatization," with boundaries that may be formed from the pleural line or a pleural effusion if present and the aerated lung, potentially forming an irregular scattered line if the consolidation is limited (shred sign) or a regular line if the whole lobe is involved. The LUS is logically capable in detecting superficial pneumonia, but it remains, however, doubtful in detecting deep alveolar lesions [39]. Consolidation is defined as an isoechoic tissue-like structure, which is caused by the loss of lung aeration. [4, 27] Power Doppler sometimes is used in order to differentiate tissue-like structures (e.g., echoic pleural effusion) from consolidation. The shred sign is specific for consolidation. B-lines are well-defined hyperechoic comet-tail artifacts, arising from pleural line and spreading vertically indefinitely, erasing A-lines and moving with the lung sliding when lung sliding is present. It indicates partial loss of lung aeration. Lung ultrasound using Doppler or contrast-enhanced sonography visualizes regional pulmonary blood flow within lung consolidations, thereby providing critical information about the etiology of the disease [27]. CXR does not provide any information about regional vascularization. The ultrasound detection of a dynamic air bronchogram is reported to be useful for differentiating obstructive atelectasis from pneumonia [27]. Several studies have demonstrated the superiority of lung ultrasound over CXR for diagnosing lung consolidation, particularly when portable CXR technique is used [30]. Therefore, the use of lung ultrasound can significantly reduce the number of chest radiographs and CT scans and decreases patients' radiation exposure. It is easily repeatable at the bedside and provides more accurate diagnostic information than CXR in critically ill and emergency patients with lung consolidation.

In this study, we did a systematic review and meta-analysis for the diagnostic accuracy of radiological exam (CXR/CT) and lung ultrasound in relation to diagnosis of pneumonia. In comparison with previous systematic review published addressing this issue [4, 42], our study included more primary studies and subjects compared to previously published systematic reviews.

In our study, we found that lung ultrasound had a high LR, sensitivity, and specificity for the diagnosis of pneumonia. That represents a strong diagnostic accuracy measure with high precision as expressed by the relatively narrow 95% CI. It is important to emphasize that this high diagnostic accuracy can be operator-dependent [34]. The lung scan should be performed by well-trained operators in at least 6 zones to be able to achieve such high diagnostic accuracy [36]. However, in relation to CXR, previous 2 meta-analyses agrees about the superiority of ultrasound over portable CXR [4, 42].

This study emphasizes the role of lung ultrasound as an accurate technique for diagnosing pneumonia compared to chest radiological imaging. This comes in agreement with the multiple reports published for LUS use in multiple settings and new indication [43–47]. In addition, it can help in reducing the movement of patients to the radiology department for CT particularly in unstable mechanical ventilated patient.

## Limitation

Moderate-to-high degree of inconsistency/heterogeneity was observed which puts some caution for the interpretation of this study. The reason of heterogeneity can be due to differences in the population or in the reference standard (CXR and CT scan).

The study did not aim to investigate clinical end-point to prove/disprove LUS as a useful diagnostic strategy. That requires another SR of preferably RCT to elicit potential benefits of using the strategy of ultrasound diagnosis over radiological diagnosis. It will require examining several clinical outcomes such as earlier start of treatment, more effective management, reducing costs, reducing need for endoscope, and reducing complication such as cross-infection. These clinical end-points were not addressed, as the focus was to establish pooled diagnostic accuracy rather than estimating effectiveness between comparative diagnostic strategies. However, our study managed to estimate high pooled diagnostic accuracy of this tool, which may justify its use.

In addition, we did not do comparison between LUS and chest X-ray in the general population (adults and children). That will require individual patient data (IPD) which are not available in the published studies. However, IPD meta-analysis has a robust methodology and peculiar characteristics that can be considered in this topic as potential future research.

## Conclusion

Lung ultrasound can play a major and valuable role in the diagnosis of pneumonia with high diagnostic accuracy. Moreover, it can be an alternative to chest X-ray and thoracic CT in several conditions. LUS can be used at the bedside easily, safely, and repetitively. Using LUS in Emergency department, ICUs, and medical wards after adequate training can be considered as a disruptive technology in this field.

#### Abbreviations

LUS: lung ultrasound; CT: computerized axial tomography; X-Ray: X-radiation; LR: likelihood ratio; DF: degree of freedom; MeSH: medical subheadings; CXR: chest computerized axial tomography scan; QUADAS: quality assessment of primary diagnostic accuracy studies.

#### Authors' contributions

ME: study protocol, methods, discussion, and overview of completion of the manuscript. MAAS: contribution in introduction, results, and discussion. WHAM: method and result. SAA: introduction, statistical analysis. All authors read and approved the final manuscript.

#### Author details

[1] King Saud bin Abdulaziz University for Health Sciences, Riyadh, Kingdom of Saudi Arabia. [2] Emergency Medicine, College of Public Health and Health Informatics, King Saud bin Abdulaziz University for Health Sciences, Riyadh, Kingdom of Saudi Arabia. [3] National & Gulf Center for Evidence Based Health Practice (NGCEBHP), King Saud bin Abdulaziz University for Health Sciences (KSAUHS), Riyadh, Kingdom of Saudi Arabia. [4] KSAUHS, Ministry of National Guard-Health Affairs, King Abdullah International Medical Research Center, Riyadh, Kingdom of Saudi Arabia.

#### References

1. Peden M (2008) World report on child injury prevention: World Health Organization
2. Almirall J, Bolibar I, Vidal J, Sauca G, Coll P, Niklasson B et al (2000) Epidemiology of community-acquired pneumonia in adults: a population-based study. Eur Respir J 15(4):757–763
3. Meehan TP, Fine MJ, Krumholz HM, Scinto JD, Galusha DH, Mockalis JT et al (1997) Quality of care, process, and outcomes in elderly patients with pneumonia. JAMA 278(23):2080–2084
4. Chavez MA, Shams N, Ellington LE, Naithani N, Gilman RH, Steinhoff MC et al (2014) Lung ultrasound for the diagnosis of pneumonia in adults: a systematic review and meta-analysis. Respir Res 15(50):1465–9921
5. Mayaud C (2011) Pneumonia is the leading cause of death of infectious origin. La Revue du praticien 61(8):1061
6. Van der Eerden M, Vlaspolder F, De Graaff C, Groot T, Jansen H, Boersma W (2005) Value of intensive diagnostic microbiological investigation in low-and high-risk patients with community-acquired pneumonia. Eur J Clin Microbiol Infect Dis 24(4):241–249
7. Wahidi MM, Rocha AT, Hollingsworth JW, Govert JA, Feller-Kopman D, Ernst A (2005) Contraindications and safety of transbronchial lung biopsy via flexible bronchoscopy. Respiration 72(3):285–295
8. Henschke CI, Yankelevitz DF, Wand A, Davis SD, Shiau M (1996) Accuracy and efficacy of chest radiography in the intensive care unit. Radiol Clini North Am 34(1):21–31
9. Lichtenstein D, Peyrouset O (2006) Is lung ultrasound superior to CT? The example of a CT occult necrotizing pneumonia. Intensive Care Med 32(2):334–335
10. Rubinowitz AN, Siegel MD, Tocino I (2007) Thoracic imaging in the ICU. Crit Care Clin 23(3):539–573
11. Yu C-J, Yang P-C, Chang D, Luh K (1992) Diagnostic and therapeutic use of chest sonography: value in critically ill patients. AJR Am J Roentgenol 159(4):695–701
12. Oba Y, Zaza T (2010) Abandoning daily routine chest radiography in the intensive care unit: meta-analysis 1. Radiology 255(2):386–395
13. Lichtenstein DA (2009) Ultrasound examination of the lungs in the intensive care unit. Pediatric Crit Care Medi 10(6):693–698
14. Beckh S, Bolcskei PL, Lessnau K-D (2002) Real-time chest ultrasonographya comprehensive review for the pulmonologist. CHEST J 122(5):1759–1773
15. Gryminski J, Krakówka P, Lypacewicz G (1976) The diagnosis of pleural effusion by ultrasonic and radiologic techniques. CHEST J 70(1):33–37
16. Reißig A, Kroegel C (2003) Transthoracic sonography of diffuse parenchymal lung disease the role of comet tail artifacts. J Ultrasound Med 22(2):173–180
17. Volpicelli G, Elbarbary M, Blaivas M, Lichtenstein DA, Mathis G, Kirkpatrick AW et al (2012) International evidence-based recommendations for point-of-care lung ultrasound. Intensive Care Med 38(4):577–591
18. Koenig SJ, Narasimhan M, Mayo PH (2011) Thoracic ultrasonography for the pulmonary specialist thoracic ultrasonography. CHEST J 140(5):1332–1341
19. Lichtenstein D, Goldstein I, Mourgeon E, Cluzel P, Grenier P, Rouby J-J (2004) Comparative diagnostic performances of auscultation, chest radiography, and lung ultrasonography in acute respiratory distress syndrome. Anesthesiology 100(1):9–15
20. Whiting PF, Rutjes AW, Westwood ME, Mallett S, Deeks JJ, Reitsma JB et al (2011) QUADAS-2: a revised tool for the quality assessment of diagnostic accuracy studies. Ann Intern Med 155(8):529–536
21. Zamora J, Muriel A, Khan K, Coomarasamy A (2006) Meta-DiSc: a software for meta-analysis of test accuracy data. BMC Med Res Methodol 6:31
22. Deeks JJ, Macaskill P, Irwig L (2005) The performance of tests of publication bias and other sample size effects in systematic reviews of diagnostic test accuracy was assessed. J Clin Epidemiol 58(9):882–893 **(Epub 2005/08/09)**
23. Iuri D, De Candia A, Bazzocchi M (2009) Evaluation of the lung in children with suspected pneumonia: usefulness of ultrasonography. Radiol Med (Torino) 114(2):321–330
24. Unluer E, Karagoz A, Senturk G, Karaman M, Olow K, Bayata S (2013) Bedside lung ultrasonography for diagnosis of pneumonia. Hong Kong J Emerg Med 20(2):98
25. El Dien HMS, ElLatif DAA (2013) The value of bedside lung ultrasonography in diagnosis of neonatal pneumonia. Egypt J Radiol Nuclear Med 44(2):339–347
26. Caiulo VA, Gargani L, Caiulo S, Fisicaro A, Moramarco F, Latini G et al (2013) Lung ultrasound characteristics of community-acquired pneumonia in hospitalized children. Pediatric Pulmonol 48(3):280–287
27. Benci A, Caremani M, Menchetti D, Magnolfi A (1996) Sonographic diagnosis of pneumonia and bronchopneumonia. Eur J Ultrasound 4(3):169–176
28. Lichtenstein DA, Lascols N, Mezière G, Gepner A (2004) Ultrasound diagnosis of alveolar consolidation in the critically ill. Intensive Care Med 30(2):276–281
29. Lichtenstein DA, Meziere GA (2008) Relevance of lung ultrasound in the diagnosis of acute respiratory failure. CHEST J 134(1):117–125
30. Parlamento S, Copetti R, Di Bartolomeo S (2009) Evaluation of lung ultrasound for the diagnosis of pneumonia in the ED. Am J Emerg Med 27(4):379–384
31. Cortellaro F, Colombo S, Coen D, Duca PG (2012) Lung ultrasound is an accurate diagnostic tool for the diagnosis of pneumonia in the emergency department. Emerg Med J 29(1):19–23
32. Xirouchaki N, Magkanas E, Vaporidi K, Kondili E, Plataki M, Patrianakos A et al (2011) Lung ultrasound in critically ill patients: comparison with bedside chest radiography. Intensive Care Med 37(9):1488–1493
33. Reissig A, Copetti R, Mathis G, Mempel C, Schuler A, Zechner P et al (2012) Lung ultrasound in the diagnosis and follow-up of community-acquired pneumonia: a prospective, multicenter, diagnostic accuracy study. CHEST J 142(4):965–972
34. Testa A, Soldati G, Copetti R, Giannuzzi R, Portale G, Gentiloni-Silveri N (2012) Early recognition of the 2009 pandemic influenza A (H1N1) pneumonia by chest ultrasound. Crit Care 16(1):R30
35. Shah VP, Tunik MG, Tsung JW (2013) Prospective evaluation of point-of-care ultrasonography for the diagnosis of pneumonia in children and young adults. JAMA Pediatr 167(2):119–125
36. Copetti R, Cattarossi L (2008) Ultrasound diagnosis of pneumonia in children. Radiol Med (Torino) 113(2):190–198

37. Nafae R, Eman SR, Mohamad NA, El-Ghamry R, Ragheb AS (2013) Adjuvant role of lung ultrasound in the diagnosis of pneumonia in intensive care unit-patients. Egypt J Chest Dis Tuberc 62(2):281–285
38. Liu X-L, Lian R, Tao Y-K, Gu C-D, Zhang G-Q (2014) Lung ultrasonography: an effective way to diagnose community-acquired pneumonia. Emerg Med J **(emermed-2013-203039)**
39. Esposito S, Papa SS, Borzani I, Pinzani R, Giannitto C, Consonni D et al (2014) Performance of lung ultrasonography in children with community-acquired pneumonia. Ital J Pediatr 40:37
40. Nazerian P, Volpicelli G, Vanni S, Gigli C, Betti L, Bartolucci M et al (2015) Accuracy of lung ultrasound for the diagnosis of consolidations when compared to chest computed tomography. Am J Emerg Med 33(5):620–625
41. Bourcier J-E, Paquet J, Seinger M, Gallard E, Redonnet J-P, Cheddadi F et al (2014) Performance comparison of lung ultrasound and chest X-ray for the diagnosis of pneumonia in the ED. Am J Emerg Med 32(2):115–118
42. Ye X, Xiao H, Chen B, Zhang S (2015) Accuracy of lung ultrasonography versus chest radiography for the diagnosis of adult community-acquired pneumonia: review of the literature and meta-analysis. PLoS ONE 10(6):e0130066
43. Sartori S, Tombesi P (2010) Emerging roles for transthoracic ultrasonography in pulmonary diseases. World J Radiol 2(6):203
44. Lichtenstein DA (2014) Lung ultrasound in the critically ill. Ann Intensive Care. 4(1):2110–5820
45. Volpicelli G, Zanobetti M (2015) Lung ultrasound and pulmonary consolidations. Am J Emerg Med 33(9):1307–1308. doi:10.1016/j.ajem.2015.04.020 **(Epub 2015 Apr 16)**
46. Lichtenstein D (2014) Lung ultrasound in the critically ill. Curr Opin Crit Care 20(3):315–322
47. Remérand F, Dellamonica J, Mao Z, Ferrari F, Bouhemad B, Jianxin Y et al (2010) Multiplane ultrasound approach to quantify pleural effusion at the bedside. Intensive Care Med 36(4):656–664

8

# An easy-to-build, low-budget point-of-care ultrasound simulator: from Linux to a web-based solution

Domagoj Damjanovic[1], Ulrich Goebel[1], Benedikt Fischer[2], Martin Huth[2], Hartmut Breger[2], Hartmut Buerkle[1] and Axel Schmutz[1*]

**Abstract**

**Background:** Hands-on training in point-of-care ultrasound (POC-US) should ideally comprise bedside teaching, as well as simulated clinical scenarios. High-fidelity phantoms and portable ultrasound simulation systems are commercially available, however, at considerable costs. This limits their suitability for medical schools. A Linux-based software for Emergency Department Ultrasound Simulation (edus2TM) was developed by Kulyk and Olszynski in 2011. Its feasibility for POC-US education has been well-documented, and shows good acceptance. An important limitation to an even more widespread use of edus2, however, may be due to the need for a virtual machine for WINDOWS® systems. Our aim was to adapt the original software toward an HTML-based solution, thus making it affordable and applicable in any simulation setting.

**Methods:** We created an HTML browser-based ultrasound simulation application, which reads the input of different sensors, triggering an ultrasound video to be displayed on a respective device. RFID tags, NFC tags, and QR Codes™ have been integrated into training phantoms or were attached to standardized patients. The RFID antenna was hidden in a mock ultrasound probe. The application is independent from the respective device.

**Results:** Our application was used successfully with different trigger/scanner combinations and mounted readily into simulated training scenarios. The application runs independently from operating systems or electronic devices.

**Conclusion:** This low-cost, browser-based ultrasound simulator is easy-to-build, very adaptive, and independent from operating systems. It has the potential to facilitate POC-US training throughout the world, especially in resource-limited areas.

**Keywords:** Ultrasonography, Point-of-care systems, Simulation training

## Background

Point-of-care ultrasound (POC-US) has been shown to improve the diagnostic accuracy of the initial clinical assessment of critically ill patients [1]. The use of focused sonography may identify patients with an acute life-threatening condition missed at primary assessment [2]. In the expanding field of POC-US and its wide, but highly user-dependent applicability in emergency situations, adequate training is essential. Hence, training comprises bedside teaching, as well as simulated clinical scenarios, such as advanced life support or trauma resuscitation.

High-fidelity phantoms, as well as portable ultrasound simulation systems are commercially available [3]. However, their application implicates considerable costs, which limits their suitability for resource-limited settings like developing countries as well as for medical schools. University of Freiburg Medical School educates more than 300 third- and fourth-year medical students each year, going through curricular trainings in emergency medicine, as well as anesthesia. To achieve a reasonable

*Correspondence: axel.schmutz@uniklinik-freiburg.de
[1] Department of Anesthesiology and Critical Care, Medical Center-University of Freiburg, Faculty of Medicine, University of Freiburg, Hugstetter Strasse 55, 79106 Freiburg, Germany
Full list of author information is available at the end of the article

student-ultrasound phantom ratio, this would afford the purchase or upgrade of at least three more high-fidelity phantoms only for the curricular training itself. Furthermore, to offer modern concepts of blended learning would require making even more simulators available to students.

In 2011, Kulyk and Olszynski introduced the portable emergency department ultrasound simulator (edus2TM), an easy-to-build, low-cost bedside ultrasound simulator, that allows for integration into high-fidelity simulation scenarios [4]. The machine consists of a laptop computer and a Radio-Frequency Identification (RFID) antenna, hidden in a mock ultrasound probe. RFID tags (cards, points, stickers) attached to phantoms, or standardized patients may then trigger a video sequence, displayed on the laptop and showing the particular ultrasound findings. Thus, pathological POC-US findings can be simulated easily with any phantom or patient. As a result, not only image interpretation on a screen, but also to some extent image acquisition can be trained within real-time settings: the probe has to be held in the right place to retrieve the information (landmarking). The corresponding video files are stored on the laptop computer itself. Unfortunately, the software is LINUX based; this affords a virtual machine to allow its use with WINDOWS®. With these restrictions, specific hard- and software has to be used. The concept was published open source by the authors, including technical instructions and a set of sample videos to start with [5]. Another, more up-to-date technology was created by Ostergren. The "Awesome Ultrasound Simulator" is an iOS mobile application, where two smartphones are combined, with one of them displaying the videos, the other serves as a remote control for choosing them [6]. This solution is a freely accessible resource as well, and has successfully been used in the Trauma Resuscitation Using in situ Simulation Team Training (TRUST) study by Petrosoniak and coworkers [7]. It is, however, only available for Apple™ devices, and dependent on a second remote operator to trigger the videos. Following the abovementioned authors' intention, our aim was to adapt the original edus2TM software toward an HTML-based solution, independent of operating systems or devices, thus making it affordable and applicable in any simulation setting.

## Methods

Anonymized point-of-care ultrasound video clips from patients, showing individual and unequivocal pathologies have been recorded and stored in a database. Together with our departments' IT section, we aimed to create a browser-based application written in Hypertext Markup Language (HTML5). This in turn reads the input from a sensor as a keystroke to start displaying ultrasound video clips. Sensors should be RFID antennas, Near-Field Communication (NFC), or Quick Response Codes™ (QR Codes™). The input of the sensor initiates the particular pre-recorded ultrasound video clip on the respective device (e.g., Laptop, Tablet, Smartphone) with any operating system (Mac OS, Android, Windows, Raspian, SUSE, etc.). Access to the pre-recorded videos should be possible wherever they are stored (computer main store, hard drive disk, database server, cloud, etc.). RFID tags were hidden under the artificial skin of a megacode mannequin (ALS Simulator, Laerdal™) or attached to a patient and then masked, as shown in Additional file Digital Content (Additional file 2: SDC video 2). Multiple scans are possible by placement of several RFID tags either on the mannequin or on the patient. Every set of tags can be linked to different profiles, so that several scenarios may be employed using the same hardware. Figure 1 gives an overview of the whole simulation concept and summarizes the different triggers used. As an example, Fig. 2 shows in detail how the RFID antenna was mounted into a self-designed 3D printed mock ultrasound probe (Fig. 2). Video clips provided in the Additional file Digital Content illustrate the concept using a mobile phone (Additional file 1: SDC video 1) or a tablet (Additional file 2: SDC video 2). The different profiles are again chosen by the respective tags, which in SDC video 1 are called P1-P3. Additional file 3: SDC video 3 demonstrates the scanning of an NFC tag directly with a mobile phone, without the need for an additional ultrasound probe. Figure 3 shows a mobile phone which is used as a handheld ultrasound simulator, compared to a commercially available device (General Electric Healthcare, Vscan dual™, courtesy, GE).

An open access version of the simulator application is available at the following URL: https://drive.google.com/file/d/0B7FPzgyHC6cGZHpBa3BFNlpfLVk/view.

You can use the simulator in your own institution and implement own or other pre-recorded ultrasound video clips.

## Results

We successfully created an HTML5-based ultrasound simulator which is independent from the operating system as well as the displaying device, appearing on laptops, personal computer workstations as well as smartphones and tablets with any operating system. It was able to display the corresponding video triggered by RFID tags as well as by Near-Field Communication or QR code detection instantly. The students could replay the ultrasound video clip if necessary. Adding new video clips to the selected file storage worked well, be it in the device itself, a cloud data storage or a video streaming platform.

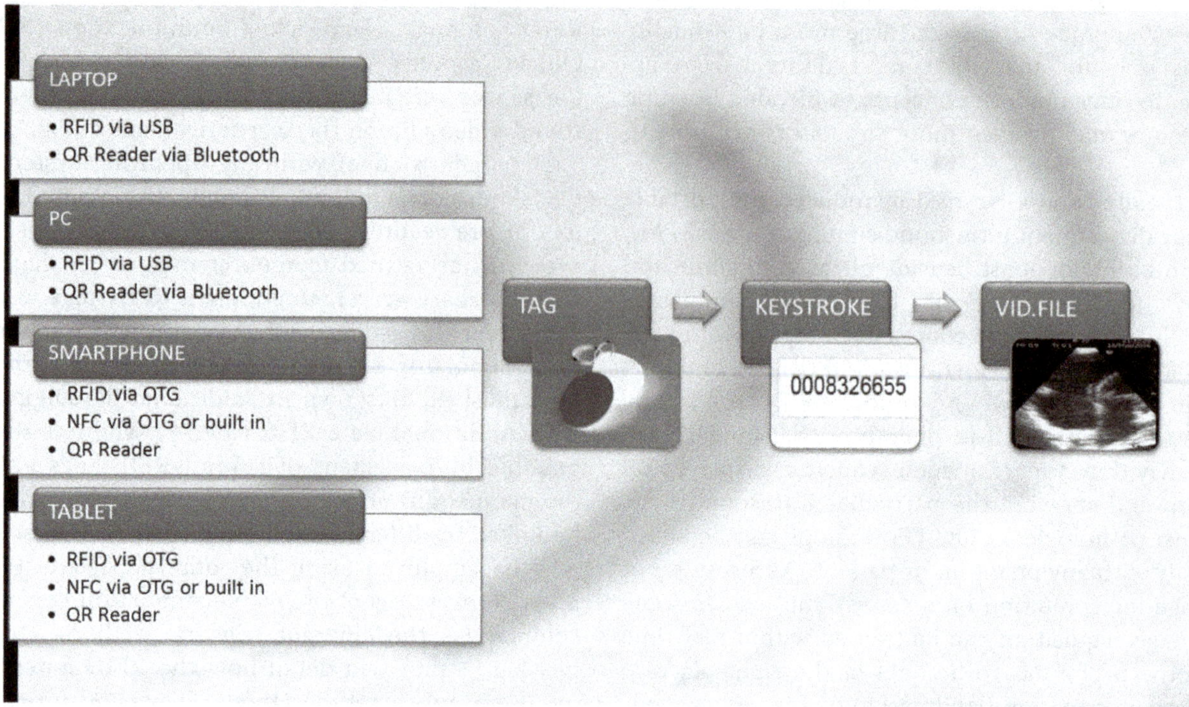


**Fig. 1** Different devices such as laptop computers, desktop computers/PCs, smartphones as well as tablets can be used to display video files, that is, ultrasound loops, respectively. These are triggered by tags, the content of which is read as a keystroke. *RFID* radio-frequency identification, *USB* universal serial bus, *QR* quick response, *OTG* on the go, *NFC* near-field communication. VID. FILE video of ultrasound loop stored as a separate file

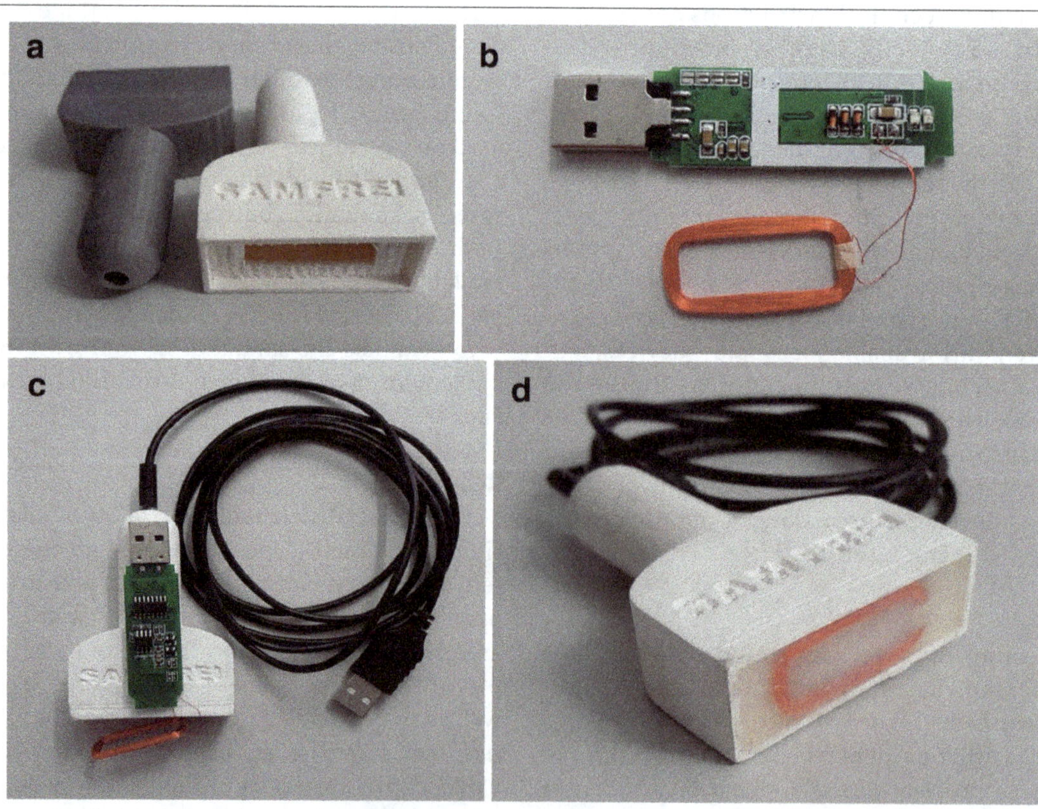


**Fig. 2** Three-dimensional printed mock ultrasound probe with RFID antenna. **a** Raw material as printed. **b** The partly disassembled RFID antenna, which originally has USB-stick format. **c** How the antenna is built into the housing. **d** The complete probe with USB wire

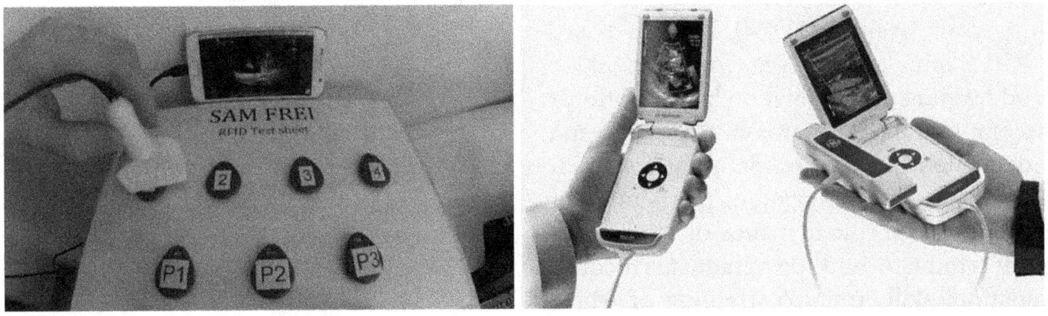


**Fig. 3** *Left panel* shows the simulator using a mobile phone for the display of a specific ultrasound loop video, *Right panel* shows a commercially available handheld point-of-care ultrasound device (VSCAN DUAL, courtesy General Electric). Please note the three different profile switches, tag P1, P2, and P3 which allow for different findings to be displayed with the same tag *1*, *2*, *3*, or *4*, respectively

The total costs for a set of RFID Tags, an RFID antenna, a 3D-printed ultrasound probe, and a USB wire were well below 100 EUR, which is only a minor fraction the cost of commercially available simulated ultrasound systems. Working time for acquisition, adjustment, and review of the video material are not included, however.

## Discussion

The main findings of this study are (a) it is feasible to convert the edus2 software into an HTML browser-based application, (b) this—in combination with a mock US probe—makes ultrasound training and simulation affordable in developing countries, since (c) our software solution may be used on any operating system (Mac OS®, Android, WINDOWS®, etc.) and on any gadget available (smartphone, tablet, PC, etc.).

Considering the capabilities of our readily available ultrasound simulator at only a fraction of the cost of commercially available solutions, it might be especially relevant for medical education and training in developing countries. These can be remote environments or poor areas in the developing world with a lack of imaging modalities other than ultrasound [8–12]. Of note, acute surges in availability of imaging services can also occur in developed healthcare systems, with emergency ultrasound filling the gap. An impressive illustration of this is the report from the Boston bombings, where POC-US significantly aided in the management of mass casualties [13].

The high adaptability of the system allows for customization according to the requirements of the respective teaching facility. If there is no opportunity to acquire video material by oneself, there are several freely accessible video libraries for this purpose [14].

Due to its low cost and independence of hardware solutions, our simulator allows to be employed for blended learning in our own medical school in a broad manner, which has the potential to spare time and resource. Learners can not only prepare themselves with conventional e-learning material, but also train more aspects of image acquisition, with a unique haptic experience. The latter very much adds to the imaging skills, compared to the sole use of screen-based training choosing videos on the displaying device manually [5]. Given the steep learning curves, quite specific for POC-US, a rapid translation of the clinical skills augmented by such training efforts into clinical routine may be expected [15–17].

When using QR Codes™ as triggers, which can be downloaded and printed out, no additional hardware, i.e., sets of RFID or NFC tags, has to be distributed. Thus, the system can remotely be made available for download. Some minor technical details are subject to our further investigation and development, such as the design of the application surface. Furthermore, strategies for accurate review and quality control of the teaching material have to be implemented. Programming and indexing tags with their corresponding video clips may be time consuming, as it is for any ultrasound video loop editing for educational purposes. As some mobile devices failed to feed battery power to the RFID antennas, the capability of using different triggering solutions provides a useful backup plan. Finally, the sole triggering of a video clip to be displayed does not encompass probe manipulation and image optimization skills as commercially available systems do, which is another field of further technical development for the system. Furthermore, the video output format of ultrasound machines and the anonymizing function varies. Several different file types and codecs may hamper their universal utilization for an ultrasound simulation library. This can easily be overcome using free file converters. Altogether, despite some minor technical issues, we did not want to withhold this important technical advance from publication, since we are convinced, that it will have a considerable impact on worldwide training in POC-US.

## Conclusion

We created a universally available HTML browser-based solution for POC-US simulation at very low cost, which makes ultrasound training and simulation broadly affordable also in developing countries. It was easy to set up and use, running independently from the operating system or displaying device. In medical education, this simulator can be adapted easily to specific demands of the respective setting: undergraduate and postgraduate medical education, simulation, skills training, training of whole POC-US protocols and blended learning. Although the system itself is "low cost," the technique enables incorporation into high-fidelity simulation, and it enables trainees to learn the indications of ultrasound, learn precise image interpretation, and finally integrate the findings into patient management. We expect our simulator to enhance clinical competence, facilitate health care professionals' education, and enable research purposes in this important emergency care diagnostic tool.

## Additional files

**Additional file 1.** Mp4, video of cell-phone used as mock handheld ultrasound machine.

**Additional file 2.** Mp4, video of a tablet-pc used as mock handheld ultrasound machine.

**Additional file 3.** Mp4, video with NFC-tags and QR-codes used as ultrasound video triggers.

### Abbreviations

POC-US: point-of-care ultrasound; edus2TM: Emergency Department Ultrasound Simulation; HTML: Hypertext Markup Language; RFID: radio-frequency identification; NFC: near-field communication; QR Codes™: quick response codes™; SDC: supplementary digital content.

### Authors' contributions

DD developed the idea for the simulator. MH, BF, and HB developed the browser application. DD, MH, and BF manufactured the mock probe. DD and AS wrote the manuscript, and UG and HB revised the manuscript. All authors contributed substantially to this work and all of them revised and agreed to the final version of the manuscript. They all agree to be accountable for all aspects of the work. All authors read and approved the final manuscript.

### Author details

[1] Department of Anesthesiology and Critical Care, Medical Center-University of Freiburg, Faculty of Medicine, University of Freiburg, Hugstetter Strasse 55, 79106 Freiburg, Germany. [2] Information Technology Section, Department of Anesthesiology and Critical Care, Medical Center-University of Freiburg, Faculty of Medicine, University of Freiburg, 79106 Freiburg, Germany.

### Acknowledgements

We want to thank our medical educators who helped implementing the concept into single teaching sessions: Thomas Ahne, Michael Buechling, Leonardo Eisert, Susanne Langer, Martina Laub, Oliver Marx, Daniel Petraschka, Tomas Sander, Carolin Schuetz, Luc Seywert, Johannes Spaeth, Felix Ulbrich, as well as our student tutors and peer-to-peer teachers Lisa Artner, Jascha S Heider, Tobias Seufert, and Sophia Reithmeier.

Furthermore, we want to express our gratitude to Paul Kulyk and Paul Olszynski, the developers of the original EDUS2, for their dedicated work and the open source publication, making it available to the world, which gave us the technical starting point.

### References

1. Bernier-Jean A, Albert M, Shiloh AL, Eisen LA, Williamson D, Beaulieu Y (2015) The diagnostic and therapeutic impact of point-of-care ultrasonography in the intensive care unit. J Intensive Care Med. doi:10.1177/0885066615606682
2. Laursen CB, Sloth E, Lassen AT et al (2012) Focused sonographic examination of the heart, lungs and deep veins in an unselected population of acute admitted patients with respiratory symptoms: a protocol for a prospective, blinded, randomised controlled trial. BMJ Open. doi:10.1136/bmjopen-2012-001369
3. Laerdal. SonoSim®. http://www.laerdal.com/us/UltrasoundSolution. Accessed 9 Oct 2016
4. Kulyk P, Olszynski P (2016) Emergency Department Ultrasound Simulator. http://www.edus2.com/. Accessed 9 Oct 2016
5. Olszynski PA, Harris T, Renihan P, D'Eon M, Premkumar K (2016) Ultrasound during critical care simulation: a randomized crossover study. CJEM. 18(3):183–190. doi:10.1017/cem.2015.87
6. Östergren P (2016) Awesome Ultrasound Simulator. http://ultrasound-simulator.com/. Accessed 9 Oct 2016
7. Petrosoniak A, Gray A, Fan M et al (2016) MP036: Trauma Resuscitation Using in situ Simulation Team Training (TRUST): a novel approach to latent safety threat identification in trauma care. CJEM. 18(S1):S78–S79. doi:10.1017/cem.2016.177
8. The PURE initiative: point-of-care ultrasound in resource-limited environments: dedicated to improving ultrasound education in the developing world. http://www.pureultrasound.org. Accessed 8 Oct 2016
9. McNeil CR, McManus J, Mehta S (2009) The accuracy of portable ultrasonography to diagnose fractures in an austere environment. Prehosp Emerg Care. 13(1):50–52. doi:10.1080/10903120802474513
10. Shorter M, Macias DJ (2012) Portable handheld ultrasound in austere environments: use in the Haiti disaster. Prehosp Disaster Med. 27(2):172–177. doi:10.1017/S1049023X12000611
11. Whitfield DA, Portouw SJ (2012) Retinal detachment due to facial gunshot wound: the utility of ultrasonography in a medically austere environment. J Emerg Med 42(6):678–681. doi:10.1016/j.jemermed.2011.06.010
12. Zhang S, Zhu D, Wan Z, Cao Y (2014) Utility of point-of-care ultrasound in acute management triage of earthquake injury. Am J Emerg Med 32(1):92–95. doi:10.1016/j.ajem.2013.10.009
13. Kimberly HH, Stone MB (2013) Clinician-performed ultrasonography during the Boston marathon bombing mass casualty incident. Ann Emerg Med 62(2):199–200. doi:10.1016/j.annemergmed.2013.05.014
14. SonoCloud—Videos. http://sonocloud.org/videos/. Accessed 9 Oct 2016
15. Chenkin J, McCartney CJL, Jelic T, Romano M, Heslop C, Bandiera G (2015) Defining the learning curve of point-of-care ultrasound for confirming endotracheal tube placement by emergency physicians. Crit Ultrasound J 7(1):14. doi:10.1186/s13089-015-0031-7
16. Beaulieu Y, Laprise R, Drolet P et al (2015) Bedside ultrasound training using web-based e-learning and simulation early in the curriculum of residents. Crit Ultrasound J 7:1. doi:10.1186/s13089-014-0018-9
17. Cantisani V, Dietrich CF, Badea R et al (2016) EFSUMB statement on medical student education in ultrasound short version. Ultraschall Med 37(1):100–102. doi:10.1055/s-0035-1566959

# 9

# Point-of-care ultrasound and Doppler ultrasound evaluation of vascular injuries in penetrating and blunt trauma

Miguel Angel Montorfano[1*], Fernando Pla[1], Leonardo Vera[1], Omar Cardillo[1], Stefano Geniere Nigra[2] and Lisandro Miguel Montorfano[1]

**Abstract**

**Background:** The aim of this study is to describe point-of-care ultrasound and Color flow Duplex Doppler characteristics of penetrating and blunt trauma-related vascular injuries of the limbs and neck.

**Methods:** Penetrating and blunt trauma-related vascular injuries such as vein disruption, intimal flap, deep vein thrombosis, arterial dissection, pseudoaneurysm, and arteriovenous fistulae are discussed in this manuscript. Images of the most significant lesions of our personal clinical experience are presented to illustrate point-of-care ultrasound and Color flow Duplex Doppler ultrasound findings.

**Results:** Penetrating and blunt trauma-related vascular injuries represent a big challenge. While patients with hard signs of arterial damage must be sent immediately to surgical exploration, when there are soft signs or no clear signs of vascular injury at the physical examination, and the patient is stable, imaging investigation and observation can be useful in the diagnosis and management of these patients. Although angiography is the gold standard of the imaging methods, point-of-care ultrasound and Color flow Duplex Doppler ultrasound are widely available, cheaper, noninvasive, and faster to obtain. They can provide bedside valuable information for the identification of some vascular injuries allowing to an integrated management of the trauma patient, enriched by the use of ultrasound.

**Conclusions:** Point-of-care ultrasound and Color flow Duplex Doppler examination are increasingly used in the decision making process of trauma-related vascular injuries.

**Keywords:** Doppler sonography, Color flow Duplex Doppler, Critical ultrasound, Point-of-care ultrasound, Vascular injury, Trauma

## Background

Injuries are an important public health problem worldwide. More than 5 million people die each year as a result of injuries. This accounts for 9% of the world deaths, nearly 1.7 times the number of fatalities that result from HIV/AIDS, tuberculosis, and malaria combined. Among the causes of injury are traffic accidents, interpersonal violence, burns, drowning, falls, and poisonings. A quarter of the deaths are the result of traffic injuries, while suicide and homicide account for nearly another quarter.

For every person who died as a result of violence, many more are injured, causing a rise in costs in health care systems and in a massive burden in national economies [1]. Moreover, violence exacts a high cost on global development [2].

More than 90% of injury-related deaths occur in low- and middle-income countries and in remote locations.

Increase in urban crime and violence are affecting the lives of millions of people in Latin America.

*Correspondence: miguel.montorfano@winfocus.org
[1] Present Address: Department of Ultrasound, Clemente Álvarez Emergency Hospital, Av. Pellegrini 3205, 2000 Rosario, Santa Fe, Argentina
Full list of author information is available at the end of the article

The Pan American Health Organization called violence in Latin America "the social pandemic of the 20th century" [3].

Social inequality and substantial increase in the size of drug markets are considered major contributing factors to the levels of violence in Latin America. Of the world's 50 most dangerous cities, 43 are located in Latin America and the Caribbean.

Although the main goal must be to prevent injuries and violence from happening, a quick and rapid diagnosis and treatment are essential to prevent fatalities and reduce disabilities [1].

Vascular injuries represent less than 3% of all traumatic findings, yet they are associated with potentially severe complications [4–9]. If not recognized and treated fast, injuries to major arteries and veins may have devastating consequences resulting in amputations or even death. Knowing the mechanism of the trauma is of extreme importance for making the correct diagnosis. Although blunt trauma is a common cause of acute trauma presentation in the civil population worldwide, the increasing urban violence in our region has produced a rise of penetrating trauma produced by gun shot and stab wounds that deserve especial considerations (Fig. 1). Most vascular injuries are caused by penetrating trauma, such as gunshot wounds, stabbing, and blast injuries [6]. Blunt trauma causes significant soft tissue injury, while vascular disorders are less frequent [4]. Nonetheless, also in blunt trauma, vascular injuries need to be ruled out, especially in patients with displaced long bone fractures, crush injuries, and patients with prolonged immobilization [4–7]. Blunt trauma is more often associated with partial or complete vascular occlusion, arterial dissections, and intimal flaps, while penetrating trauma can also cause pseudoaneurysms, arteriovenous fistulas, and vein thrombosis [10–13].

The majority of vascular injuries are located in the extremities. Vascular injuries present a great challenge to emergency physicians because some vascular lesions may not be immediately identified with clinical evaluation and monitoring of vital signs.

The presence of "hard signs" in the physical examination" (such as pulsatile external bleeding, expanding haematoma, absent distal pulses, cold/pale limb, palpable thrill, or audible bruit) is an indication of immediate surgical intervention.

When the site or presence of a vascular injury is less obvious, the patient is stable and there are no signs or just soft signs of vascular injuries (such as peripheral nerve deficit, history of moderate hemorrhage at scene, a reduced but palpable pulse, or an injury in proximity to a major artery) imaging investigation and observation can be useful in the diagnosis and management of these patients. [4, 14].

Angiography is the gold standard for the evaluation of trauma-related vascular injuries; however, other noninvasive imaging methods such as computer tomography angiogram, magnetic resonance angiography, and Doppler ultrasound have emerged in recent years as valid alternatives [15].

Color flow Duplex Doppler is a widely available and reliable method with high sensitivity (95–97%), specificity (95–98%), and accuracy (98%) in assessment of peripheral vascular injuries [15, 16].

Bergstein et al. compared Color flow Doppler with arteriography in 67 patients without obvious vascular injuries. Using arteriography as the gold standard, Color flow Doppler had a specificity of 99%, sensitivity of 50%,

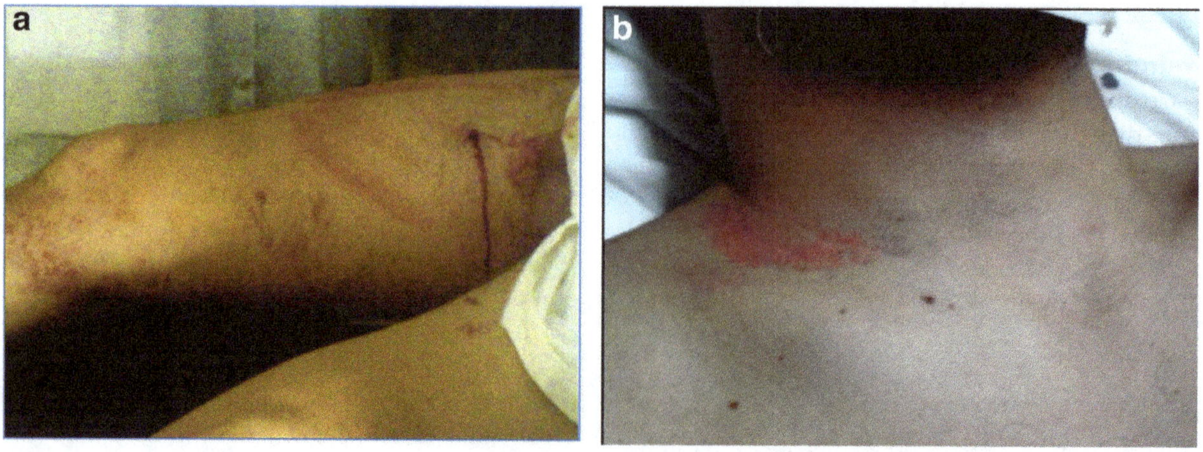

**Fig. 1** **a** Penetrating wound in the leg: gun shot wound. **b** Blunt trauma of the neck

and negative and positive predictive values of 66 and 7%, respectively [16].

Fry et al. described 100% sensitivity and specificity of Duplex Doppler compared with the conventional arteriography and operative exploration [17].

In a recent study, Mohd Wani et al. evaluate with Color flow Duplex Doppler 150 patients with soft signs of vascular injury of the limbs. The patients with features of vascular injury on Color Doppler (110 patients) were subjected to exploration, while patients who had normal Doppler (40 patients) were subjected to CT- angiography. Color flow Doppler had a sensitivity of 94% and specificity of 82.5% in diagnosis of vascular injury compared with CT angiography and surgical exploration [18].

Point-of-care ultrasound is widely available in trauma centers, emergency departments and is increasingly being used in the prehospital setting and in remote locations. In many cases, it is the first diagnostic method available. In these scenarios, it is used for a whole body examination, from head to toe, allowing to an integrated management of the trauma patient [19].

In the extremities and neck Point of care ultrasound is used for the diagnosis of fractures, hematomas, and the identification of foreign bodies [20]. At the same time we propose that, in stable patients without hard signs of vascular damage, it could be of great help for a prompt bedside diagnosis, characterization, and monitoring of trauma-related vascular injuries.

### The technique

Vascular injuries of the extremities and neck must be investigated with high-frequency linear transducers because a higher resolution and a lower penetration are commonly needed. There are some exceptions, such as patients with large hematomas and super obese patients, in which a convex probe with higher penetration is recommended. When evaluating vascular injuries, we have to explore the region of the trauma, and transversal and longitudinal scans of the vessels should be performed with B-mode. Proximal and distal flows should be investigated with Color flow Duplex Doppler ultrasound. For comparative purposes, both limbs and both sides of the neck should be evaluated.

Normal veins usually are oval in shape and completely compressible with a controlled pressure of the probe. The pulsed wave Doppler analysis shows a continuous flow pattern with respiratory variations.

Normal arteries are round in shape, with an echogenic wall, and noncompressible with the probe. Arteries of the extremities show a triphasic pattern in the pulsed Doppler spectrum. The triphasic pattern has a first positive phase related with the systole of the left ventricle, a second negative phase related with the closure of the aortic valve, and a third positive phase produced by the elasticity of the arterial walls. The loss of this triphasic pattern is always pathologic [21, 22]. The absence of triphasic pattern can be acute (traumatic injury or obstruction) or chronic (atherosclerosis, diabetes, aging).

Although in trauma patients, the presence of obesity, large hematomas, subcutaneous air, or large open wounds of the skin can represent a technical limitation to the penetration of the sound waves, with point-of-care ultrasound and Color flow Duplex Doppler is possible to accurately rule in or rule out trauma-related vascular injuries, [15, 16, 23, 24].

The aim of this study is to review and describe point-of-care ultrasound and Doppler ultrasound characteristics of penetrating and blunt trauma-related vascular injuries of the limbs and neck, such as vein rupture, intimal flap, deep vein thrombosis, arterial dissection, pseudoaneurysm, and arteriovenous fistulae. A bedside identification of these lesions can help to a better care of these patients. Images of most significant lesions are presented to illustrate point-of-care ultrasound and Doppler ultrasound findings.

#### *Pathologic sonographic patterns*

In patients with clinical suspicion of a vascular injury, point-of-care ultrasound and Doppler ultrasound are used to answer 2 basic questions:

1. Does the patient have a vascular lesion? Yes or no?
2. If the answer is yes: what kind of lesion?

Ultrasound can rapidly rule out vascular injuries after trauma at the bedside (Figs. 2, 3, 4).

When there is a trauma-related vascular lesion three basic patterns can be identified:

- Venous injuries
- Arterial injuries
- Mixed arterial and venous injuries

#### *Venous injuries*

Normal veins are anechoic and easily totally compressible by ultrasound transducers [21, 22, 25]. Traumatized veins may suffer partial or complete disruption, intimal injury, or post-traumatic thrombosis and this may alter the normal characteristics of these vessels. In complete disruption, it might be difficult to identify the site of injury due to shrinkage of injured veins or vein compression by the resultant hematoma. The presence of hematoma in the anatomical site where a major large caliber vein is supposed to be seen without a clear visualization of the vein is a strong indicator of complete vein rupture. In some blunt trauma patients, the ultrasonographic

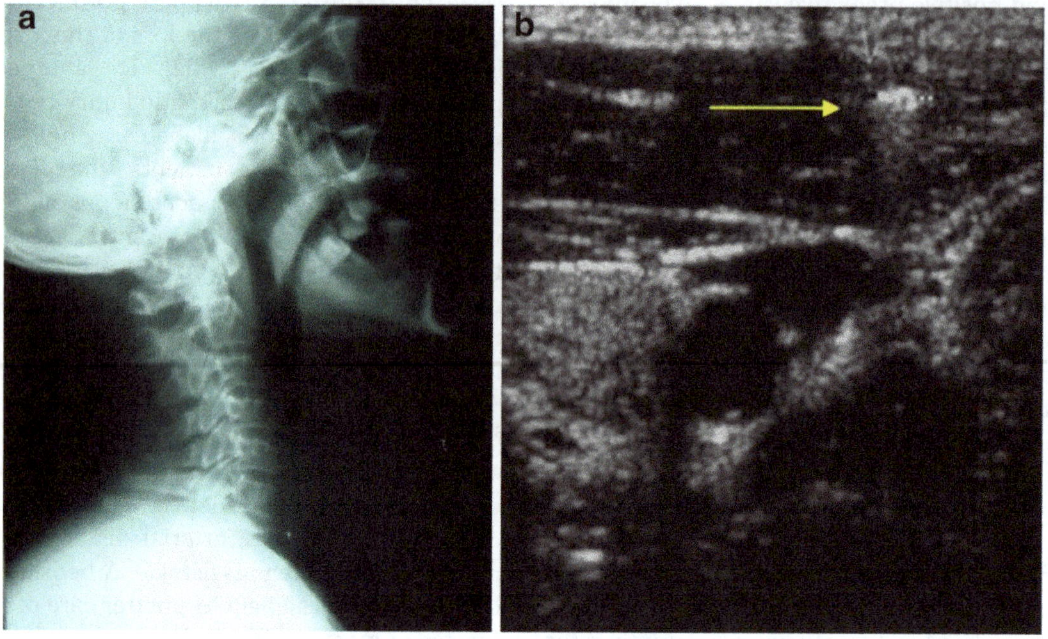


**Fig. 2** No vascular compromise: B mode. **a** X ray showing a bullit in the base of the neck. **b** Mode showing the bullit in the esternocleidomastoid muscle. No vascular compromise of the jugular vein nor the carotid artery

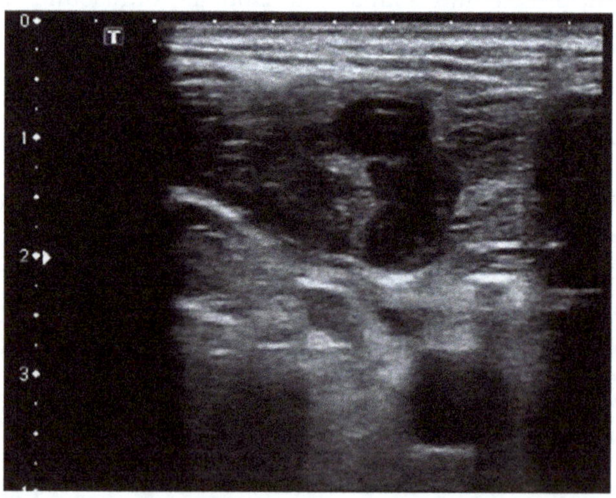


**Fig. 3** Soft tissue hematoma of the left side of the neck. No vascular injury

identification of a venous intimal flap injury may occur (Fig. 5).

Other common injury in trauma patients is vein thrombosis. When present, it usually appears after minutes or hours after the trauma. For the identification and diagnosis of venous thrombosis, we can use the compression technique and the Color Duplex Doppler evaluation [25–30].

In cases of acute thrombosis, the vein appears dilated, anechoic, and is not compressible (Fig. 6). In chronic thrombosis, the thrombus appears more echogenic and the vein is not dilated. Occasionally, in chronic thrombosis, the vein is partially collapsible, due to partial thrombosis or, in chronic thrombosis, because of the presence of channels within the thrombus, that leave the blood pass through (thrombus channeling or tunneling) (Fig. 7).

Color Duplex Doppler evaluation will show the presence or absence of blood flow and the direction and velocity of the flow. In normal veins, the flow is continuous and spontaneous at rest and the velocity varies with respiration, increasing during inspiration, and decreasing during expiration or when a Valsalva maneuver is performed. The active compression of distal segments of the legs will cause an increase or "augmentation" of the velocity of the venous flow (Fig. 8). In case of partial thrombosis, the flow may be normal or pathologic, losing the variability during respiration. In total occlusive thrombosis, there will be complete absence of flow in color Doppler and in the spectral analysis.

### *Arterial injuries*

In most cases, blunt and penetrating traumas cause only a slight wall irregularity (Fig. 9). When a serious injury occurs, intimal detachments, pseudoaneurysms, or arteriovenous fistula may occur.

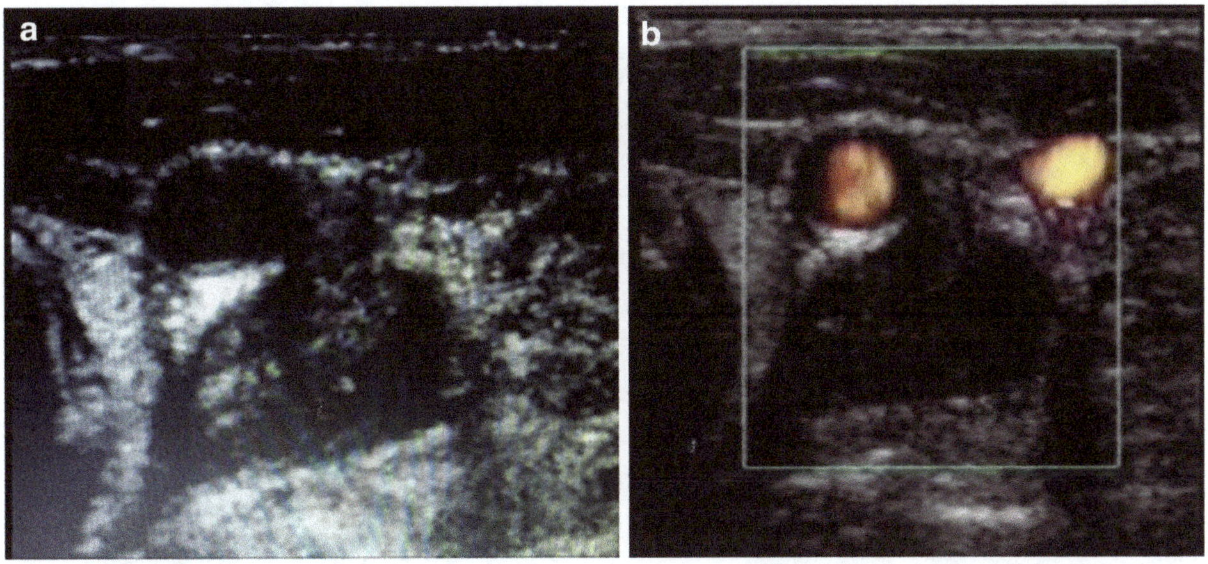


**Fig. 4** Perivascular hematoma. Knife penetrating wound in the *left side* of the neck**. a** Transverse view of the neck showing an hypoecoic hematoma between carotid and yugular vein. **b** Power Doppler showing indemnity of carotid and yugular with the hemathoma between the two vessels

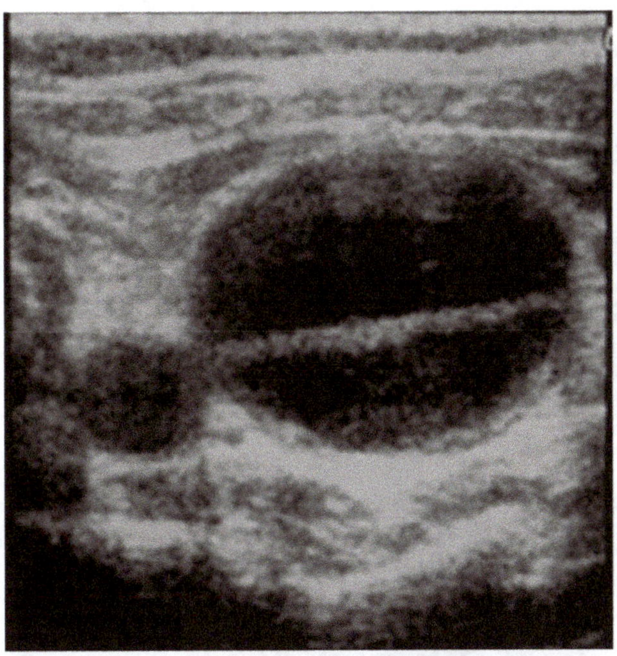

**Fig. 5** Blunt trauma to the neck. Transverse view of the *left side* of the neck showing the carotid artery and a dilated jugular vein with with detachment of the wall

Regarding ***intimal flaps***, they appear as thin, echogenic structures swimming within the vessel lumen (Fig. 10). In some cases, depending on the size of the intimal flap, PWD and CFD may show turbulence and irregular flow (Fig. 11). The usual approach for most cases is to *wait and see*, supplemented or not with antiplatelet medication, and a strict follow-up [31, 32]. Endovascular management of intimal defects has also been proposed [32] Occasionally, these injuries can progress to arterial thrombosis. The presence of arterial thrombosis is observed in B-mode as echogenic material occupying arterial lumen. Doppler examination may show no flow both in PWD and CFD mode (Fig. 12).

A ***pseudoaneurysm*** is produced by the partial rupture of an artery wall, which causes accumulation of periarterial blood, surrounded and contained by the adventitia, hematomas, or soft tissue. It is always in communication with the arterial lumen by a small portion called pseudoaneurysm neck. The most common cause is an interventional medical procedure [15, 33]. Penetrating trauma, by gunshot or stab wound, is other very common cause [34, 35]. Using the B-mode, the presence of

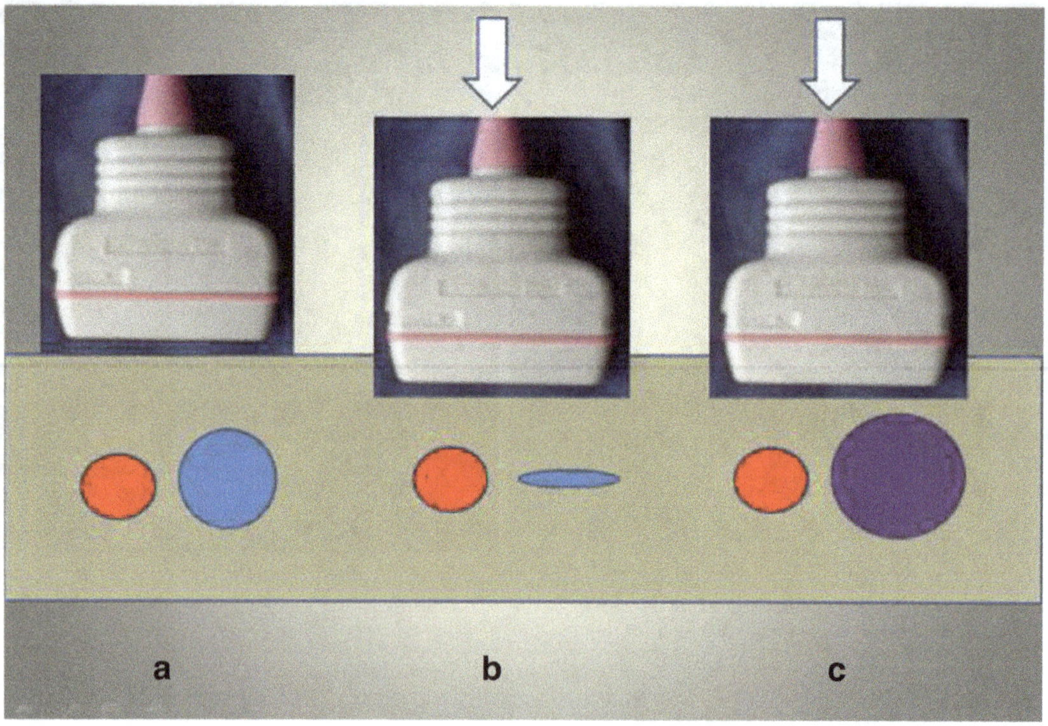


**Fig. 6** Schematic representation of the compression vein technique. **a** Without compression, **b** compressive normal vein, **c** non compressive venous thrombosis

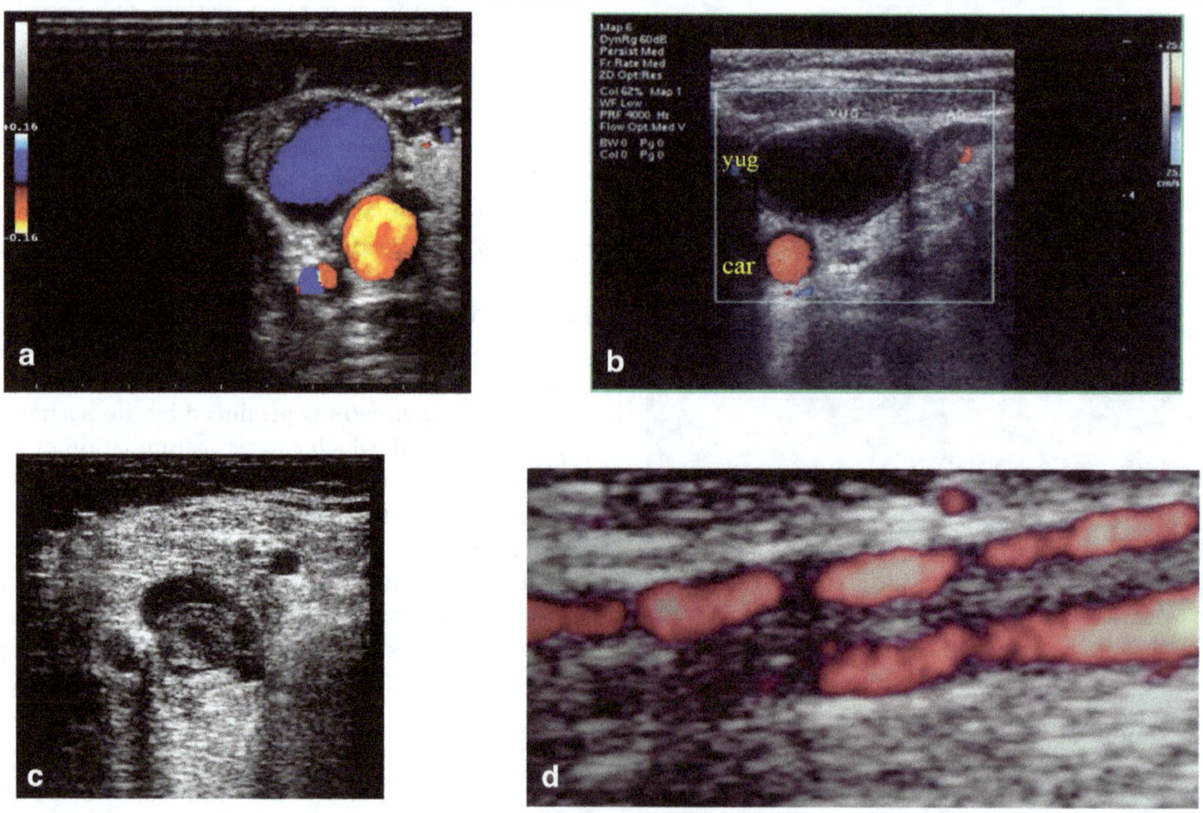


**Fig. 7** Venous thrombosis. **a** Partial thrombosis of right yugular vein: color Doppler (jugular vein in *blue*, carotid artery in *red*). **b** Complete acute hypoechoic thrombosis of left jugular vein (yug): transverse view. Carotid artery is seen in *red* (car). **c** Post trauma partial venous thrombosis. **d** Chronic thrombosis: partial recanalization: multiple color tunnels are seen inside the thrombus

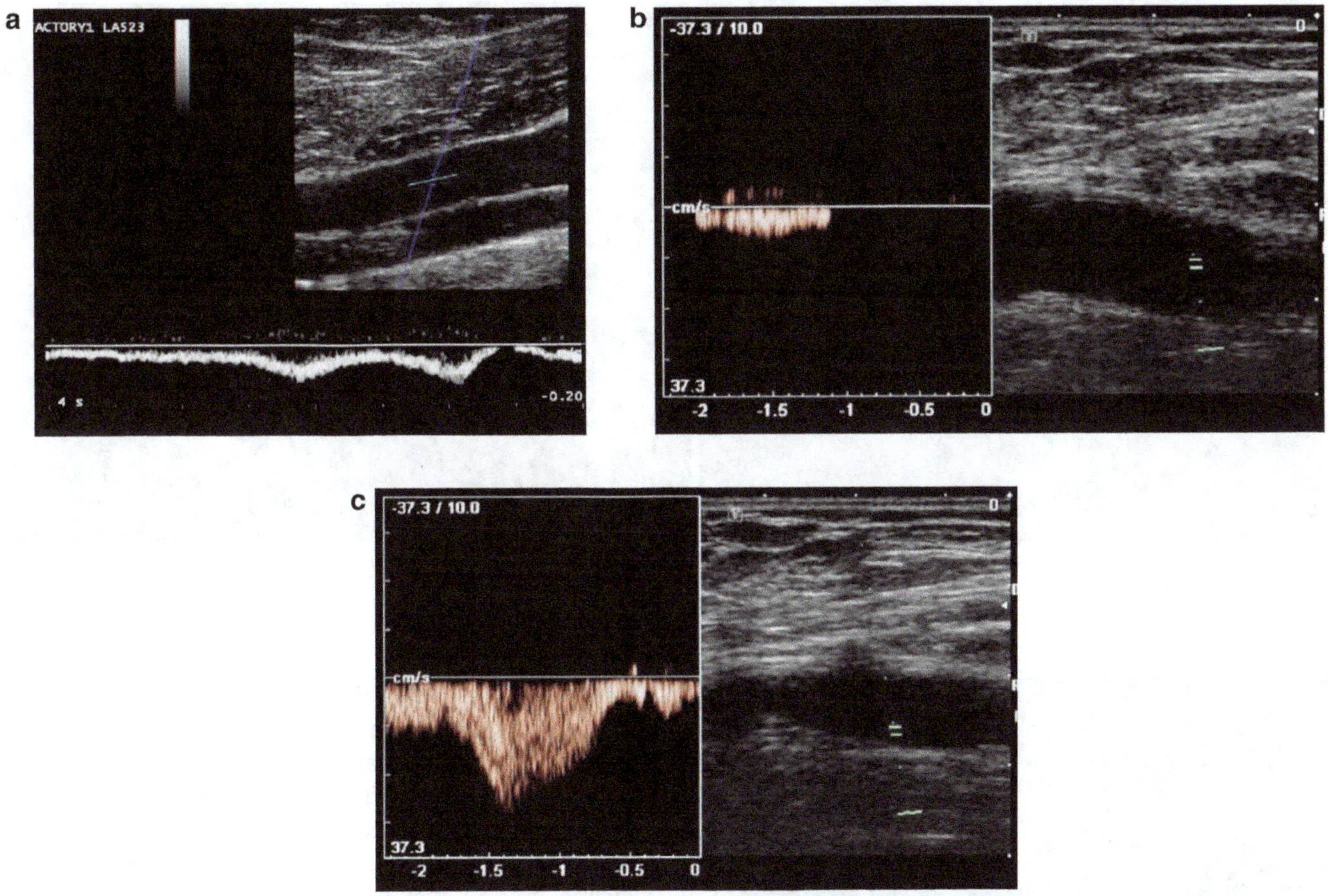


**Fig. 8** Normal spectral Doppler venous flow. **a** respiratory variability, **b** a proximal compression or a Valsalva maneuver cause stop of the flow, **c** the distal compression of the vein cause an increase of the velocity of the flow (augmentation)

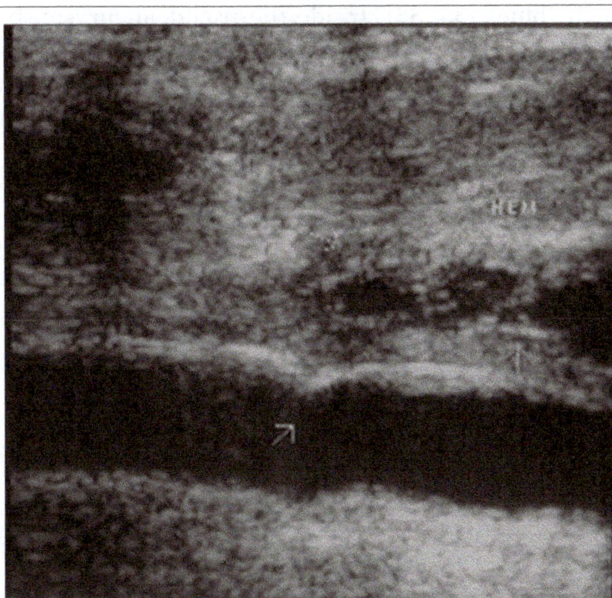


**Fig. 9** B mode of carotid artery after a penetrating wound caused by a knife: soft tissues edema and irregularity of the anterior wall of the carotid artery is clearly observed

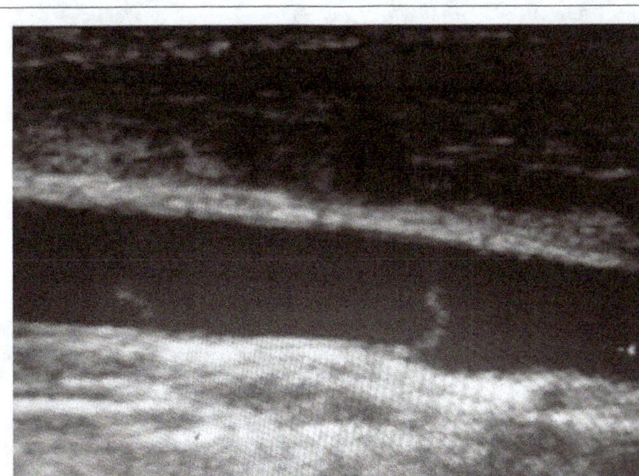

**Fig. 10** Post traumatic carotid artery intimal flap. B mode. Echogenic flap into the lumen

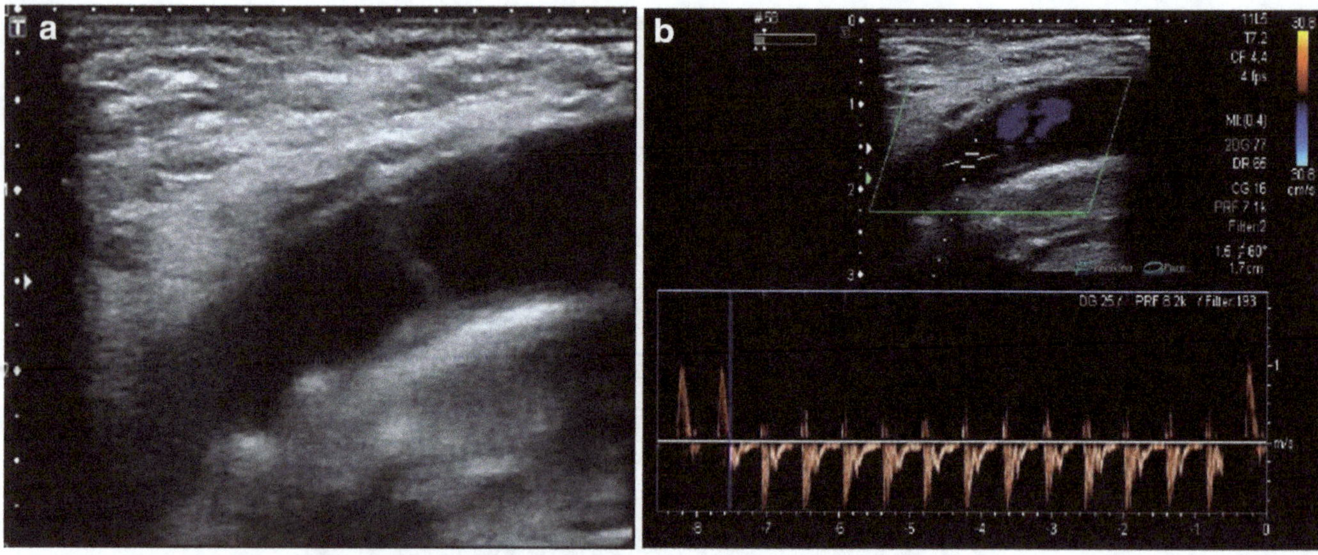


**Fig. 11** Post traumatic femoral artery intimal flap. **a** B mode. Small echogenic flap into the lumen. **b** Turbulent flow with change of direction of the flow was seen moving the sample volume near the moving flap

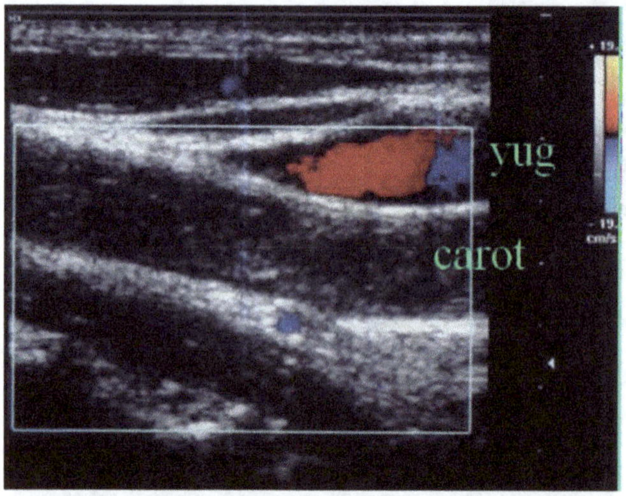


**Fig. 12** Complete post traumatic carotid artery thrombosis. Longitudinal view of the neck shows abscence of flow in the carotid artery (carot). The jugular vein is partially visualized (in *red* and *blue*)

an anechoic or hypoechoic image, similar to a hematoma, but containing moving echoes (pulsatile hematoma), may be observed. Occasionally, it can swell during systole. The lumen can be partially filled by echogenic structures due to the presence of thrombus. When using CFD evaluation, the diagnosis is made by showing the typical swirling motion that causes a colorized yin–yang sign (Fig. 13). This sign is cause by the circular motion of the blood inside the pseudoaneurysm cavity. During systole, the flow goes towards the pseudoaneurysm cavity (red) and during diastole the blood moves back to the arterial lumen (blue) [33, 35]. Inside the pseudoaneurysm, turbulent flow is recorded with the spectral analysis. If we place the sample volume on the neck of the pseudoaneurysm, we might be able to see a characteristic flow pattern known as "to-and-fro." This is a bidirectional flow caused by the continuous entry and exit of blood from the artery

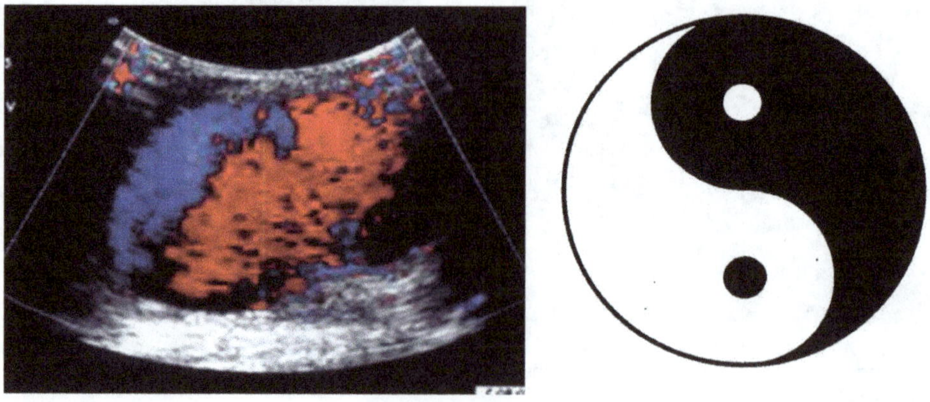

**Fig. 13** Pseudoaneurism: color Doppler aspect: colorized yin yang sign

to the pseudoaneurysm (Figs. 14, 15, 16). Ultrasound is also used to treat of iatrogenic femoral pseudoaneurysm. Ultrasound-assisted arterial compression, thrombin injection, and further monitoring have demonstrated to have high efficacy and low complications rates [36, 37].

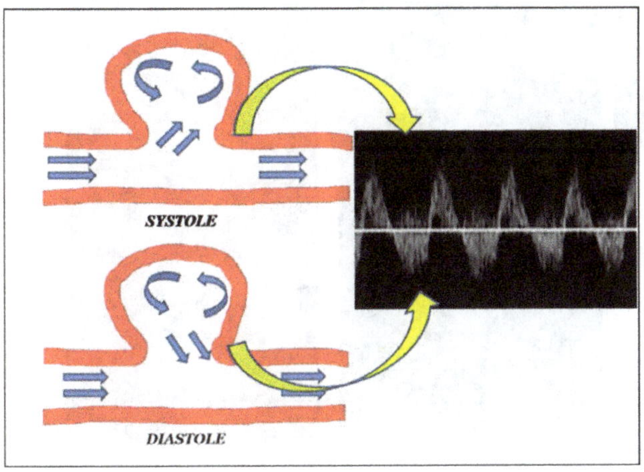


**Fig. 14** Schematic representation of the movement of the flow into a pseudoaneurism causing a characteristic biphasic flow in the neck of the PA

***Mixed arterial and venous injuries***

An ***Arteriovenous fistula*** (AVF) is a permanent communication between an artery and a vein. Depending of the size, it may cause hemodynamic alterations with cardiac effects [38, 39]. It can be congenital or acquired (i.e., traumatic, iatrogenic) [40, 41]. The vein caliber and local venous pressure usually increases due to different pressure between arteries and the veins. These modifications are followed by a phenomenon called arterialization of the flow and the vessel. It is unusual to diagnose AVF soon after trauma. A murmur and thrill on the site of the fistula may be present. With B-mode, the presence of an anechoic, anfractuous structure communicating the vein and artery may be seen. CFD examination may reveal the presence of a color mosaic (aliasing), due to the presence of multiple velocities inside the fistula, causing high flow turbulence. The pulsed Doppler spectral analysis may show high systolic and diastolic velocities with

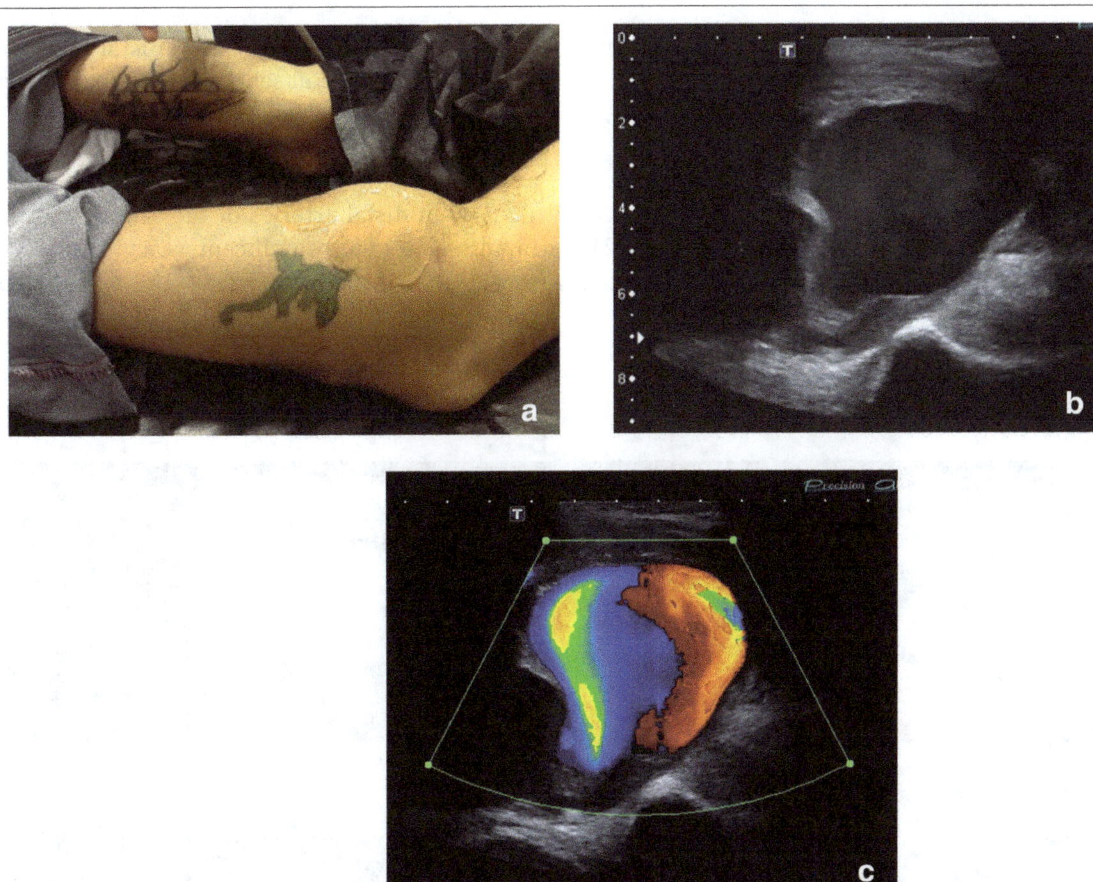


**Fig. 15** Popliteal pseudoaneurism (gun shot wound one week before). **a** Left popliteal mass. **b** B mode: hipoechoic liquid image with swirling movements in real time. **c** Color Doppler: Yin Yang colorized sign

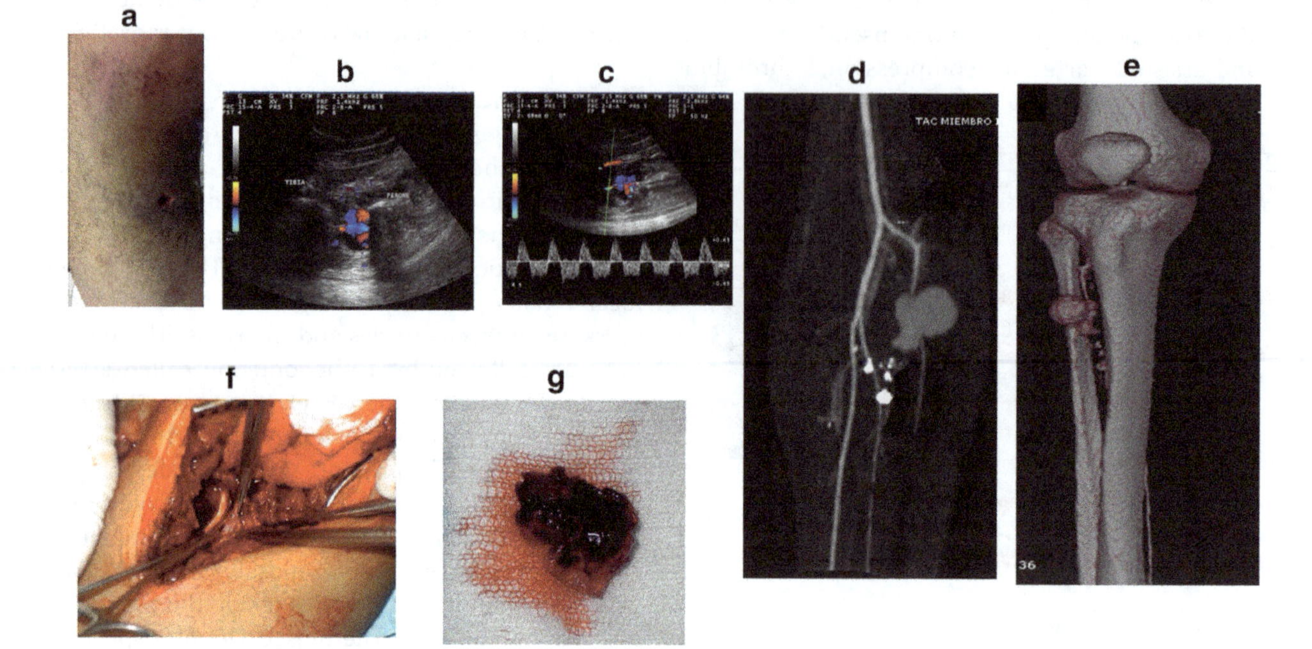


**Fig. 16** Pseudoaneurism: Gun shot gun wound in the *right leg* with an arterial tibial pseudoaneurism. **a** Penetrating wound, **b** pseudo aneurism: color Doppler, **c** pulsed Doppler with the sample volume at the neck of the pseudoaneurism: bidirectional flow (to and fro), **d** CT angiography showing the pseudoaneurism and the metallic foreign bodies, **e** CT: 3D reconstruction, **f** surgical repairment, **g** intraoperative photography of the resected pseudoaneurysm

loss of systolic windows due to the wide velocity range (Figs. 17, 18).

### Distal flow analysis

The presence of triphasic flow in the distal arteries of the lower extremities may be interpreted as an indication of absence of lesion in the proximal arteries [21] (Fig. 19). Arterial injuries of the lower limbs, (being acute or chronic) can cause distal alteration of the flow (Fig. 20). The absence of flow or the presence of a biphasic or monophasic flow may be considered pathologic and further investigation may be necessary [42]. If an arterial injury is suspected, the detection of triphasic flow in distal arteries of the lower limbs may help to rapidly rule out a significant vascular injury with 100% sensitivity (Montórfano et al. The FAST D protocol: A

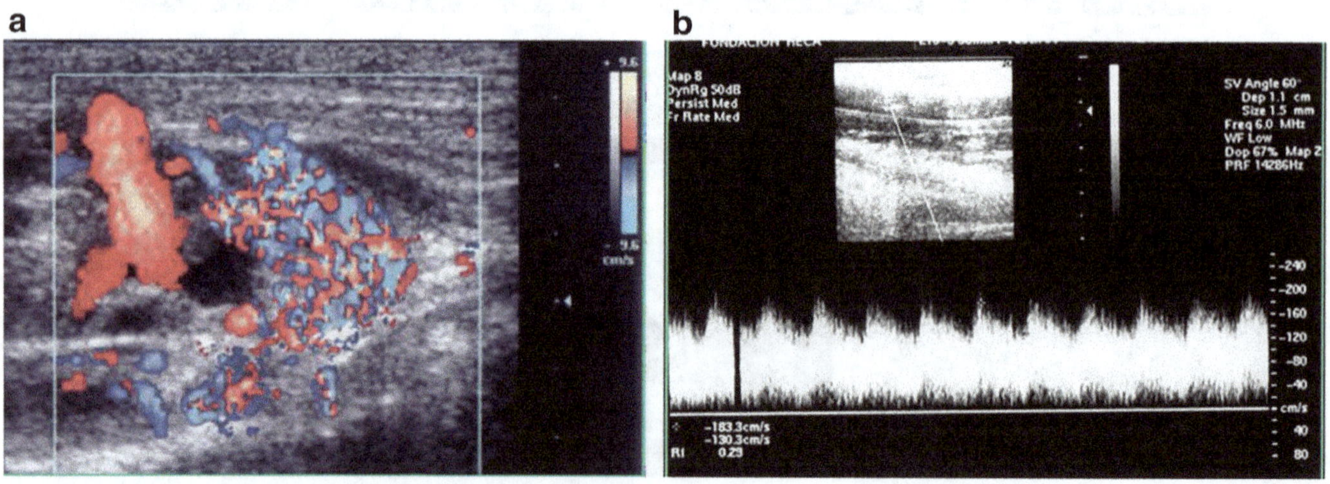


**Fig. 17** Arterio venous fistula. **a** Color Doppler aspect: mosaic of colours representing multiple different velocities. **b** Spectral analysis: high systolic and diastolic velocities

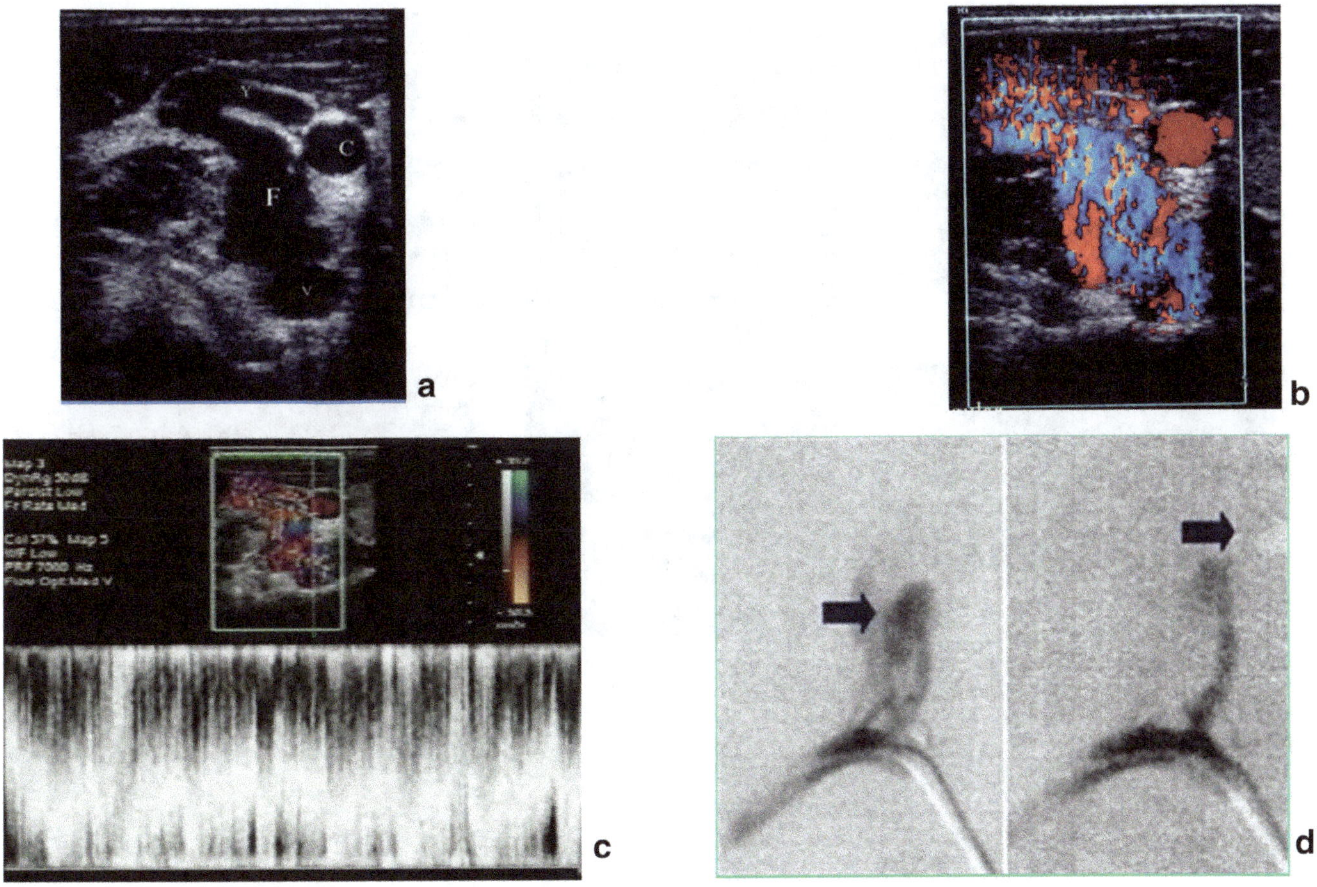

**Fig. 18** Arterio venous fistula: gun shot wound in the *right side* of the neck. Arteriovenous traumatic fistula between right yugular vein and right vertebral artery. **a** B mode: anechoic image connecting right yugular vein with the right vertebral artery. *C* carotid artery, *V* vertebral artery, *Y* yugular vein, *F* fistula. **b** Color Doppler: mosaic of colours representing different velocities. Color in soft tissues surrounding the FAV representing the thrill. **c** Pulse Doppler: spectral analysis with hight velocities spectrum and turbulent flow. **d** Angiographic findings

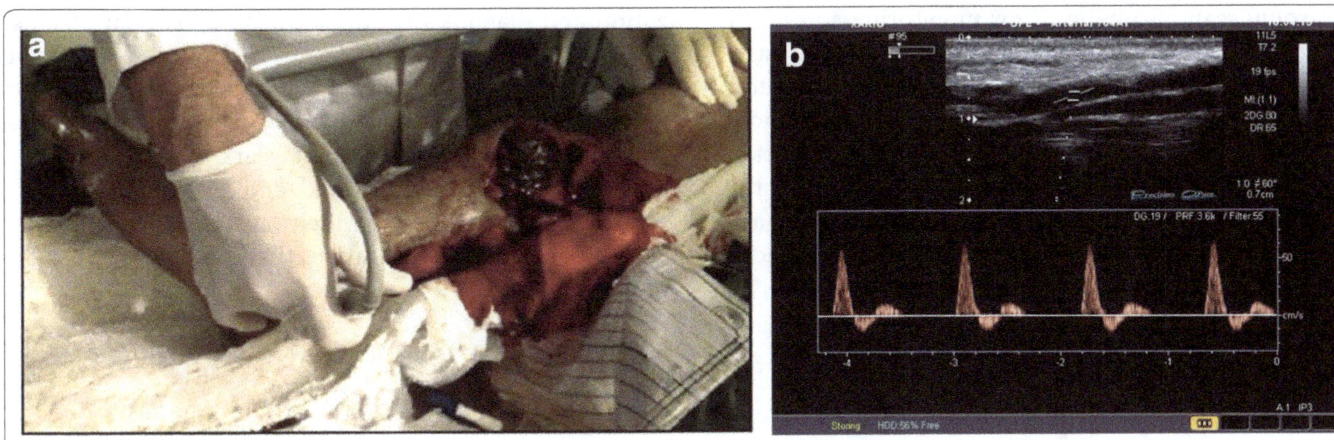

**Fig. 19** Open fracture of the tibia. **a** Displaced long bone fracture with segment exposure. Exploration of distal pulses. **b** Normal triphasic flow

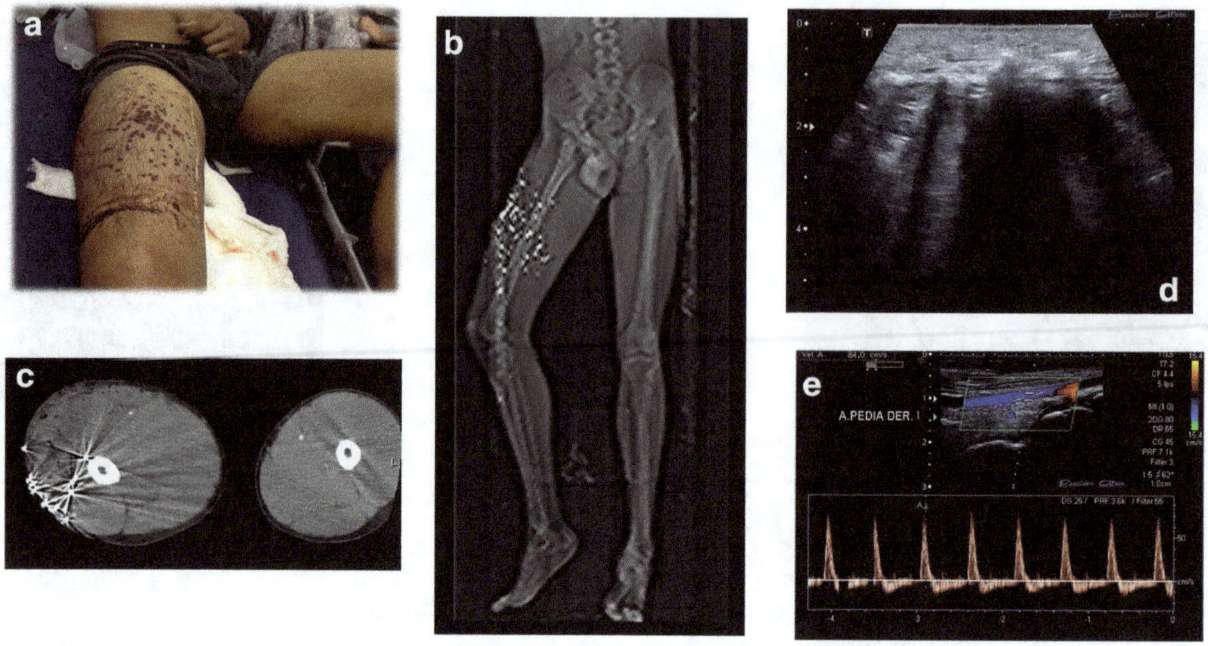


**Fig. 20** External compression. **a** Multiple penetrating gun shot wounds in the right tight. **b** CT scan. **c** CT multiple bullets. Increase diameter of the right tight. **d** Ultrasound showed the metallic foreign bodies with acoustic shadow and edema of the soft tissues. **e** Color Doppler showed no vascular lesion in the right tight Pulse wave Doppler showed lost of the triphasic normal flow in distal arteries caused by external compression of the arteries cause by edema and tumefaction

simple method to rule out traumatic vascular injuries of the lower extremities. Submitted to Critical Ultrasound Journal).

### *Eco Doppler ultrasound monitoring*

B-mode ultrasound and Color flow Duplex Doppler ultrasound can also be used for monitoring and follow-up after endovascular or surgical treatment of vascular injuries [41, 43–46]. B-mode evaluation is useful for monitoring the soft tissue surrounding the lesion, and for ruling in and ruling out hematomas and fluid collections. The Color flow Duplex Doppler technique is used for the evaluation of blood flow patterns in the anastomotic area, proximal and distal flow characteristics, the presence of pathological flow variation, and eventual occlusions [21] (Fig. 21).

## Conclusions

When there are no hard signs of vascular injury and the patient is stable, imaging methods can aid in the localization and diagnosis of trauma-related vascular lesions. While angiography still remains the gold standard for the assessment of traumatic vascular injuries of the limbs and neck, other less invasive imaging modalities have gained popularity in the recent years and are routinely used. Point-of-care ultrasound and Color flow duplex Doppler ultrasound are widely available, noninvasive, sensible and specific techniques that can be used bedside,

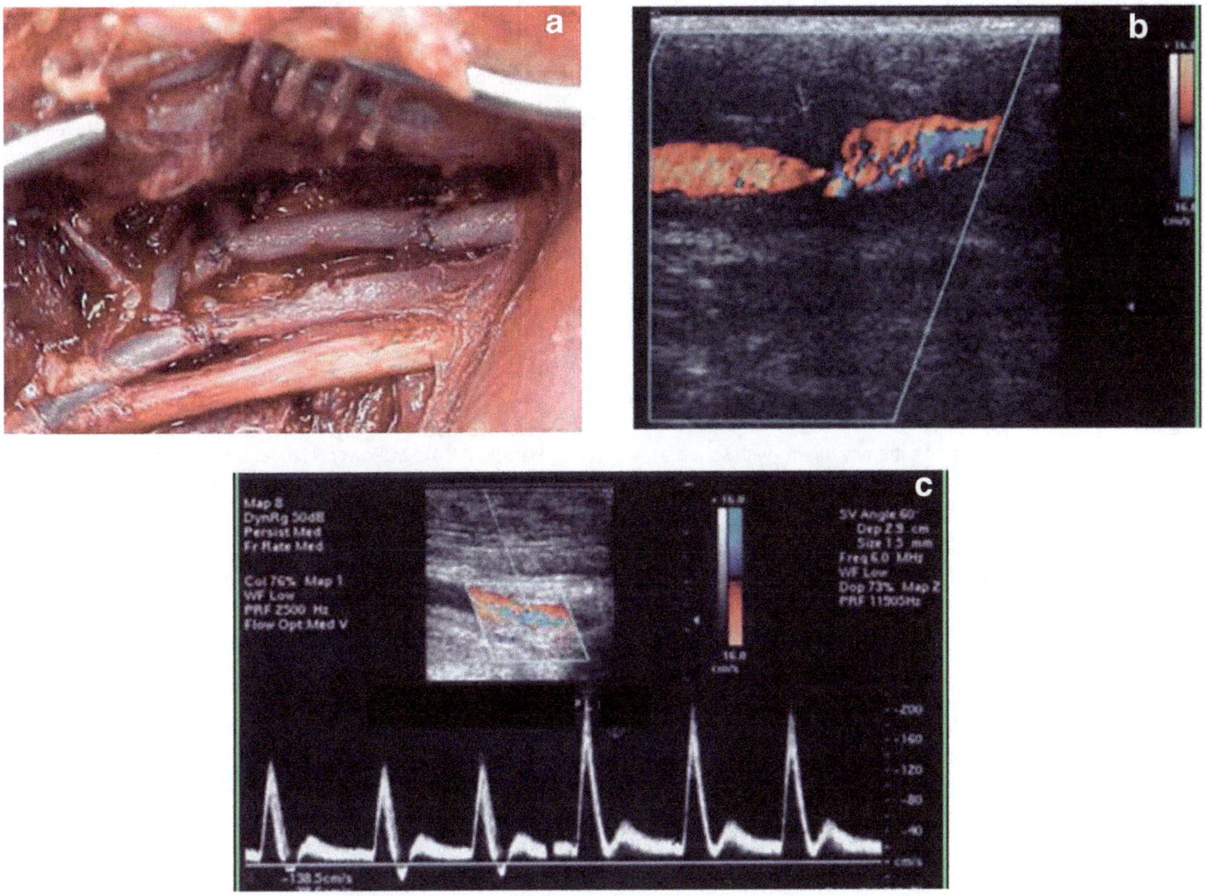


**Fig. 21** Gun shot femoral artery injury. Post operative follow up. **a** Surgical repairment with vein interposition. **b** Color flow: stenosis with turbulent flow in the anastomosis. **c** Increase of the velocity at the level of the stenosis in the pulsed Doppler spectrum

as a first approach for a prompt diagnosis and follow-up of trauma-related vascular injuries, and for an integrated management of trauma patients.

### Authors' contributions

MAM: Manuscript writing and final review, provided figures. FP: Manuscript writing. LV: Manuscript writing. OC: Manuscript writing. SGN: Manuscript writing and edition. LMM: Manuscript writing and edition. All authors read and approved the final manuscript.


### Author details

[1] Present Address: Department of Ultrasound, Clemente Álvarez Emergency Hospital, Av. Pellegrini 3205, 2000 Rosario, Santa Fe, Argentina. [2] Emergency Medicine Residency, University of Pavia, Strada Nuova 65, 27100 Pavia, Italy.



### Acknowledgements

Not applicable.


### References


1. WHO—World Health Organization (2014) Injuries and violence, the facts
2. Skarpedas S et al (2009). The costs of violence. Social Development Department. The World Bank
3. Chelala C (1997) Violence in the Americas: The Social Pandemic of the 20th Century. Pan American Health Organization, Washington, DC
4. Rozycki GS et al (2003) Blunt vascular trauma in extremities: diagnosis, management and outcome. J Trauma 55:814–824
5. Soto GS et al (2004) Trauma vascular periférico. Cuad Cir 18:91–97
6. Martín Trenor A (2005) Traumatismos vasculares periféricos. Rev Med Univ Navarra 49(2):24–31
7. Torres Carranza SA (2006) Trauma vascular de las extremidades y un poco de su historia. Trauma 9(3):83–86
8. Suárez CA et al (2007) Heridas por armas de fuego y traumas vasculares: una ventana a la violencia civil en Caracas. Gac Méd Caracas 115(4):304–312
9. Sonneborn R et al (2002) Vascular trauma in Latin America. A regional survey. Surg Clin North Am 82:189–194
10. Fogelman MJ, Stewart RD (1956) Penetrating wounds of the neck. Am J Surg 91:581–593
11. Campbell FC, Robbs JV (1980) Penetrating injuries of the neck: a prospective study of 108 patients. Br J Surg 67:582–586

12. Willis BK et al (1994) The incidence of vertebral artery injury after midcervical spine fracture or subluxation. Neurosurgery 34:435–442
13. Hoff SJ et al (1994) Analysis of blunt and penetrating injury of the innominate and subclavian arteries. Am Surg 60:151–154
14. Frykberg ER (1995) Advances in the diagnosis and treatment of extremity vascular trauma. Surg Clin North Am 75:207–223
15. Gaitini D et al (2008) Sonographic evaluation of vascular injuries. J Ultrasound Med 27:95–107
16. Bergstein JM, Blair JF, Edwards J et al (1992) Pitfalls in the use of color-flow duplex ultrasound for screening of suspected arterial injuries in penetrated extremities. J Trauma 33:395–402
17. Fry WR, Smith RS, Sayers DV, Henderson VJ, Morabito DJ, Tsoi EK et al (1993) The success of duplex ultrasonographic scanning in diagnosis of extremity vascular proximity trauma. Arch Surg 128(12):1368–1372
18. Wani ML, Sheikh MT, Nayeem-ul-Hassan A, Irshad I, Ahangar AG, Ganie FM, Sheikh MT, Wani SN (2014) Int Cardiovasc Res J 8 (1)
19. Neri L, Storti E, Lichtenstein D (2007) Towards an ultrasound curriculum. Crit Care Med 35(5):S290–S304
20. Lyon M, Blaivas M (2003) Evaluation of extremity trauma with sonography. J Ultrasound Med 22:625–630
21. Polak J (1992) Peripheral vascular sonography. A practical guide. Williams & Wilkins, Philadelphia
22. Noble VE et al (2007) Manual of emergency and critical care ultrasound. Cambridge University Press, Cambridge
23. Schwartz M, Weaver F, Yellin A, Ralls P (1993) The utility of Color flow Doppler examination in penetrating extremity arterial trauma. Am Surg 59:375–378
24. Schoder M, Prokof M, Lammer J (2002) Traumatic injuries: imaging and intervention of large arterial trauma. Eur Radiol 12:1617–1631
25. Lensing et al (1997) A comparison of compression ultrasound with Color Doppler ultrasound for the diagnosis of symptomless postoperative deep vein thrombosis. Arch Int Med 157:765–768
26. Birdwell et al (1998) The clinical validity of normal compression ultrasonography in outpatients suspected of having deep venous thrombosis. Ann Intern Med 128:1–7
27. Burnside PR et al (2008) Systematic review of emergency physician-performed ultrasonography for lower-extremity deep vein thrombosis. Acad Emerg Med 15:493–498
28. Blaivas M, Lambert MJ, Harwood RA et al (2000) Lower-extremity Doppler for deep venous thrombosis—can emergency physicians be accurate and fast? Acad Emerg Med 7:120–126
29. Theodoro DL, Blaivas M, Duggal D et al (2002) Emergency physician-performed lower extremity doppler results in significant time savings. Acad Emerg Med 9:541
30. Bernardi E et al (2008) Serial 2-point ultrasonography plus D-dimer vs whole-leg color-coded Doppler ultrasonography for diagnosing suspected symptomatic deep vein thrombosis: a randomized controlled trial. JAMA 300(14):1653–1659
31. Hernández-Maldonado JJ, Padberg FT Jr, Teehan E, Neville R, DeFouw D, Durán WN, Hobson RW (1993) Arterial intimal flaps: a comparison of primary repair, aspirin, and endovascular excision in an experimental model. J Trauma 34(4):565–569; (discussion 569–70).
32. Jr Neville RF, Yasuhara H, Watanabe BI, Canady J, Durán W, Hobson RW (1991) Endovascular management of arterial intimal defects: an experimental comparison by arteriography, angioscopy, and intravascular ultrasonography. J Vasc Surg 13(4):496–502
33. Mitchell DG, Needleman L, Bezzi M, Goldberg BB et al (1987) Femoral artery pseudoaneurysm: diagnosis with conventional duplex and Color Doppler US. Radiology 165:687–690
34. Olinde AJ (1989) Traumatic subclavian axillary artery aneurysm. J Vasc Surg 11:848–849
35. Yetkin U, Gurbuz A (2003) Post-traumatic pseudoaneurysm of the brachial artery and its surgical treatment. Tex Heart Inst J 30:293–297
36. Vázquez V et al (2003) Utilidad de la inyección de trombina dirigida por ecografía en los seudoaneurismas femorales iatrogénicos después del fracaso de la compresión. Med Clin (Barc) 121(2):53–57
37. Eisenberg L et al (1999) Sonographically guided compression repair of pseudoaneurysms: further experience from a single institution. AJR Am J Roentgenol 173:1567–1573
38. Li JC et al (2002) Diagnostic criteria for locating acquired arteriovenous fistulas with color Doppler sonography. J Clin Ultrasound 30(6):336–342
39. Bowers AL et al (2008) Traumatic lower extremity arteriovenous fistulae in children. Orthopedics 31:6
40. Turnipseed WD, Hurschler C, Vanderby R Jr (1995) The effects of elevated compartment pressure on tibial arteriovenous flow and relationship of mechanical and biochemical characteristics of fascia to genesis of chronic anterior compartment syndrome. J Vasc Surg 21:810–816
41. Scalea TM, Sclafani SJ (1991) Angiographically placed balloons for arterial control. A description of a technique. J Trauma 31:1671–1677
42. Robbs JV, Carrim AA, Kadwa AM, Mars M (1994) Traumatic arterio-venous fistula: experience with 202 patients. Br J Surg 81:1296–1299
43. Kang SS et al (2000) Expanded indications for ultrasound-guided thrombin injection of pseudoaneurysms. J Vasc Surg 31:289–298
44. Magge D, Farber A, Vladimir F, Woodson J, Collins K, Shaw P, Gibbons G (2008) Diagnosis and management of traumatic pseudoaneurysm of the carotid artery: case report and review of the literature. Vascular 16(6):350–355
45. Hanson JM, Atri M, Power N (2008) Ultrasound-guided thrombin injection of iatrogenic groin pseudoaneurysm: Doppler features and technical tips. Br J Radiol 81:154–163
46. Fusonie GE, Edwards JD, Reed AB (2004) Covered stent exclusion of blunt traumatic carotid artery pseudoaneurysm: case report and review of the literature. Ann Vasc Surg 18(3):376–379

# 10

# One-month outcomes of patients with SARS-CoV-2 infection and their relationships with lung ultrasound signs

Thiago Thomaz Mafort[1,2], Rogério Rufino[1,2], Claudia Henrique da Costa[1,2], Mariana Soares da Cal[1], Laura Braga Monnerat[1], Patrícia Frascari Litrento[1], Laura Lizeth Zuluaga Parra[1], Arthur de Sá Earp de Souza Marinho[1] and Agnaldo José Lopes[1,2,3*]

**Abstract**

**Background:** The role of lung ultrasound (LUS) in evaluating the mid- and long-term prognoses of patients with COVID-19 pneumonia is not yet known. The objectives of this study were to evaluate associations between LUS signs at the time of screening and clinical outcomes 1 month after LUS and to assess LUS signs at the time of presentation with known risk factors for COVID-19 pneumonia.

**Methods:** This was a retrospective study of data prospectively collected 1 month after LUS screening of 447 adult patients diagnosed with COVID-19 pneumonia. Sonographic examination was performed in screening tents with the participants seated. The LUS signs (B-lines > 2, coalescent B-lines, and subpleural consolidations) were captured in six areas of each hemithorax and a LUS aeration score was calculated; in addition, the categories of disease probability based on patterns of LUS findings (high-probability, intermediate-probability, alternate, and low-probability patterns) were evaluated. The LUS signs at patients' initial evaluation were related to the following outcomes: symptomatology, the need for hospitalization or invasive mechanical ventilation (IMV), and COVID-19-related death.

**Results:** According to the evaluations performed 1 month after LUS screening, 36 patients were hospitalised, eight of whom required intensive care unit (ICU) admission and three of whom died. The presence of coalescent B-lines was associated with the need for hospitalization ($p = 0.008$). The presence of subpleural consolidations was associated with dyspnoea ($p < 0.0001$), cough ($p = 0.003$), the need for hospitalization ($p < 0.0001$), the need for ICU admission ($p < 0.0001$), and death ($p = 0.002$). A higher aeration score was associated with dyspnoea ($p < 0.0001$), the need for hospitalization ($p < 0.0001$), the need for ICU admission ($p < 0.0001$), and death ($p = 0.003$). In addition, patients with a high-probability LUS pattern had a higher aeration score ($p < 0.0001$) and more dyspnoea ($p = 0.024$) and more often required hospitalization ($p < 0.0001$) and ICU admission ($p = 0.031$).

**Conclusions:** In patients with COVID-19 pneumonia, LUS signs were related to respiratory symptoms 1 month after LUS screening. Strong relationships were identified between LUS signs and the need for hospitalization and death.

**Keywords:** COVID-19, SARS-CoV-2, Lung ultrasound, Pneumonia, 1-month outcomes

## Background

In the lungs, infection by severe acute respiratory syndrome coronavirus 2 (SARS-CoV-2) is characterized by severe pneumonia and/or acute respiratory distress syndrome (ARDS) in approximately 20% of patients, and mid- and long-term respiratory complications are

*Correspondence: agnaldolopes.uerj@gmail.com
[1] Department of Pulmonology, Piquet Carneiro Policlinic, State University of Rio de Janeiro, Av. Mal. Rondon, 381, São Francisco Xavier, Rio de Janeiro 20950-003, Brazil
Full list of author information is available at the end of the article

beginning to be described [1]. However, data from previous coronavirus outbreaks, such as SARS and Middle East respiratory syndrome, suggest that some patients will have these complications after the acute phase of the disease [2]. The possible pulmonary sequelae include pulmonary vascular disease and interstitial lung disease; however, many other respiratory manifestations and changes in pulmonary function can be observed [3, 4].

Amid the coronavirus disease 2019 (COVID-19) pandemic and given the frequent lung involvement observed, new tools are needed to evaluate affected patients and to identify data with potential prognostic implications. Because lung ultrasound (LUS) is a fast test, it has been increasingly used as an alternative imaging method, and evidence supports its ability to identify lung lesions in COVID-19 [5–7]. In fact, LUS can be useful at various times, from screening for early diagnosis of lung involvement to decision-making about intensive care unit (ICU) treatment and respiratory support (e.g., mechanical ventilation, prone positioning, positive end-expiratory pressure, recruitment manoeuvres) [8–12]. Because of the strong association between LUS and computed tomography (CT) findings, LUS may be effective for diagnosing peripherally distributed lesions, which are characteristic of SARS-CoV-2 infection [13, 14]. In addition, LUS can identify the persistence of subclinical residual lung damage in COVID-19, even if patients meet the discharge criteria [15].

With the increasing number of patients who have survived COVID-19 worldwide, the most effective follow-up strategies for these patients must be determined. However, few studies have explored the follow-up of such patients after the acute phase of the disease. Severe disease is known to be associated with a higher probability of disability, and patients requiring ICU admission have been observed to have worse mid- and long-term outcomes, with physiological impairment and persistent radiological changes, than those not requiring ICU admission [3]. Because LUS has been increasingly used in the diagnosis of COVID-19 pneumonia, evidence of the prognostic role of LUS should be extended to the management of COVID-19 pneumonia. Thus, the objectives of this study were to evaluate associations between LUS signs at patients' initial evaluation as a screening tool for pulmonary involvement due to COVID-19 and clinical outcomes 1 month after LUS and to assess LUS signs at the time of presentation with known risk factors for COVID-19 pneumonia.

## Materials and methods

### Participants

This was a retrospective study of data prospectively collected from LUS examinations performed on patients aged ≥ 18 years with fever and/or acute respiratory symptoms (dyspnoea, cough, and/or coryza) and diagnosed with COVID-19 confirmed by reverse-transcription polymerase chain reaction (RT-PCR). The patients were screened in tents installed in the courtyard of Piquet Carneiro Policlinic, State University of Rio de Janeiro, Rio de Janeiro, Brazil. Patients with LUS exams showing no pathological signs (absence of significant multiple and coalescent B-lines, absence of peripheral and large consolidations) were excluded. The results were analysed at the time of the initial LUS examination, and a clinical follow-up was conducted by phone 1 month after the initial LUS test. The outcomes studied included symptomatology, the need for hospitalization, the need for invasive mechanical ventilation (IMV), and COVID-19-related death. The study was approved by the National Research Ethics Committee of Brazil under number CAAE-30135320.0.0000.5259. All participants read the protocol and agreed to participate in the study.

### Lung ultrasound

We used an Aplio XG device (Toshiba Medical Systems, Tokyo, Japan) for the LUS examinations; the device was coupled to a 7.5–10-MHz multifrequency linear transducer or a 3.5- to 5-MHz convex transducer in B mode. The convex transducer was routinely used for analysis, while the linear transducer was used only when doubts remained regarding the analysis of the pleural surface. All LUS evaluations were carried out by a team of 6 pulmonologists employed at the policlinic with experience in the method (three with 13 years of experience, two with 11 years of experience, and one with 8 years of experience in ultrasound at the screening site). The LUS exams were performed with the participants in a sitting position since they were all outpatients and had no ventilatory or haemodynamic instability (individuals with respiratory symptoms were examined in screening tents). All LUS evaluations were performed by two examiners using a standard data collection form, and when disagreements occurred between the examiners, an agreement was reached through a collective discussion. Although no standard has been established with respect to specific scanning protocols, LUS signs were captured in six areas of each hemithorax following a 12-zone protocol [16, 17] as follows: two anterior, two lateral, and two posterior areas (Fig. 1). Each intercostal space of the upper and lower parts of the anterior, lateral, and posterior regions of the left and right chest walls were carefully examined. When evaluating pathological LUS signs, we searched for the following findings: B-lines > 2 (hyperechoic vertical artefacts arising from the pleural line, extending to the bottom of the screen without fading, and vacillating with lung movement, which occurs when the lung loses

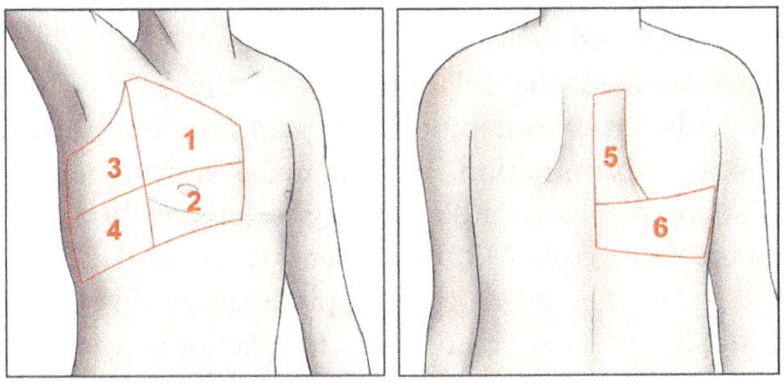


**Fig. 1** Representation of the 12 zones on the chest. **a** The anterior and axillary zones; **b** the posterior zones. The zones 1 and 2 are limited by the parasternal and anterior axillary lines. The zones 3 and 4 are limited by the anterior axillary and posterior axillary lines. Finally, the zones 5 and 6 are limited by the paravertebral and posterior axillary lines and by the contour of the scapula

normal aeration but is not completely consolidated), coalescent B-lines (coalescence of many vertical artefacts to form more extended echogenic patterns corresponding to severe lung aeration loss), and subpleural consolidations (hypoechoic areas that appear as the subpleural density approaches the density of solid tissue, suggesting subpleural fluid-filled alveoli) [14, 18]. These abnormalities were evaluated separately and in combination to obtain an aeration score. To obtain the aeration score, we used a score for each area ranging from 0 to 3 according to the LUS sign as follows: B-lines > 2, 1 point; coalescent B-lines, 2 points; and consolidations, 3 points; the aeration score was calculated as the sum of these points and ranged between 0 and 36 [19]. In addition, we evaluated categories of disease probability based on patterns of LUS findings (high-probability, intermediate-probability, alternate, and low-probability patterns) [20–22].

### Statistical analysis

A nonparametric method was applied because the variables did not have a Gaussian distribution as indicated by rejection of the null hypothesis of a normal distribution by the Shapiro–Wilk test and graphical analysis of histograms. Thus, the most appropriate measures for summarizing the results were quartiles (the medians and interquartile ranges) for numerical data and the frequency (percentage) for categorical data. For numerical data, associations between pathological LUS signs, clinical findings detected 1 month after LUS, and poor outcomes were evaluated by the Mann–Whitney test for comparisons between two subgroups or Kruskal–Wallis ANOVA for comparisons between three subgroups (Dunn's multiple comparison test was applied to identify which subgroups differed significantly from each other). For categorical data, associations were evaluated using the Chi-square or Fisher's exact test. The significance level adopted was 5%. Statistical analysis was performed using the statistical software SAS 6.11 (SAS Institute, Inc., Cary, NC, USA).

**Table 1** Sample characteristics at the time of diagnosis of pneumonia due to COVID-19 by LUS

| Variables | Values |
|---|---|
| Demographic data | |
| Age (years) | 40 (34–50) |
| Female sex | 305 (68.2%) |
| BMI (kg/m$^2$) | 28.7 (35.5–32.7) |
| Comorbidities | |
| Hypertension | 98 (21.9%) |
| Diabetes | 52 (11.6) |
| Asthma | 35 (7.8) |
| CHF | 28 (6.3) |
| COPD | 3 (0.67) |
| Others | 110 (24.6) |
| Signs on lung ultrasound | |
| B-lines > 2 | 349 (78.1%) |
| Coalescent B-lines | 228 (51%) |
| Subpleural consolidations | 59 (13.2%) |
| Aeration score | 4 (2–7) |

Data are expressed as the median (interquartile range) or number (%)

*BMI* body mass index, *CHF* chronic heart failure, *COPD* chronic obstructive pulmonary disease

## Results

Among the 460 patients eligible for inclusion in the study, 13 were lost to follow-up because they could not be reached by telephone. Among the 447 participants with COVID-19 pneumonia diagnosed by LUS included in the study, 305 (68.2%) were women, and the median age was 40 (34–50) years. The median time since symptom onset was 5 (2–7) days. The most prevalent comorbidities in this sample were hypertension (98, 21.9%) and diabetes (52, 11.6%). On LUS, the most frequent pathological sign was B-lines > 2, and the median aeration score at the time of COVID-19 pneumonia diagnosis was 4 (2–7). The demographic and clinical characteristics of the sample and the LUS data at the time of diagnosing pulmonary involvement are provided in Table 1.

According to the evaluations performed 1 month after LUS screening for COVID-19 pneumonia, 36 (8.1%) patients required hospitalization due to pulmonary complications, with a median length of stay of 7 (4–10) days; among those who required hospitalization, 8 (1.8%) required admission to the ICU, and 3 (0.7%) died. In the sample studied 1 month after the initial evaluation, 121 (27.1%) reported general fatigue, while 62 (13.9%) complained of dyspnoea. Cough and fever were reported by 39 (8.7%) and 3 (0.7%) patients, respectively.

We evaluated associations between LUS findings at the time of screening, clinical outcomes, and the presence of symptoms 1 month after LUS. In this analysis, the presence of B-lines > 2 was not associated with any clinical finding or outcome. However, the presence of coalescent B-lines was associated with older age ($p=0.035$), a higher body mass index ($p=0.027$), diabetes ($p=0.027$), dyspnoea ($p=0.037$), and the need for hospitalization ($p=0.008$). The presence of subpleural consolidations on LUS was associated with diabetes ($p=0.002$), chronic heart failure (CHF, $p=0.021$), general fatigue ($p=0.013$), dyspnoea ($p<0.0001$), cough ($p=0.003$), fever ($p=0.043$), the need for hospitalization ($p<0.0001$), the need for ICU admission ($p<0.0001$), and death ($p=0.002$) (Fig. 2).

We evaluated the relationships of the LUS aeration score with clinical outcomes and symptoms 1 month after ultrasound examination. In this analysis, a higher aeration score was associated with hypertension ($p=0.032$), diabetes ($p=0.0001$), dyspnoea ($p<0.0001$), cough ($p=0.041$), the need for hospitalization ($p<0.0001$), the need for ICU admission ($p<0.0001$), and death ($p=0.003$) (Fig. 3).

Additionally, we evaluated categories of the probability of COVID-19 based on patterns of LUS signals. In this analysis, 234 cases (52.3%) had high-probability patterns, 180 cases (40.3%) had intermediate-probability patterns, and 33 cases (7.4%) had alternate LUS patterns; no participant had low-probability patterns. Although

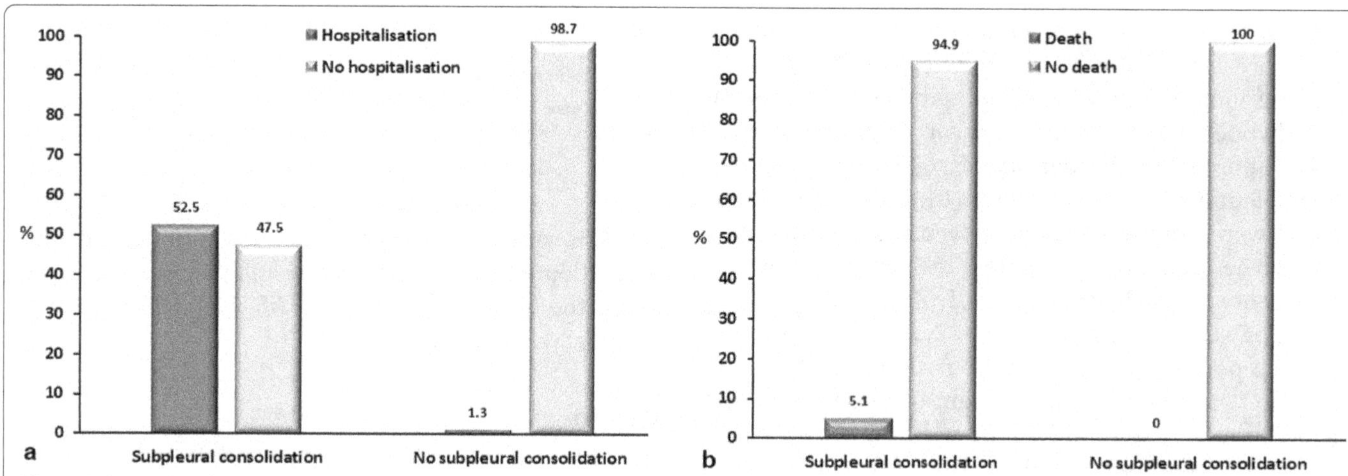


**Fig. 2** Relationships between the presence of subpleural consolidation on lung ultrasound and the outcomes of **a** hospitalization ($p<0.0001$) and **b** death ($p=0.002$)

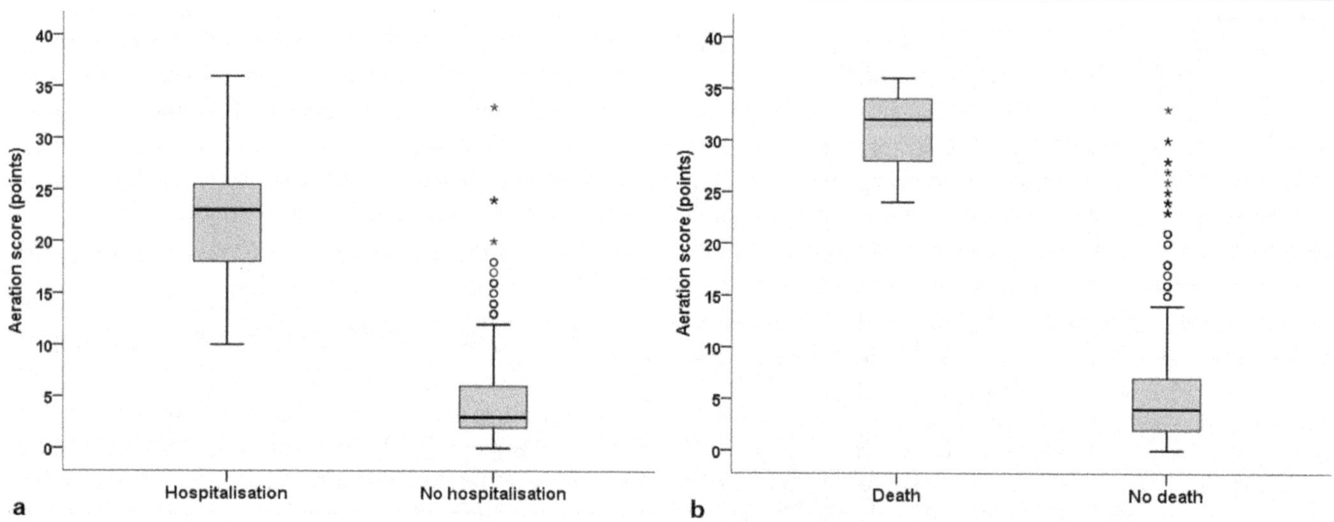


**Fig. 3** Relationships between the aeration score on lung ultrasound and the outcomes of **a** hospitalization ($p<0.0001$) and **b** death ($p=0.003$)

all participants were positive for COVID-19 by RT-PCR, the alternate LUS patterns were as follows: chronic heart failure ($n=18$), bacterial pneumonia ($n=6$), tuberculosis sequelae ($n=4$), systemic sclerosis ($n=3$), and rheumatoid arthritis ($n=2$). Interestingly, we observed that patients with a high-probability LUS pattern had a higher aeration score ($p<0.0001$) and more dyspnoea ($p=0.024$) and more often required hospitalization ($p<0.0001$) and ICU admission ($p=0.031$) (Table 2).

## Discussion

LUS has played a critical role in the pandemic caused by SARS-CoV-2, with growing evidence of its usefulness both to screen for lung involvement and to evaluate disease severity. Sequential LUS has also been used as an efficient tool to monitor the progression of lung lesions in individuals with more severe lung disease. Despite all these indications, the prognostic power of LUS in COVID-19 is also important to evaluate. Here, we searched for correlations between pathological LUS signs and patient outcomes. The main results of the present study were that 1 month after LUS screening, LUS signs (especially subpleural consolidations) were associated with the presence of persistent respiratory symptoms and general fatigue. The LUS findings strongly predicted the need for hospitalization (including in the ICU) and death. In addition, the LUS aeration score was correlated with the persistence of respiratory manifestations at 1 month after ultrasound examination. Finally, we also observed a strong relationship between aeration scores and poor outcomes, such as the need for hospitalization (including in the ICU) and death. To our knowledge, this study is the first to evaluate the relationship between pathological LUS signs and 1-month clinical outcomes.

The mid- and long-term complications of COVID-19, including those related to the respiratory system, should be identified, and affected patients require follow-ups by appropriate services. In the present study, we observed that respiratory manifestations (such as dyspnoea and cough) and systemic manifestations (such as fever and general fatigue) were associated with LUS signs diagnosed 1 month before the prospective evaluation. Since ultrasound equipment is increasingly available and LUS can be performed at the bedside within a few minutes and in patients with mild disease or even in unstable patients [23], we believe that these interrelationships may be of great clinical interest in the context of the COVID-19 pandemic. Although LUS signs may not be specific for COVID-19 compared to some other lung diseases, the identification of certain patterns in the epidemiological context of the pandemic can certainly help clinicians to identify individuals likely to exhibit worsening clinical conditions and to develop sequelae after resolution of the acute phase of the disease [24, 25].

The clinical significance of B-lines depends mainly on their quantity (the number of B-lines per area examined and the presence or absence of confluent B-lines) and is usually associated with interstitial syndromes [2]. As the disease progresses, the air content decreases and lung density and the number of B-lines increase, leading to confluent areas equivalent to ground-glass opacities (GGOs) on CT [2, 24]. In the present study, we observed that coalescent B-lines were associated with older age, obesity, and diabetes, which are considered risk factors for COVID-19 exacerbation [4, 26, 27]. However,

**Table 2** Comparisons between disease probability categories based on LUS signal patterns

| Variables | High-probability pattern ($n=234$) | Intermediate-probability pattern ($n=180$) | Alternate pattern ($n=33$) | $p$-value |
|---|---|---|---|---|
| LUS aeration score | 7 (4–13.3)[a,b] | 2 (1–2)[b] | 3 (1–4) | **<0.0001** |
| Symptoms 1 month after LUS | | | | |
| General fatigue | 61 (26.1) | 48 (26.7) | 12 (36.4) | 0.47 |
| Dyspnoea | 39 (16.7)[a] | 16 (8.9) | 7 (21.2) | **0.024** |
| Cough | 21 (8.9) | 9 (5) | 9 (27.3) | 0.29 |
| Fever | 2 (0.9) | 1 (0.6) | 0 (0) | 0.99 |
| Poor outcomes | | | | |
| Need for hospitalization | 36 (15.4)[a,b] | 0 (0) | 0 (0) | **<0.0001** |
| Need for ICU admission | 8 (3.4)[a] | 0 (0) | 0 (0) | **0.031** |
| Death | 3 (1.3) | 0 (0) | 0 (0) | 0.41 |

Data are expressed as the number (%) except for the aeration score, which is expressed as the median (interquartile range)

Bold values indicate significant differences

*ICU* intensive care unit

[a] Significantly different from the intermediate-probability pattern

[b] Significantly different from the alternate pattern

the strongest associations with persistent respiratory symptoms 1 month after LUS were observed for previously diagnosed subpleural consolidations. In fact, as the pneumonic process progresses in COVID-19, lung density increases even more because of alveolar infiltration with inflammatory cells, causing loss of aeration and consolidation areas [2, 24]. Thus, the finding of subpleural consolidations on LUS may not only predict worsening of symptoms in the course of the disease [23] but may also indicate a more severe course in terms of pulmonary sequelae in SARS-CoV-2 infection.

The use of a scoring system to assess pathological LUS signs in patients infected with SARS-CoV-2 has been increasingly widespread during the pandemic [11, 28]. In our study, we observed that the LUS aeration score was strongly related to dyspnoea and cough 1 month after ultrasound screening. Interestingly, Lichter et al. [29] evaluated 120 consecutive patients with COVID-19 who underwent LUS within 24 h after admission. These authors observed that clinical deterioration was associated with increased follow-up LUS scores, mainly due to loss of aeration in anterior lung segments. Using an LUS scoring system and the need for supplemental oxygen at the time of examination, Manivel et al. [30] proposed a protocol to assist clinicians with decision-making in patients with COVID-19 and to facilitate provision planning within emergency departments. Because our study examined 1-month outcomes, we think that our results provide additional evidence that the LUS score can be used as a prediction tool for clinical outcomes of the disease after the acute phase and can be used as an additional tool for clinical reasoning.

In COVID-19, lung lesions play a key role in determining the clinical course and prognosis [31]. In this sense, one of the objectives of the current study was to evaluate the correlations of LUS findings with poor outcomes. We observed that the pathological LUS signs (particularly subpleural consolidations) and a higher aeration score were associated with the need for hospitalization, the need for ICU admission, and death. In line with our findings, some researchers have observed that early LUS signs (including the LUS score) are effective for assessing the need for prolonged hospitalization [15, 32]. Other studies have shown the potential of LUS to stratify early risk in COVID-19 patients who visit emergency departments according to mortality risk and the need for IMV, with this risk being higher in individuals with more pathological lung areas [29, 33, 34]. Given the scarcity of equipment and trained health professionals, the use of a relatively simple diagnostic procedure that does not use ionizing radiation, such as LUS, may have clinical and public health implications [34]. In contrast to studies evaluating short-term consequences, our study assessed 1-month outcomes, which may have important implications from the perspective of utilizing scarce resources in disadvantaged socioeconomic areas.

When using LUS, the criteria for positivity must be defined considering the possibility of alternative diagnoses and levels of probability [20, 21]. Because LUS signs are nonspecific, LUS cannot be used alone to establish a definitive diagnosis of COVID-19 infection [35]. In fact, almost 10% of our cases had LUS patterns more consistent with other diagnoses (including cardiogenic pulmonary oedema and bacterial pneumonia), although the diagnosis of COVID-19 was confirmed in all participants by RT-PCR. Importantly, our study showed that patients with high-probability LUS patterns had higher aeration scores and more dyspnoea 1 month after LUS screening and more often required hospitalization and ICU admission. Although more studies are needed, the use of categories of the probability of COVID-19 pneumonia can be an interesting strategy to predict the evolution of the disease in the short and medium term.

Several limitations in our study should be noted. First, our study was conducted at a single reference centre during the screening of COVID-19 pneumonia; therefore, generalization of our results to other periods of the pandemic should be executed with caution. However, with the emergence of the second wave of the pandemic in many regions of the world, the role of LUS may become even more prominent in the process of implementing local and global measures efficiently. Second, ultrasound evaluates only approximately 1/16 of the total lung and detects only changes closely related to the pleural surface [36]; therefore, other chest imaging methods may have a greater prognostic role than LUS. Third, we performed only a single evaluation by LUS; serial LUS examinations can be useful for tracking the clinical trajectory of an apparently unpredictable disease course, thus improving the prediction of clinical outcomes.

## Conclusion

In patients with COVID-19 pneumonia, LUS signs, including the aeration score, were related to respiratory and systemic symptoms 1 month after ultrasound screening examination. In these patients, a strong relationship was also found between LUS findings and poor outcomes, such as the need for hospitalization (including in the ICU) and death. Future studies should evaluate the relationship between LUS signs at the time of diagnosing lung involvement and long-term consequences.

#### Abbreviations

SARS-CoV-2: Severe acute respiratory syndrome coronavirus 2; ARDS: Acute respiratory distress syndrome; COVID-19: Coronavirus disease 2019; LUS: Lung ultrasound; ICU: Intensive care unit; CT: Computed tomography; RT-PCR:

Reverse-transcription polymerase chain reaction; IMV: Invasive mechanical ventilation; GGO: Ground-glass opacities.

**Acknowledgements**
Not applicable.

**Authors' contributions**
TTM, RR, CHC, and AJL developed the hypothesis. All authors were involved in the literature search and refinement of the hypothesis. TTM, MSC, LBM, PFL, LLZP, and ASESM performed and interpreted imaging exams and collected data. AJL prepared the initial draft of the manuscript. All authors read and approved the final manuscript.

**Author details**
[1] Department of Pulmonology, Piquet Carneiro Policlinic, State University of Rio de Janeiro, Av. Mal. Rondon, 381, São Francisco Xavier, Rio de Janeiro 20950-003, Brazil. [2] Postgraduate Programme in Medical Sciences, School of Medical Sciences, State University of Rio de Janeiro, Av. Prof. Manuel de Abreu, 444, 2° andar, Vila Isabel, Rio de Janeiro 20550-170, Brazil. [3] Rehabilitation Sciences Post-Graduation Programme, Augusto Motta University Centre (UNISUAM), Rua Dona Isabel, 94, Bonsucesso, Rio de Janeiro 21032-060, Brazil.

**References**

1. Chen N, Zhou M, Dong X et al (2020) Epidemiological and clinical characteristics of 99 cases of 2019 novel coronavirus pneumonia in Wuhan, China: a descriptive study. Lancet 395:507–513. https://doi.org/10.1016/S0140-6736(20)30211-7
2. Allinovi M, Parise A, Giacalone M et al (2020) Lung ultrasound may support diagnosis and monitoring of COVID-19 pneumonia. Ultrasound Med Biol 46:2908–2917. https://doi.org/10.1016/j.ultrasmedbio.2020.07.018
3. George PM, Barratt SL, Condliffe R et al (2020) Respiratory follow-up of patients with COVID-19 pneumonia. Thorax 75:1009–1016. https://doi.org/10.1136/thoraxjnl-2020-215314
4. Mo X, Jian W, Su Z et al (2020) Abnormal pulmonary function in COVID-19 patients at time of hospital discharge. Eur Respir J 55:2001217. https://doi.org/10.1183/13993003.01217-2020
5. Smargiassi A, Soldati G, Torri E et al (2021) Lung ultrasound for COVID-19 patchy pneumonia. J Ultrasound Med 40:521–528. https://doi.org/10.1002/jum.15428
6. Fonsi GB, Sapienza P, Brachini G et al (2020) Is lung ultrasound imaging a worthwhile procedure for severe acute respiratory syndrome coronavirus 2 pneumonia detection? J Ultrasound Med. https://doi.org/10.1002/jum.15487 (**Epub ahead of print**)
7. Zhu F, Zhao X, Wang T et al (2020) Ultrasonic characteristics and severity assessment of lung ultrasound in COVID-19 pneumonia in Wuhan, China: a retrospective, observational study. Engineering. https://doi.org/10.1016/j.eng.2020.09.007 (**Epub ahead of print**)
8. Lopes AJ, Mafort TT, da Costa CH et al (2020) Comparison between lung ultrasound and computed tomographic findings in patients with COVID-19 pneumonia. J Ultrasound Med. https://doi.org/10.1002/jum.15521 (**Epub ahead of print**)
9. Mafort TT, Lopes AJ, da Costa CH et al (2020) Changes in lung ultrasound of symptomatic healthcare professionals with COVID-19 pneumonia and their association with clinical findings. J Clin Ultrasound 48:515–521. https://doi.org/10.1002/jcu.22905
10. Zieleskiewicz L, Markarian T, Lopez A et al (2020) Comparative study of lung ultrasound and chest computed tomography scan in the assessment of severity of confirmed COVID-19 pneumonia. Intensive Care Med 46:1707–1713. https://doi.org/10.1007/s00134-020-06186-0
11. Perrone T, Soldati G, Padovini L (2020) A new lung ultrasound protocol able to predict worsening in patients affected by severe acute respiratory syndrome coronavirus 2 pneumonia. J Ultrasound Med. https://doi.org/10.1002/jum.15548 (**Epub ahead of print**)
12. Hussain A, Via G, Melniker L et al (2020) Multi-organ point-of-care ultrasound for COVID-19 (PoCUS4COVID): international expert consensus. Crit Care 24:702. https://doi.org/10.1186/s13054-020-03369-5
13. Bernheim A, Mei X, Huang M et al (2020) Chest CT findings in coronavirus disease-19 (COVID-19): relationship to duration of infection. Radiology 295:200463. https://doi.org/10.1148/radiol.2020200463
14. Sultan LR, Sehgal CM (2020) A review of early experience in lung ultrasound in the diagnosis and management of COVID-19. Ultrasound Med Biol 46:2530–2545. https://doi.org/10.1016/j.ultrasmedbio.2020.05.012
15. Gaspardone C, Meloni C, Preda A et al (2021) Lung ultrasound in COVID-19 a role beyond the acute phase? J Ultrasound Med 40:503–511. https://doi.org/10.1002/jum.15425
16. Soummer A, Perbet S, Brisson H et al (2012) Ultrasound assessment of lung aeration loss during a successful weaning trial predicts postextubation distress. Crit Care Med 40:2064–2072. https://doi.org/10.1097/CCM.0b013e31824e68ae
17. Tung-Chen Y, Algora-Martín A, Llamas-Fuentes R et al (2021) Point-of-care ultrasonography in the initial characterization of patients with COVID-19. Med Clin. https://doi.org/10.1016/j.medcli.2020.12.007 (**Epub ahead of print**)
18. Saraogi A (2015) Lung ultrasound: present and future. Lung India 32:250–257. https://doi.org/10.4103/0970-2113.156245
19. Tung-Chen Y, de Gracia MM, Díez-Tascón A et al (2020) Correlation between chest computed tomography and lung ultrasonography in patients with coronavirus disease 2019 (COVID-19). Ultrasound Med Biol 46:2918–2926. https://doi.org/10.1016/j.ultrasmedbio.2020.07.003
20. Volpicelli G, Lamorte A, Villén T (2020) What's new in lung ultrasound during the COVID-19 pandemic. Intensive Care Med 46:1445–1448. https://doi.org/10.1007/s00134-020-06048-9
21. Millington SJ, Koenig S, Mayo P et al (2021) Lung ultrasound for patients with coronavirus disease 2019 pulmonary disease. Chest 159:205–211. https://doi.org/10.1016/j.chest.2020.08.2054
22. Volpicelli G, Gargani L, Perlini S et al (2021) Lung ultrasound for the early diagnosis of COVID-19 pneumonia: an international multicenter study. Intensive Care Med. https://doi.org/10.1007/s00134-021-06373-7 (**Epub ahead of print**)
23. Tung-Chen Y (2020) Lung ultrasound in the monitoring of COVID-19 infection. Clin Med 20:e62–e65. https://doi.org/10.7861/clinmed.2020-0123
24. Vetrugno L, Baciarello M, Bignami E et al (2020) The "pandemic" increase in lung ultrasound use in response to Covid-19: can we complement computed tomography findings? A narrative review Ultrasound J 12:39. https://doi.org/10.1186/s13089-020-00185-4
25. Convissar DL, Gibson LE, Berra L et al (2020) Application of lung ultrasound during the COVID-19 pandemic: a narrative review. Anesth Analg 131:345–350. https://doi.org/10.1213/ANE.0000000000004929
26. Zheng Z, Peng F, Xu B et al (2020) Risk factors of critical & mortal COVID-19 cases: a systematic literature review and meta-analysis. J Infect 81:e16–e25. https://doi.org/10.1016/j.jinf.2020.04.021
27. Korakas E, Ikonomidis I, Kousathana F et al (2020) Obesity and COVID-19: immune and metabolic derangement as a possible link to adverse clinical outcomes. Am J Physiol Endocrinol Metab 319:E105–E109. https://doi.org/10.1152/ajpendo.00198.2020
28. Vetrugno L, Bove T, Orso D et al (2020) Our Italian experience using lung ultrasound for identification, grading and serial follow-up of severity of lung involvement for management of patients with COVID-19. Echocardiography 37:625–627. https://doi.org/10.1111/echo.14664
29. Lichter Y, Topilsky Y, Taieb P et al (2020) Lung ultrasound predicts clinical course and outcomes in COVID-19 patients. Intensive Care Med 46:1873–1883. https://doi.org/10.1007/s00134-020-06212-1
30. Manivel V, Lesnewski A, Shamim S et al (2020) CLUE: COVID-19 lung ultrasound in emergency department. Emerg Med Australas 32:694–696. https://doi.org/10.1111/1742-6723.13546
31. Istvan-Adorjan S, Ágoston G, Varga A et al (2020) Pathophysiological background and clinical practice of lung ultrasound in COVID-19 patients: a short review. Anatol J Cardiol 24:76–80. https://doi.org/10.14744/AnatolJCardiol.2020.33645
32. Jin YH, Cai L, Cheng ZS et al (2020) A rapid advice guideline for the diagnosis and treatment of 2019 novel coronavirus (2019-nCoV) infected pneumonia (standard version). Mil Med Res 7:4. https://doi.org/10.1186/s40779-020-0233-6

33. Brahier T, Meuwly J-Y, Pantet O et al (2020) Lung ultrasonography for risk stratification in patients with COVID-19: a prospective observational cohort study. Clin Infect Dis. https://doi.org/10.1093/cid/ciaa1408 (**Epub ahead of print**)
34. Bonadia N, Carnicelli A, Piano A et al (2020) Lung ultrasound findings are associated with mortality and need for intensive care admission in COVID-19 patients evaluated in the emergency department. Ultrasound Med Biol 46:2927–2937. https://doi.org/10.1016/j.ultrasmedbio.2020.07.005
35. Volpicelli G, Gargani L (2020) Sonographic signs and patterns of COVID-19 pneumonia. Ultrasound J 12:22. https://doi.org/10.1186/s13089-020-00171-w
36. Serafino MD, Notaro M, Rea G et al (2020) The lung ultrasound: facts or artifacts? In the era of COVID-19 outbreak. Radiol Med 125:738–753. https://doi.org/10.1007/s11547-020-01236-5

# 11

# Prospective evaluation of cardiac ultrasound performance by general internal medicine physicians during a 6-month faculty development curriculum

Christopher J. Smith[1*], Abdulrahman Morad[2], Christopher Balwanz[2], Elizabeth Lyden[3] and Tabatha Matthias[1]

**Abstract**

**Background:** Point-of-care (POCUS) education is rapidly expanding within medical schools and internal medicine residency programs, but lack of trained faculty is a major barrier. While POCUS training can improve short-term outcomes, knowledge and skills rapidly decay without deliberate practice and feedback. The purpose of this study was to evaluate the performance of focused cardiac ultrasound (FCU) by volunteer general internal medicine (GIM) faculty participating in a longitudinal POCUS curriculum.

**Methods:** Participants: Nine GIM clinician-educators participated in a 6-month POCUS curriculum. Faculty performance was compared to three cardiology fellows. Three diagnostic cardiac sonographers (DCS) were also evaluated and served as the gold standard. Evaluation: the primary outcome was a FCU efficiency score, calculated by dividing image quality score by exam duration. FCU exams were conducted on three standardized patients after completion of an introductory workshop, at 3 months, and at 6 months. Two blinded cardiologists scored the exams. Analysis: mean efficiency scores were compared using a linear mixed effects model, followed by pairwise comparisons using Tukey's test.

**Results:** GIM faculty's FCU efficiency scores were maintained over the 6-month period (2.2, SE 1.0 vs. 3.8, SE 1.0, $p = 0.076$). Their scores at each session were similar to cardiology fellows ($p > 0.69$), but inferior to DCSs ($p < 0.0001$).

**Conclusion:** GIM faculty participating in a POCUS curriculum maintained their FCU performance over 6 months with efficiency scores comparable to experienced cardiology fellows.

**Keywords:** Point-of-care ultrasound, Faculty development, Internal Medicine

## Background

Point-of-care ultrasound (POCUS) is clinician-performed ultrasonography used to guide real-time diagnostic and management decisions. POCUS training is rapidly expanding in undergraduate and graduate medical education. Twenty-eight percent of medical schools offer POCUS curricula [1], including several well-established, vertically-integrated programs [2–4]. A survey of Association of Program Directors in Internal Medicine members found that 25% of respondents reported formal POCUS curricula, with another 25% planning to implement programs within a year [5]. Educational leaders in these studies identified faculty development as a major barrier to broader adoption of POCUS training [1, 5].

Despite the increasing need for POCUS-trained faculty in medical education, limited research has investigated training programs for general internal medicine (GIM) faculty. One 10-week faculty program resulted in improved self-reported confidence and exam scores, but image acquisition skills were not assessed [6].

*Correspondence: csmithj@unmc.edu
[1] Section of Hospital Medicine, Division of General Internal Medicine, Department of Internal Medicine, University of Nebraska Medical Center, 986430 Nebraska Medical Center, Omaha, NE, USA
Full list of author information is available at the end of the article

POCUS training can improve short-term outcomes, but knowledge and skills decay without ongoing support. A study of internal medicine physicians who completed a 3-year POCUS curriculum during residency demonstrated poor retention of cardiac ultrasound skills after more than 1 year of nonuse [7]. Surgical residents and medical students who participated in a 2-h cardiac ultrasound course had significant decay in their knowledge and skills within 1 month [8]. Studies of internal medicine residents found knowledge deteriorated in the months following workshop-based training [9], but that longitudinal support prevented knowledge decay [10].

This study investigated the impact of a longitudinal POCUS curriculum on GIM faculty's performance of focused cardiac ultrasound (FCU). We hypothesized that at the end of the study period, GIM faculty performance of FCU would be resilient to skills decay and comparable to cardiology fellows' performance.

## Methods

### Participants and setting

Nine volunteer GIM clinician-educators at an academic health center participated in a 6-month POCUS curriculum with a goal of developing core faculty for a residency program. Faculty did not receive protected time from other duties. Figure 1 illustrates the structure and content of the faculty development curriculum, including elements that were eligible for continuing medical education (CME) credit. The introductory workshop was required, but all other curricular elements were voluntary. Subsequent lectures and workshops were scheduled to accommodate as many participants as possible. Before these sessions, participants were asked to review relevant online modules from free open-access medical education resources. Modules were typically 10–15 min in duration. In-person didactics were recorded and posted to an online learning management system for asynchronous review. Peer-group practice was arranged by group members.

GIM faculty performance was compared to three senior cardiology fellows who had completed level 1 echocardiography training [11], including performance of 75 comprehensive echocardiographic studies. Three registered diagnostic cardiac sonographers (DCS) served as the gold standard.

### Evaluation

We scored FCU exams using a validated image acquisition assessment tool [12]. As in the validation study, our primary outcome was an FCU efficiency score, calculated by dividing an image quality score by exam duration in minutes. The original 68-point image quality score was modified to 66-points, as two scoring items were not taught (inferior vena cava M-mode and respiratory variation measurement). The scoring instrument was comprised of two sections. The first section included scoring of anatomic structures and image optimization (appropriate depth, gain, and centering) in the following views: parasternal long axis; parasternal short-axis aortic valve, mitral valve, mid-papillary, and apex; apical four chamber; subcostal long axis; and subcostal inferior vena cava (IVC). The second section scored the overall diagnostic image quality of the exam for common clinical questions, such as left ventricular systolic function. Assessments took place after completion of an 8-h introductory workshop (baseline), at 3 months, and at 6 months. FCU exams were performed on the same three standardized patients (SPs) at each session. The research team chose SPs that represented a cross-section of typical IM patients (two women, age 48–79 years, body mass index 23–39 kg/m$^2$). One SP had a hiatal hernia, which was not known prior to the research sessions. Using cart-sized point-of-care ultrasound machines (Sparq; Philips Healthcare, Andover, MA), participants captured video

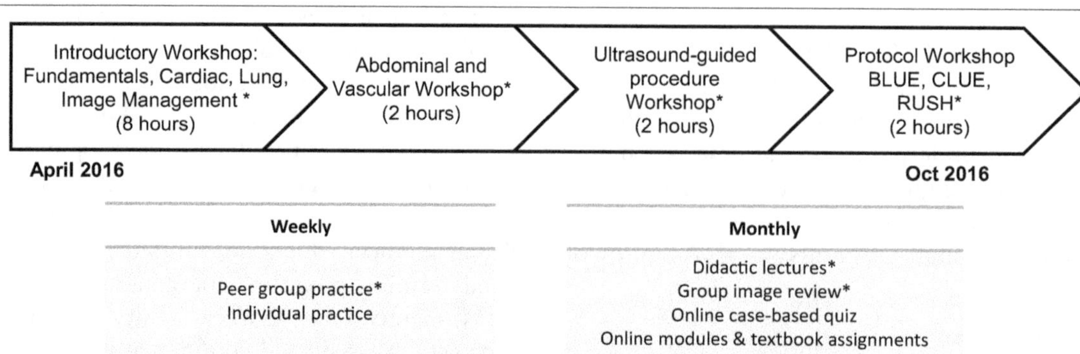


**Fig. 1** Curricular elements of 6-month point-of-care ultrasound curriculum for internal medicine faculty. *Curricular elements that qualified for CME credits. *BLUE* bedside lung ultrasound in emergency, *CLUE* cardiopulmonary limited ultrasound examination, *RUSH* rapid ultrasound for shock and hypotension

loops in the required views, outlined above. Before each session, written instructions were provided to participants, facilitators, and SPs (Additional file 1: Appendix S1). The machines used for the assessment were the same as those available to GIM faculty during their curriculum. Before each assessment session, the cardiology fellows and DCS received an in-person tutorial on machine set-up and knobology. Two board-certified cardiologists scored the FCU exams. They were blinded to participant group, SP, and exam session. Prior to scoring research images, they scored three pilot exams together to ensure similar application of the scoring instrument. They then independently scored two pilot exams, resulting in nearly identical scores (53 vs. 52 and 41.5 vs. 42.5 points).

### Analysis

Mean FCU efficiency scores, image quality total score, image quality sub-group scores, and exam duration were compared using a linear mixed effects model with random effects for SP and participant and fixed effects for session and group (GIM faculty, cardiology fellows, and DCSs). If the interaction of group and session were statistically significant, Tukey's test was performed to make pairwise comparisons of the mean scores between the three groups for each session. If the interaction of group and session was not significant, pairwise comparisons were performed between the groups (combining sessions) and between the sessions (combining groups). Model adjusted means and standard errors (SE) were used for descriptive statistics. Spearman correlation coefficients were used to assess the association of total CME hours with efficiency score. $p < 0.05$ was considered statistically significant. Statistics were calculated using SAS Version 9.4 software (SAS Inc., Cary, NC). The University of Nebraska Medical Center Institutional Review Board approved the study (163-16-EX).

## Results

Four of nine GIM faculty were female (44%) and eight (89%) had no prior POCUS training. Eight participants (89%) completed all three sessions. Faculty earned an average of 30.6 CME hours (SD 8.6 h) over the 6 months. The average attendance at voluntary curricular components (workshops, didactics, and image review sessions) over the 6 months was 68% (range 38–88%). FCU efficiency score data are displayed in Table 1. GIM faculty efficiency scores were maintained over the 6-month study period (baseline 2.2, SE 1.0 vs. 6 months 3.8, SE 1.0, $p = 0.076$). There was no difference between mean GIM faculty and cardiology fellow efficiency scores during any of the three assessment sessions (Fig. 2). DCSs performed significantly better than GIM faculty and cardiology fellows during all three assessments ($p < 0.0001$).

GIM faculty image quality scores were sustained between the baseline and 6-month evaluations (36.7, SE 5.2 vs. 39.7, SE 5.3, $p = .34$). In the linear mixed effect model analysis, there was no significant interaction between group and session for image quality score ($p = 0.73$), so pairwise comparison was made combining the three sessions. Overall, cardiology fellows had a higher mean image quality score than GIM faculty (50.6, SE 6.0 vs. 40.8, SE 5.0, $p = 0.037$). Table 2 displays the image quality scores for each exam sub-section. GIM faculty and cardiology fellow sub-group scores were comparable for the parasternal long axis and subcostal long axis views, as well as for overall diagnostic quality. Cardiology fellow scores were significantly higher for the parasternal short axis, apical four chamber, and subcostal IVC.

GIM faculty's exam duration decreased during the study period (baseline 17.5 min, SE 1.5 vs. 6 months 13.0, SE 1.5 min, $p < .001$). Combining the three sessions, GIM faculty and cardiology fellow exam duration were comparable across the three sessions (faculty 15.3 min, SE 1.4 vs. fellows 13.8 min, SE 1.8, $p = 0.64$).

**Table 1 Focused cardiac ultrasound efficiency scores for participant groups throughout the 6-month study period**

| Baseline | | | 3 months | | | 6 months | | |
|---|---|---|---|---|---|---|---|---|
| GIM | CF | *p* | GIM | CF | *p* | GIM | CF | *p* |
| 2.2 (1.0) | 3.7 (1.2) | 0.69 | 3.3 (1.0) | 4.7 (1.2) | 0.77 | 3.8 (1.0) | 4.4 (1.2) | 1.00 |
| GIM | DCS | *p* | GIM | DCS | *p* | GIM | DCS | *p* |
| 2.2 (1.0) | 11.7 (1.2) | <0.001 | 3.3 (1.01) | 16.0 (1.2) | <0.001 | 3.8 (1.0) | 14.3 (1.2) | <0.001 |
| CF | DCS | *p* | CF | DCS | *p* | CF | DCS | *p* |
| 3.7 (1.2) | 11.7 (1.2) | <0.001 | 4.7 (1.16) | 16.0 (1.2) | <0.001 | 4.4 (1.2) | 14.32 (1.2) | <0.001 |

Data reported as model-adjusted means (SE). Comparisons reported using adjusted *p* value

*GIM* general internal medicine faculty, *CF* cardiology fellows, *DCS* diagnostic cardiac sonographers, *SE* standard error

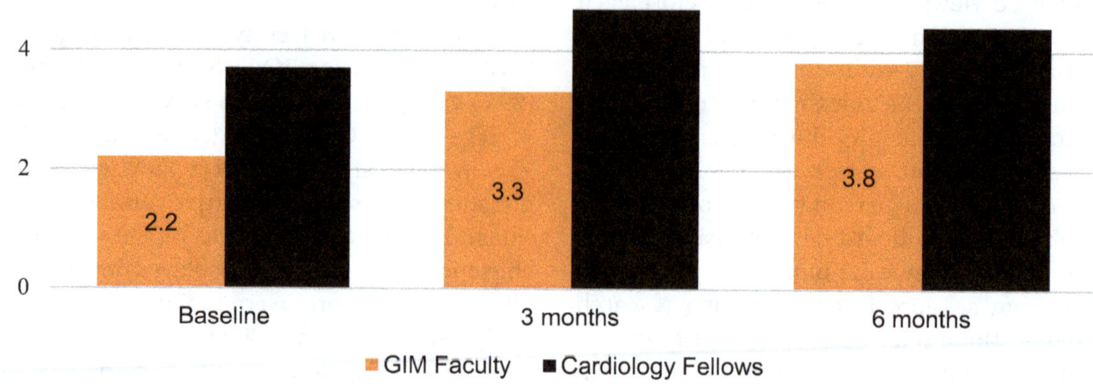


**Fig. 2** Focused cardiac ultrasound efficiency scores for GIM faculty and cardiology fellows. Baseline line assessment occurred after GIM faculty completed an introductory point-of-care ultrasound workshop. There were no significant differences between the two groups at any of the three assessments

**Table 2 Focused cardiac ultrasound image quality scores for general internal medicine (GIM) faculty and cardiology fellows**

| | Maximum score | GIM faculty | Cardiology fellows | *p* value |
|---|---|---|---|---|
| Parasternal long | 12 | 8.7 (0.7) | 9.6 (0.9) | 0.50 |
| Parasternal short | 18 | 11.0 (0.9) | 14.5 (1.3) | 0.04 |
| Apical | 10 | 6.0 (0.8) | 8.1 (1.0) | 0.04 |
| Subcostal long | 8 | 4.2 (1.3) | 5.2 (1.4) | 0.46 |
| Subcostal IVC | 6 | 2.5 (1.0) | 3.6 (1.0) | 0.03 |
| Diagnostic quality | 12 | 8.6 (1.0) | 9.5 (1.2) | 0.52 |
| Total | 66 | 40.8[a] (5.0) | 50.6 (6.0) | 0.04 |

Data reported as model-adjusted means (SE) combining the three assessment sessions. Comparisons reported using adjusted *p* value

*GIM* general internal medicine faculty, *SE* standard error

[a] Model adjusted mean reported, so total does not equal sum of individual sub-sections

## Discussion

GIM faculty participating in a voluntary, multi-modal curriculum maintained their FCU acquisition skills over a 6-month period. GIM faculty efficiency scores were similar to those previously reported by critical care physicians with American Society of Echocardiography level III certification (although the latter performed FCU on mechanically ventilated patients) [12]. Our findings highlight the importance of longitudinal support when teaching FCU to novice faculty. FCU performance requires integration of a complex set of psychomotor skills, which cannot be mastered without regular practice and feedback. Prior studies of novice cardiology fellows [13] and hospitalists [14] found that FCU skills can be developed in weeks to months with frequent expert coaching. The duration of training required to achieve proficiency likely depends on institutional resources and needs. In the present study, GIM faculty did not have dedicated time and was concomitantly learning non-cardiac POCUS applications, requiring a longer curriculum.

Our primary outcome was a measure of efficiency, which Gaudet et al. [12] have argued is a "hallmark of expertise". Efficiency has been used as an assessment variable in prior FCU performance studies [15] and is important for several reasons. First, POCUS must be economical for integration into clinicians' daily workflow. Exam efficiency is also vital for the prompt assessment of time-sensitive clinical conditions, such as shock. Finally, task efficiency may precede improvements in performance quality. This phenomenon has been observed in prior FCU studies [12, 13] and performance research for other fine-motor skills, such as endoscopy [16].

While GIM faculty had efficiency scores similar to cardiology fellows, their total image quality scores were lower. This reason for this is likely multifactorial. GIM faculty may not have engaged in enough deliberate practice over the 6 months to advance their image acquisition skills [17]. Additionally, cardiology fellows' extensive experience in interpreting diagnostic echocardiography studies may have contributed to their superior scores. It should also be noted that our FCU protocol included views which are more technically challenging for novices [15]. Some of these views, such as apical four chambers, are excluded from commonly-used FCU exam protocols [18]. Although their total image quality scores were lower, GIM faculty performed comparably to cardiology fellows for overall diagnostic quality. This may be the most clinically relevant outcome, as the primary purpose of POCUS is to quickly gain information to guide clinical decision making.

This study adds to the existing literature in several ways. It is one of the first papers to examine the educational outcomes of a longitudinal POCUS curriculum for GIM faculty. Studies of residents and fellows may not be applicable to faculty, given differences in clinical experience, time availability, and willingness to adopt innovations [19]. Additionally, we assessed performance of a complete FCU exam protocol including all recommend views [20] and utilized a validated scoring instrument. Finally, the baseline assessment occurred *after* an intensive introductory workshop, allowing us to evaluate the impact of the longitudinal portion of the curriculum independent of the introductory training.

There are limitations to this study. It was conducted at a single institution with few participants. Repeated scanning of the same SPs may have led to higher scores due to familiarity, although this was likely limited by the 3-month washout periods. Furthermore, only the GIM faculty group showed improvement across all testing periods. We were unable to accurately track the number of exams performed by each participant during the curriculum to look for correlation with performance outcomes. Additionally, our study did not assess image interpretation skills, which typically develop more quickly than image acquisition skills [21].

In conclusion, GIM faculty participating in a longitudinal POCUS curriculum maintained their FCU acquisition skills over a 6-month period. Efficiency scores were comparable to cardiology fellows, but overall image quality was lower. Future studies will need to examine if GIM performance of FCU is sustainable beyond 6 months.

## Additional file

**Additional file 1.** Instructions for study participants, facilitators, and standardized patients.

#### Abbreviations

POCUS: point-of-care ultrasound; GIM: general internal medicine; FCU: focused cardiac ultrasound; CME: continuing medical education; DCS: diagnostic cardiac sonographer; SP: standardized patient; SE: standard error; BLUE: bedside lung ultrasound in emergency; CLUE: cardiopulmonary limited ultrasound examination; RUSH: rapic ultrasound for shock and hypotension.

#### Authors' contributions

CS and TM: study design, literature review, original writing, data collection, figure design. AM and CB: ultrasound exam scoring. EL: statistical analysis. All authors participated in manuscript editing. All authors read and approved the final manuscript.

#### Author details

[1] Section of Hospital Medicine, Division of General Internal Medicine, Department of Internal Medicine, University of Nebraska Medical Center, 986430 Nebraska Medical Center, Omaha, NE, USA. [2] Division of Cardiology, Department of Internal Medicine, University of Nebraska Medical Center, Omaha, NE, USA. [3] Department of Biostatistics, University of Nebraska Medical Center, Omaha, NE, USA.

#### Acknowledgements

The authors wish to thank Dr. Kevin Piro for his help in reviewing this paper and Dr. Kristy Carlson for assisting with figure design.

#### References

1. Dinh VA, Fu JY, Lu S et al (2016) Integration of ultrasound in medical education at United States medical schools: a national survey of directors' experiences. J Ultrasound Med 35(2):413–419. https://doi.org/10.7863/ultra.15.05073
2. Hoppmann RA, Rao VV, Poston MB et al (2011) An integrated ultrasound curriculum (iUSC) for medical students: 4-year experience. Crit Ultrasound J 3(1):1–12. https://doi.org/10.1007/s13089-011-0052-9
3. Bahner DP, Adkins EJ, Hughes D et al (2013) Integrated medical school ultrasound: development of an ultrasound vertical curriculum. Crit Ultrasound J 5(1):6. https://doi.org/10.1186/2036-7902-5-6
4. Wilson SP (2017) Implementation of a 4-year point-of-care ultrasound curriculum in a liaison committee on medical education-accredited US medical school. J Ultrasound Med 36(2):321–325. https://doi.org/10.7863/ultra.16.03068
5. Schnobrich DJ, Gladding S, Olson AP et al (2013) Point-of-care ultrasound in internal medicine: a national survey of educational leadership. J Grad Med Educ 5(3):498–502. https://doi.org/10.4300/jgme-d-12-00215.1
6. Maw A, Jalali C, Jannat-Khah D et al (2016) Faculty development in point of care ultrasound for internists. Med Educ Online 21:33287. https://doi.org/10.3402/meo.v21.33287
7. Kimura BJ (2016) Retention of ultrasound skills and training in "point-of-care" cardiac ultrasound. J Am Soc Echocardiogr 29(10):992–997. https://doi.org/10.1016/j.echo.2016.05.013
8. Yamamoto RR (2018) Rapid decay of transthoracic echocardiography skills at 1 month: a prospective observational study. J Surg Educ. https://doi.org/10.1016/j.jsurg.2017.07.011
9. Town JA et al (2016) Internal medicine residents' retention of knowledge and skills in bedside ultrasound. J Grad Med Educ 8(4):553–557. https://doi.org/10.4300/jgme-d-15-00383.1
10. Kelm DJ, Ratelle JT, Azeem N et al (2015) Longitudinal ultrasound curriculum improves long-term retention among internal medicine residents. J Grad Med Educ 7(3):454–457. https://doi.org/10.4300/jgme-14-00284.1
11. Ryan T et al (2015) COCATS 4 task force 5: training in echocardiography: endorsed by the American society of echocardiography. J Am Soc Echocardiogr 28(6):615–627. https://doi.org/10.1016/j.echo.2015.04.014
12. Gaudet J, Waechter J, McLaughlin K et al (2016) Focused critical care echocardiography: development and evaluation of an image acquisition assessment tool. Crit Care Med. https://doi.org/10.1097/ccm.0000000000001620
13. Prinz C, Dohrmann J, van Buuren F et al (2012) The importance of training in echocardiography: a validation study using pocket echocardiography. J Cardiovasc Med (Hagerstown, Md) 13(11):700–707. https://doi.org/10.2459/jcm.0b013e328356a55f
14. Lucas BP et al (2009) Diagnostic accuracy of hospitalist-performed hand-carried ultrasound echocardiography after a brief training program. J Hosp Med 4(6):340–349. https://doi.org/10.1002/jhm.438
15. Chisholm CB et al (2013) Focused cardiac ultrasound training: how much is enough? J Emerg Med 44(4):818–822. https://doi.org/10.1016/j.jemermed.2012.07.092
16. Verdaasdonk EGG et al (2007) Construct validity and assessment of the learning curve for the SIMENDO endoscopic simulator. Surg Endosc 21(8):1406–1412. https://doi.org/10.1007/s00464-006-9177-5
17. Ericsson KA (2008) Deliberate practice and acquisition of expert performance: a general overview. Acad Emerg Med 15(11):988–994. https://doi.org/10.1111/j.1553-2712.2008.00227.x
18. Kimura BJ et al (2015) Cardiac limited ultrasound examination techniques to augment the bedside cardiac physical examination. J Ultrasound Med 34(9):1683–1690. https://doi.org/10.7863/ultra.15.14.09002
19. Sahin I (2006) Detailed review of Rogers' diffusion of innovations theory and educational technology-related studies based on Rogers' theory. Turk Online J Educ Technol 5(2):14–22
20. Via G, Hussain A, Wells M et al (2014) International evidence-based recommendations for focused cardiac ultrasound. J Am Soc Echocardiogr 27(7):683.e1–683.e33. https://doi.org/10.1016/j.echo.2014.05.001

# 12

# Point-of-care transcranial Doppler by intensivists

Vincent Issac Lau[1,2*] and Robert Thomas Arntfield[1,2]

**Abstract**

In the unconscious patient, there is a diagnostic void between the neurologic physical exam, and more invasive, costly and potentially harmful investigations. Transcranial color-coded sonography and two-dimensional transcranial Doppler imaging of the brain have the potential to be a middle ground to bridge this gap for certain diagnoses. With the increasing availability of point-of-care ultrasound devices, coupled with the need for rapid diagnosis of deteriorating neurologic patients, intensivists may be trained to perform point-of-care transcranial Doppler at the bedside. The feasibility and value of this technique in the intensive care unit to help rule-in specific intra-cranial pathologies will form the focus of this article. The proposed scope for point-of-care transcranial Doppler for the intensivist will be put forth and illustrated using four representative cases: presence of midline shift, vasospasm, raised intra-cranial pressure, and progression of cerebral circulatory arrest. We will review the technical details, including methods of image acquisition and interpretation. Common pitfalls and limitations of point-of-care transcranial Doppler will also be reviewed, as they must be understood for accurate diagnoses during interpretation, as well as the drawbacks and inadequacies of the modality in general.

**Keywords:** Point-of-care ultrasound, Midline shift, Vasospasm, Intra-cranial pressure, Cerebral circulatory arrest, Neuro-critical care

## Background

In the absence of consciousness, a complete neurological exam is not always possible. Limited to the assessment of brainstem structures for neurological function (pupils, Glasgow Coma Scale, Cushing's reflex, cranial nerve reflexes/responses and respiratory pattern), the intensivist at the bedside must instead rely on other tools to characterize sub-catastrophic anatomic events, as some of the above findings can be non-specific for the etiology of decreased level of consciousness. Most typically, this involves the use of computed tomography (CT) or magnetic resonance (MR) imaging, and in many cases, an invasive intra-cranial pressure (ICP) monitoring through insertion of an intracerebral catheter. Though these tools offer great value, they also introduce well-defined risks of transport or radiation [1, 2], and risk of an invasive procedure [3, 4], as well as delays in identifying and managing time-sensitive neurologic processes [5]. A more immediate, non-invasive, bedside approach to complement these existing methods is therefore of interest.

In 1982, Aaslid et al. introduced into clinical practice the use of transcranial Doppler (TCD) ultrasonography. TCD offers a non-invasive means of evaluating intra-cranial blood vessel flow and velocity with color and spectral Doppler [6]. The utility is evident, as it remains a cornerstone for neurologists, neurosurgeons, and intensivists in the identification of vasospasm after sub-arachnoid hemorrhage [7–9]. TCD may also be used to roughly predict ICP [10–14] as well characterize the alterations in blood flow that occur during intra-cranial cerebral circulatory arrest from severely raised ICP [15], although TCD cannot be used as a surrogate for invasive ICP monitor [16, 17].

As ultrasound technology has improved, the same transcranial acoustic windows used for the Doppler assessment of the cerebral circulation may also be used to achieve two-dimensional (2D) images of the brain parenchyma. Though anatomic detail is inferior to CT imaging,

*Correspondence: vinceissaclau@gmail.com
[2] London Health Sciences Centre, Victoria Hospital Rm, D2-528, 800 Commissioners Road East, London, ON N6A 5W9, Canada
Full list of author information is available at the end of the article

resolution is sufficient to answer emergent bedside questions such as mass effect leading to midline shift [18–20] and predict adverse outcomes after stroke [21, 22]. Given phenomena such as elevated ICP, vasospasm, midline shift, and brain death are of routine concern in the intensive care unit (ICU), it is appealing to consider this skill in the hands of the intensivist at the bedside for the expedition of care. Similar to all other point-of-care (POC) ultrasound applications, immediate, round-the-clock availability and repeatability in response to interventions or clinical change are particular advantages of TCD being in the hands of the intensivist. Additionally, resource-limited settings (remote areas, low-income countries, combat field, sports arenas, etc.) where CT access is scarce may be of particular benefit to acute care providers.

Despite the widespread availability of portable ultrasound machines in the ICU (due largely to the significant uptake of point-of-care echocardiography and critical care ultrasound in the critical care community), uptake of point-of-care TCD has not been observed. In the face of barriers to uptake such as the omission of TCD from the internationally adopted critical care ultrasound competency statement [23], it is important to illustrate the potential value and influence that point-of-care TCD may yield in the hands of the intensivist. To this end, our review will highlight potential applications of point-of-care TCD and how it may be used to screen four specific entities. Through four representative cases, the reader will be briefed on the theoretical and technical aspects of intensivist-conducted TCD for expedition of care. We will also describe the common pitfalls and limitations that are common to the technique.

## Example case descriptions

All figures/tables associated with the following cases in this article are original submissions.

### Case 1: midline shift

A 58-year-old female presented with a headache and decreased level of consciousness (LOC), and is found to have diffuse SAH, intra-cranial hemorrhage (ICH), and intra-ventricular hemorrhage (IVH) from a right middle cerebral artery (MCA) aneurysm with only 2 mm of initial midline shift measured by CT head. The patient had further deterioration in her neurological status with concerns of about increasing mass effect from her hemorrhages, and a point-of-care (POC) TCD 2D image was obtained (Fig. 1a, b), which found that her midline shift had increased to 6.5 mm towards the left:

$$\text{Midline shift (MLS)} = (\text{distance A} - \text{distance B})/2$$

$$\begin{aligned}\text{Midline shift (MLS)} &= (7.41 - 6.11\ \text{cm})/2 = 1.3\ \text{cm}/2 \\ &= 0.65\ \text{cm} = 6.5\ \text{mm}\end{aligned}$$

This was later confirmed on urgent repeat CT head imaging (Fig. 1c) of 7 mm towards the left secondary to enlarging ICH.

### Case 2: vasospasm

An 83-year-old male with diffuse SAH from a right anterior-communicating (AComm) artery aneurysm (Fig. 2a), secured by coiling. Despite prophylactic nimodipine to improve outcomes in vasospasm patients, 5 days later, patient again had decreased LOC and required intubation. An urgent CT head was arranged, and an urgent bedside POC TCD (Fig. 2b) was rapidly performed, showing a mean velocity of 123 cm/s, with a Lindegaard ratio of 3.8 (Fig. 2c) which correspond with TCD signs of mild vasospasm (Additional file 1: Video 1). CT-angiogram confirmed this, including moderate vasospasm in the anterior cerebral artery (ACA) and posterior cerebral artery (PCA) territories. This prompted hypertensive

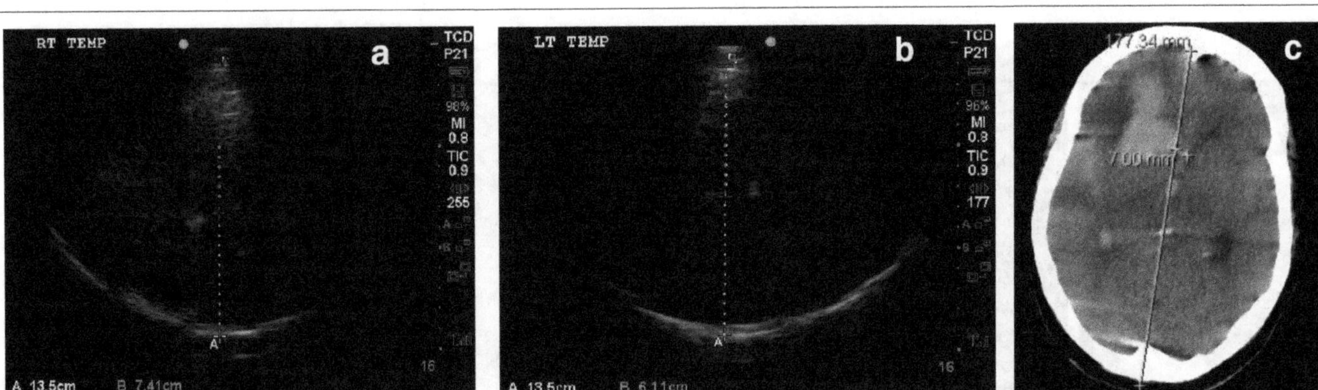


**Fig. 1** Transcranial imaging for midline shift. **a** Insonation from right temporal bone to third ventricle, representing distance A (7.41 cm). **b** Insonation from left temporal bone to third ventricle, representing distance B (6.11 cm). **c** Follow-up CT scan post TCD which reveals midline shift to be 7 mm

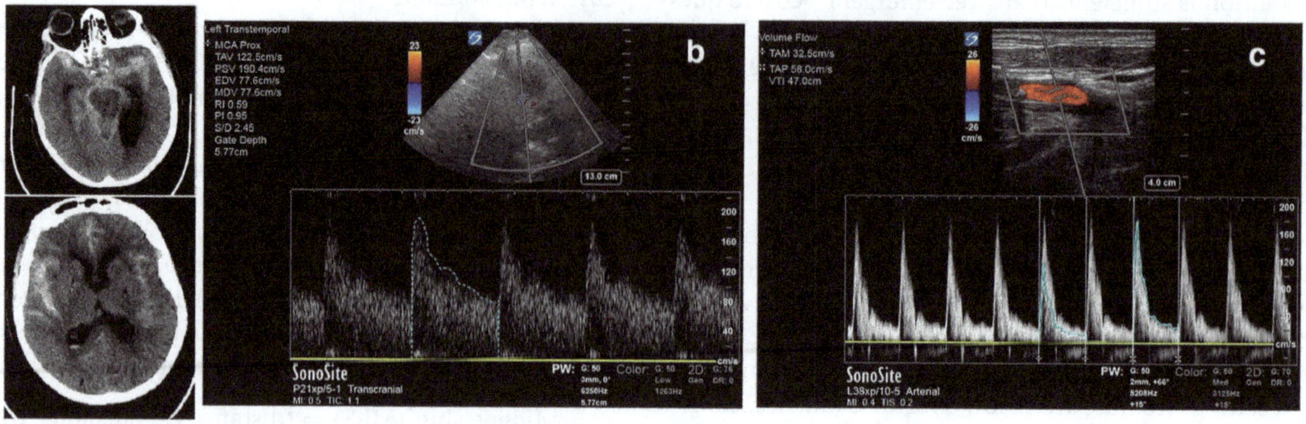


**Fig. 2** Transcranial Doppler for vasospasm following subarachnoid hemorrhage. **a** CT Head demonstrating diffuse subarachnoid hemorrhage. **b** TCD measurement of left MCA flows, demonstrating a mean MCA velocity of 123 cm/s (in-keeping with mild vasospasm). **c** Measurement of ipsilateral left ICA flows for calculation of Lindegaard ratio of 3.8 (Mean MCA/ICA velocity = 123/32.5 cm/s), which confirmed mild MCA vasospasm

therapy with vasopressors as per local neurosurgical standard of care. Follow-up serial screening TCDs and CT-As by radiology showed worsening to severe vasospasm in all vascular territories, first diagnosed on POC TCD.

**Case 3: raised intra-cranial pressure**

A 74-year-old male, previously on dual antiplatelet agents (aspirin, clopidogrel) for cardiac stents, fell down 15 stairs. He was diagnosed with traumatic brain injury (TBI) on CT head (Fig. 3a) with diffuse sub-SAH and subdural hemorrhage (SDH), with an admission GCS of 14. GCS rapidly deteriorated to three, and a POC TCD was performed immediately (Additional file 2: Video 2) as the neurosurgeon was already preparing to insert an EVD following intubation. TCD was performed simultaneously while scalp was prepped on contralateral side. Interrogation of the MCA flows (Fig. 3b) showed a pulsatility index of 4.31 (equating to an ICP of 46 mmHg by TCD). The extra-ventricular drain (EVD) was placed at the bedside for therapeutic effect and confirmed the TCD findings of ICP elevation (EVD monitor measured ICP = 42 mmHg). After appropriate neuro-resuscitative measures (osmotic therapy, vasoactive agents and ICP drainage via EVD), a follow-up POC TCD (Fig. 3c) showed decreased ICP (TCD pulsatility index = 1.65, ICP = 17 mmHg). These dynamic changes were also mirrored in agreement with the EVD monitor (EVD ICP = 16 mmHg).

**Case 4: cerebral circulatory arrest**

A 63-year-old male presented with retro-orbital headaches was diagnosed with an AComm artery aneurysm which underwent a coiling attempt. During the procedure, however, the patient had internal carotid artery (ICA) dissection, trans-mural perforation and pseudoaneurysm formation. CT head revealed diffuse SAH from aneurysmal rupture with IVH (Fig. 4a). An EVD was

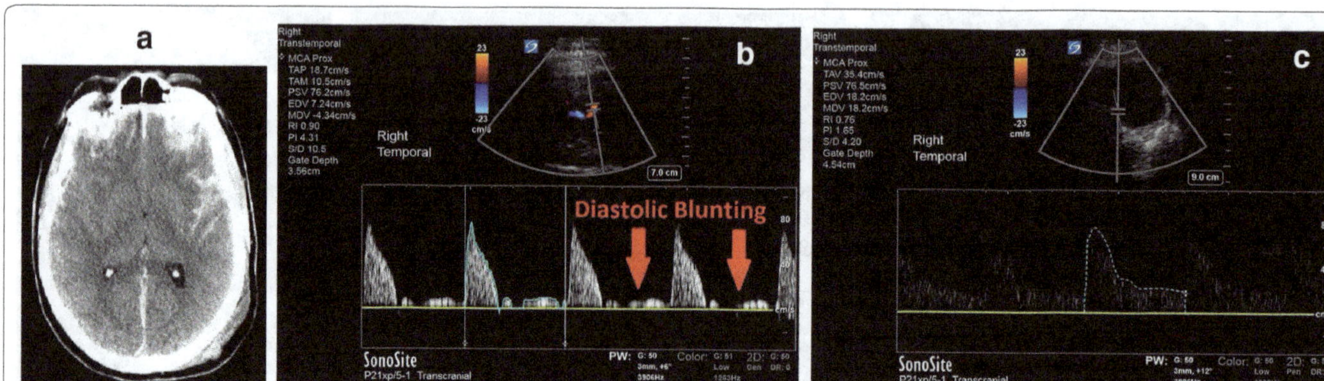


**Fig. 3** Raised intra-cranial pressure by spectral Doppler on TCD, as calculated by pulsatility index. **a** Diffuse subarachnoid hemorrhage on CT head. **b** Spectral Doppler of MCA, demonstrating diastolic blunting secondary to raised ICP (pulsatility index = 4.31, ICP = 46 mmHg). **c** Following interventions to reduce ICP, there was normalization of diastolic flow in the MCA, and resolution of high ICP (pulsatility index = 1.65, ICP = 17 mmHg)

placed immediately at bedside, which showed raised ICP (> 60 mmHg). A poor prognosis was given and goals of care changed to Do Not Resuscitate (DNR). The patient subsequently developed dilated pupils bilaterally and had hemodynamic alterations in keeping with a Cushing's response. A POC TCD was obtained serially to determine and characterize the progression to brain death through the predictable spectral Doppler evolution: diastolic blunting, diastolic flow reversal, and, finally, biphasic/oscillating flow (Fig. 4b–d).

## Methods

### Ultrasound technique

To perform a TCD or TCD image (TCDI), place your patient in the supine position with the head of bed > 30° (not always possible in ICU patients). Use a 1–5 MHz phased array ultrasound transducer with a TCD preset, or if unavailable, a cardiac preset. For either preset, the sonographer must ensure that the lowest Nyquist level should be selected (~ 20 cm/s) for color-coded duplex sonography (CDDS). Place the probe on the trans-temporal window (Fig. 5a), with the index mark pointed towards the patient's anterior/front (Fig. 5b). With the index mark orientated to screen left, identify the ipsilateral/contralateral temporal bones, and the third ventricle (a midline structure) (Fig. 5c). Decrease the depth to the distance of the third ventricle in the far-field and identify the cerebral penducles and echogenic basal cisterns. Then place a color Doppler box over the top half of the screen (near field) where the MCA is located, just lateral to the cerebral penducles. Identify the MCA as indicated by red color Doppler signal towards the probe. Then interrogate the MCA by placing the pulse wave marker on top of the MCA, and obtain the spectral Doppler waveforms (Fig. 5d). Angle correction should be utilized upon the insonation of vessels in order to adjust the pulse wave Doppler for the angle of insonation.

MCA interrogation should be obtained at 0.5 cm for the M1 segment, and 0.4 cm for the M2 segment of the MCA. Intervals at its most distal point to the bifurcation of the proximal ICA into the MCA and ACA, to screen for focal vasospasm. The trans-temporal window can also insonate the ACAs (anterior angulation, depth 6–7 cm), terminal ICAs (caudal angulation, 6–7 cm), and PCAs (posterior angulation, 5.5–7.5 cm), bilaterally. The protocol is repeated for the opposite hemisphere. Trans-orbital and trans-foraminal windows are more typical for complete diagnostic TCD, and will not be discussed as part of POC TCD.

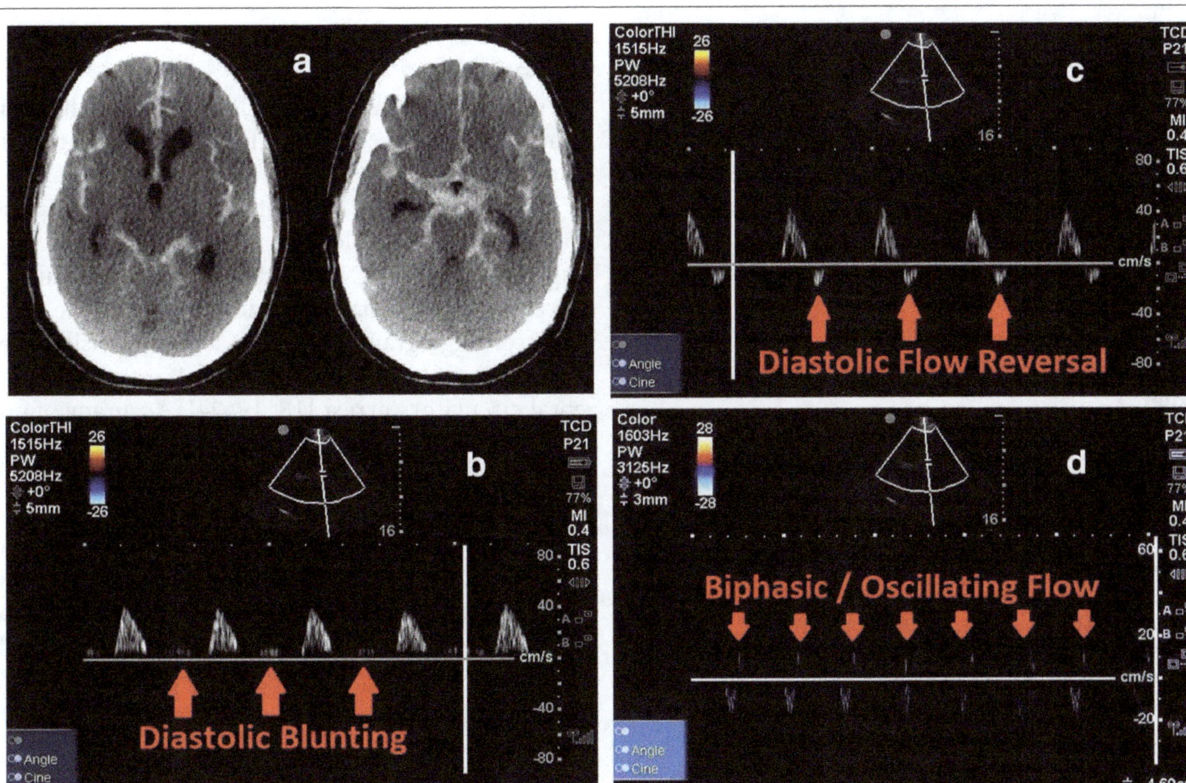


**Fig. 4** Step-wise progression of cerebral circulatory arrest. **a** CT Head demonstrating diffuse subarachnoid hemorrhage. **b** Evidence of raised ICP causing decreased diastolic flow as evidenced by blunting of the spectral Doppler signal. **c** Further progression with diastolic flow reversal as raised ICP prevents forward flow in MCA, and even induces backwards flow. **d** Biphasic and oscillating flow as evidenced by net zero flow (where systolic and diastolic flow are near equal to each other), indicating the first TCD stage of cerebral circulatory arrest

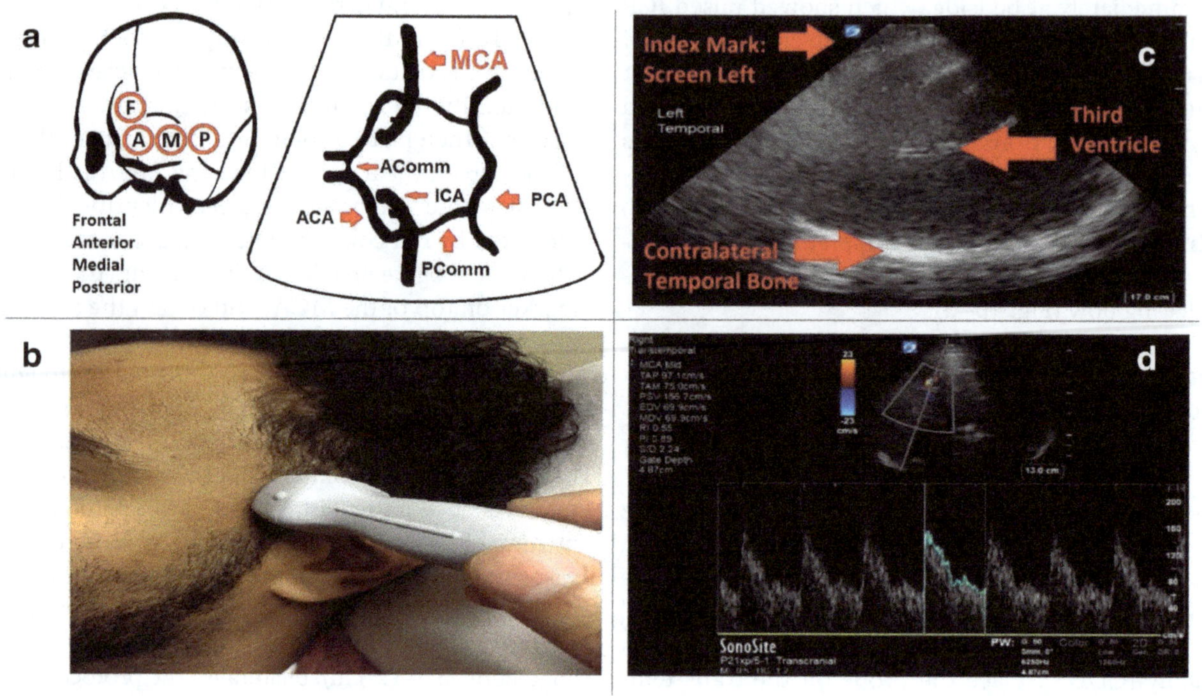


**Fig. 5** Method for acquisition of transcranial Doppler. **a** Left side shows location of the trans-temporal window and its various sections: frontal, anterior, medial, and posterior. Right side illustrates Circle of Willis, with MCA highlighted. **b** Probe index mark orientation towards the patient's anterior/front. **c** Typical 2D image of TCD from trans-temporal window with index mark to screen left, with bright echogenic contralateral temporal bone, and anechoic space of midline third ventricle. **d** Typical spectral Doppler velocity waveform from MCA, with steep systolic upstroke and step-down diastolic flow (typical mean velocity of 80 cm/s)

## Discussion

This review seeks to characterize what we feel are the four major point-of-care applications for TCD in the hands of critical care providers. There are many more additional potential indications and applications for the use of TCD at the point-of-care (full list shown in Table 1). However, outside of the four chosen POC TCD indications, the remainder are the scope of formal TCD, as they require additional training [11, 12, 18, 22, 24–32].

**Table 1 Indications for transcranial ultrasonography and Doppler**

| Indication |
|---|
| Midline shift |
| Vasospasm (post-subarachnoid hemorrhage) |
| Intra-cranial pressure (ICP) |
| Cerebral circulatory arrest (brain death) |
| Stenosis |
| Occlusion/stroke |
| Micro-emboli (transient ischemic attack or stroke) |
| Right-to-left shunts (paradoxical emboli) |
| Sickle cell hyperemia versus stenosis |
| Intra-cranial hemorrhage detection and monitoring |
| Cerebral motor vasoactivity |
| A–V malformation assessments |
| Syncope or positional vertigo |

There are several advantages to use of transcranial imaging and Doppler. It is quick, with no radiation exposure (unlike CT), and requires no patient transport (unlike MRI or CT). Additionally, unlike traditional 4-vessel angiography, TCD is a non-invasive means of monitoring for vasospasm, stenosis, stroke, ICP or cerebral circulatory arrest [18, 19, 24]. Accuracy of point-of-care TCD is unknown, the diagnostic sensitivity of TCD in the hands of expert sonographers is quite good, reaching 89–98% for the MCA [18, 19].

The four themes will be further characterized here with a focus on the technical elements as well as the value of rapid application at the bedside. As with any ultrasound modality, the acquisition of images and Doppler information is operator-dependent, and there are several limitations and pitfalls to TCD acquisition and interpretation, discussed within each topic.

## Midline shift

Diagnosis of midline shift is important both for preventing further secondary neurological injury by early neurosurgical intervention, but also neuro-prognostication.

Any amount of midline shift is considered abnormal, but poor neurological outcome can be associated with a clinically significant midline shift of as little as 0.5 cm (positive predictive value (PPV) of 78% with presence of midline shift [20, 25], as opposed to a 14% PPV without the presence of midline shift), and a twofold increase in mortality associated with greater than 1-cm midline shift (53% vs 25%) [21, 22].

Seidel et al. illustrated the use of ultrasonography for the measurement of midline shift. Reproducibility of MLS via ultrasound corresponded to $0.3 \pm 0.2$ mm in ten volunteers [20]. Measurements on ultrasound have correlated well with CT findings [20–22], and have been predictive of poor outcome from midline shift secondary to pathologies such as stroke, hemorrhage (subdural, epidural, subarachnoid), and traumatic brain injury [20–22, 25, 26].

There are two methods to quantify midline shift. One method (see Fig. 1a, b) is to measure the distance from the bilateral temporal bones to the midline third ventricle. Distance A is measured from the ipsilateral side, whereas distance B is from the contralateral side. One should also measure the full length from the ipsilateral to the contralateral temporal bone. Then use the following equation to calculate the midline shift deviation:

$$\text{Midline shift (MLS)} = (\text{distance A} - \text{distance B})/2$$

For an expedited investigation, the other method (see Fig. 1a, b) would be to measure from the ipsilateral side to the third ventricle only (distance C), and then also measure the full distance from the ipsilateral temporal bone to the contralateral temporal bone (distance D), then calculate MLS with this equation:

$$\text{Midline shift (MLS)} = \text{distance C} - (\text{distance D}/2)$$

With either method, if the MLS is positive, this means that the MLS is away from the ipsilateral side. If the MLS is negative, the MLS is toward the ipsilateral side.

Our recommendation is to utilize the first method for midline shift quantification. With 2 independent measurements from each side to assess midline shift and an internal check for correct measurements (the sum of distance A and B should equal the full distance from the ipsilateral to contralateral temporal bones), it is the least vulnerable to operator error. Clinical utilization of TCD or TCDI for midline shift also incorporates comparisons of measured cerebral blood flow velocities and pulsatility indexes between right and left anterior circulation. This will be discussed in the vasospasm and raised ICP sections, as discrepant findings and asymmetry in CBFs and PIs are a main indicator of potential midline shift.

#### Midline shift: limitations

Due to thicker cranial vaults causing higher bone attenuation, the literature states that 5–20% of patients will have difficult views leading to un-interpretable transcranial windows and images [18, 19]. MLS measurement relies heavily on finding a proper trans-temporal window. There are no data correlating angle of insonation and accuracy of transcranial US midline shift measurements. AIUM guidelines state that the upward angle of insonation should be no greater than 10–15° [7], but that may not always be possible. The presence of hydrocephalus of the third ventricle does not have much bearing on the MLS measurement, as the measurements are done to the center of the third ventricle, not to its outer walls. However, hydrocephalus does help predict the need for EVD insertion and for safe EVD removal. Kiphuth et al. observed that TCD was a reliable method for predicting the necessity for CSF drainage. In patients with external ventricular drainage (EVD), they estimated that a cut-off value of an increase of 5.5 mm in ventricle width after clamping had a high sensitivity (100%) and negative predictive value (100%). They suggested that an increase in ventricular width lower than the cut-off was an indication for a safe removal of EVD [27].

### Vasospasm

Transcranial Doppler has been studied extensively as a validated screening tool for diagnosing vasospasm [6, 7, 28–41], aiding in the management of subarachnoid hemorrhage (SAH) patients. Diagnosis of vasospasm post-SAH greatly affects prognosis, causing significant morbidity secondary to strokes from delayed cerebral ischemia, and mortality in 15–20% of patients [8, 37, 39]. Using the inverse relationship between cerebral blood vessel diameter and TCD mean velocities, we are able to quantify and subcategorize vasospasm [25, 35, 36].

Assessment of the MCA requires pulse wave spectral Doppler. The normal spectral Doppler profile of the MCA has a sharp systolic upstroke with a step-wise diastolic deceleration, with a normal mean velocity of the MCA that is usually < 80 cm/s. Mild vasospasm mean velocities are 120–159 cm/s, moderate vasospasm is 160–199 cm/s, and severe vasospasm is > 200 cm/s. These cutoffs have been derived using non-imaging traditional TCD probes as are commonly used in complete, diagnostic TCD [6, 9, 28, 36, 42]. Progressive increase of mean velocities during the early stages of SAH to predictive of vasospasm. Authors have cited a change in baseline mean velocity of > 21 cm/s per 24 h in the first 3 days to be diagnostic of vasospasm [39, 43]. Symptomatic clinical vasospasm is often only seen at mean velocities of 160 cm/s [38].

Another method of grading vasospasm severity would be the formula known as the Lindegaard ratio [36]:

$$\text{Lindegaard ratio} = \text{Ipsilateral MCA mean velocity} / \text{ipsilateral extra} - \text{Cranial ICA mean velocity}.$$

As entities other than vasospasm (e.g., hyper-dynamic flow) may increase mean velocities, the Lindegaard ratio does not grade vasospasm, but helps differentiate between hyperemia (induced by medial or endovascular treatment) versus the onset of true vasospasm. If the Lindegaard ratio > 3, this would diagnose vasospasm, as increased flow velocity would be raised in the cerebral circulation relative to the carotid circulation. A Lindegaard ratio of 3–5 would denote mild-moderate vasospasm, while a ratio > 6 would indicate severe vasospasm [36].

### Vasospasm: limitations

The diagnostic value of TCD clinical utilization to detect vasospasm is not in question. All relevant professional societies, like American Heart Association, American Society of Neuroimaging, and American Institute for Ultrasound in Medicine all recommend TCD utilization for vasospasm [7, 44–46]. Compared to CT-angiogram, the sensitivity/specificity of the MCA is quite good (~ 89–98%). However, the trans-orbital and trans-foraminal windows are less reliably insonated compared to the trans-temporal window [47], and the ACA and PCA are less sensitive and specific for vasospasm compared to the MCA. The same applies to the basilar artery and vertebral artery with lower sensitivity and specificity in the trans-foraminal window [30, 31]. Exhaustive exclusion of vasospasm calls for all cerebral vessels to be insonated. Thus, the technique as we have described it represents a screening test of the highest yield arterial territory (MCA)—of greatest value if vasospasm is identified and insufficient to exclude the possibility [6, 42].

Several factors make the diagnosis of vasospasm challenging. The clinician must be mindful that cerebral blood flow maybe influenced by many factors ($PaO_2$, $PaCO_2$, blood viscosity, collateral flow). Furthermore, operator experience is required for accurate assessment, as improper vessel identification, proximal lesions and aberrant vessel course can confound even experienced sonographers [9].

For Doppler interrogation, diagnostic TCD utilizes non-imaging probes set for measurement of spectral Doppler signs at specific distances to insonate various vessels in question. However, most radiology departments now use color-coded duplex sonography (CDDS) imaging probes with pulse wave Doppler and angle correction [48]. The advantage to using CDDS imaging probes is that insonation no longer needs a perfectly on-axis due to anatomic variations between different segments of cerebral arteries, as machines are able to solve for off-axis measurements using angle correction. The caveat is that normal velocities reported for TCD are validated for non-imaging probes and not for color-coded duplex sonography [48]. However, many radiology departments utilize CDDS instead of traditional non-imaging TCD probes despite the lack of validation prior. Absolute velocities obtained from CDDS would be underestimated, but CDDS angle correction has been shown to be no different than velocities obtained from traditional TCD [49].

### Intra-cranial pressure

TCD can be used to give a rough estimate for ICP, to help rule-in high ICP, but not as a surrogate for accurate invasive ICP monitors. As ICP increases, flow in intra-cranial vessels changes. Initially, systolic velocity increases (i.e., systolic peak flows) as increased ICP causes cerebral vessels to narrow from external pressure in the MCA. During diastole, diastolic flow becomes decreased/blunted (Fig. 3b), as raised ICP becomes the predominant external pressure opposing forward MCA flow during diastole. Raised ICP can also exceed normal forward flow during diastole, leading to diastolic flow reversal (Fig. 6) [10, 15].

Raised ICP can be estimated using the Gosling's pulsatility index, which is a reflection of peripheral resistance, which is equal to the difference between the peak systolic velocity (PSV) and end-diastolic velocity (ESV), divided by the mean velocity (MV) [10, 49–51]:

$$\text{Pulsatility index (PI)} = [\text{PSV} - \text{EDV}]/\text{MV}.$$

Bellner et al. correlated pulsatility index (PI) to ICP in clinical practice. Generally, high ICPs result in high pulsatility indices (PIs) in high-resistance vascular beds, where systolic velocity is increased relative to decreased end-diastolic velocity. This translates to an increased systolic-to-diastolic (S/D) ratio and an increased pulsatility index. A formula has been derived to convert pulsatility index into ICP (from all causes), with a sensitivity of 89%, and specificity of 92% [10].

$$\text{ICP} = (10.93 \times \text{PI}) - 1.28.$$

Based on this formula, a PI of > 2.13 would correlate to an ICP > 22 mmHg (based on new Brain Trauma Foundation guidelines cutoffs) [52], which is the clinically significant cutoff for raised ICP, and would compromise cerebral perfusion pressure (CPP) [10, 53–55], whereas normal pulsatility index (PI) is < 1.2, and corresponds to an ICP of approximately 12 mmHg (normal ICP = 5–15 mmHg) [28]. The main advantage of PI is that it is not affected by the angle of insonation [18]. This is one of many

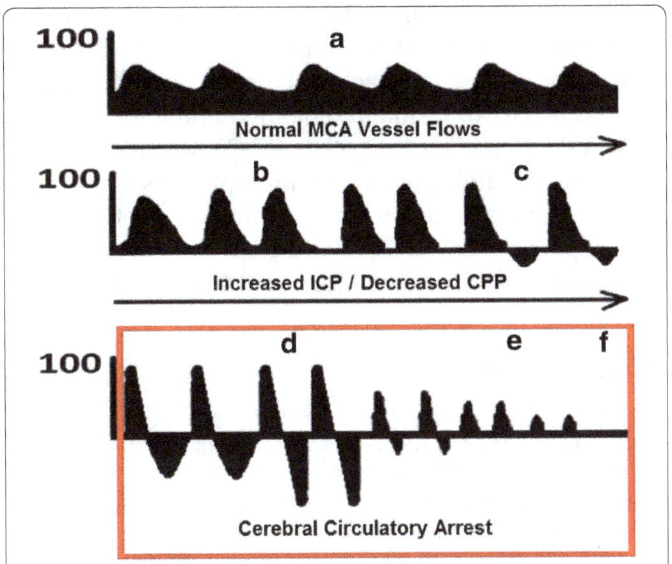


**Fig. 6** Progression of intra-cranial circulatory arrest via transcranial Doppler of middle cerebral artery flows. **a** Normal systolic upstroke with normal step-down of diastolic flow. **b** Increased peak systolic flow with decreasing diastolic flow and eventual blunting of diastolic flow. **c** Diastolic flow reversal. **d** Biphasic or oscillating flow—where diastolic flow reversal approaches equal size to systolic flow. **e** Isolated sharp systolic peak flows of < 200 ms and small systolic amplitude of < 50 cm/s. **f** Zero flow—where there was previously documented TCD flow. The red box denotes states (**d**, **e**, **f**) in which cerebral circulatory arrest can be diagnosed

TCD-derived PI formulas for estimation of ICP [12, 56–58]. Some suggest using TCD as a binary assessment for the absence of intra-cranial hypertension [12].

### Intra-cranial pressure: limitations

The main limitation of TCD PI correlation to ICP is that caution must be exercised given its wide confidence intervals when compared directly to ICP monitors [16, 17]. Other literature suggests that TCD PI is not a reliable correlate to ICP [13, 16, 17, 59–64]. Decreased $PaCO_2$ or increased arterial blood pressure (ABP) alterations can influence cerebral blood flow and PI independently of ICP. Decreases in CPP (representing an increasing trend in PI) can be from increased ICP, but also decreases in mean arterial pressure (MAP). Therefore, instead of assuming linear correlation with ICP, PI can rather be understood to be inversely proportional to mean CPP or directly proportional to ABP, and a non-linear proportion to artery/arteriole compliance in the cerebral bed, cerebrovascular resistance, and heart rate. As such, recommendations for utilization of increasing PI for following increasing ICP and decreasing CPP trends across time, rather than ICP absolute values [59].

Although not a continuous means of ICP measurement, TCD PI can be performed non-invasively serially, helping to rule in high ICP, and prompting more invasive, continuous modalities. Confounders can make PI uninterpretable for raised ICP. Lack of pulsatile flow, such as with venous–arterial (V–A) extracorporeal membrane oxygenation (ECMO) or left ventricular assist devices (LVADs), as systolic and diastolic ratios for pulsatility index would be uninterpretable for ICP and brain death. The diagnosis of vasospasm by TCD would also be more difficult given the lower flow states associated with non-pulsatile flow from an LVAD or V–A ECMO (Fig. 7).

### Cerebral circulatory arrest

Predictable, step-wise changes in cerebral blood flow may be observed as part of progression to cerebral circulatory arrest (Fig. 6): decreasing or blunted diastolic flow, oscillating flow (characterized by diastolic flow reversal), sharp systolic peak flows, and then finally, zero flow in keeping with cerebral circulatory arrest [10, 15].

Serial interrogations are often required for TCD diagnosis of cerebral circulatory arrest and brain death, including a scan preceding the onset of cerebral circulatory arrest to demonstrate the presence of prior intra-cranial flow [15, 65–67]. Cerebral circulatory arrest may be identified on TCD (red box of Fig. 6) when one of three criteria are met in bilateral blood vessels, measured at least twice, 30 min apart: (1) Net-zero oscillating waveform flow with near equal systolic forward flow and diastolic reversed flow. (2) Small sharp systolic peaks with < 50 cm/s peak systolic velocity and < 200 ms duration. (3) Disappearance of all previously seen intra-cranial flow, but extra-cranial flow still present [30, 65]. These criteria (listed in Table 2) have a sensitivity of 88%, and specificity of 98% [30].

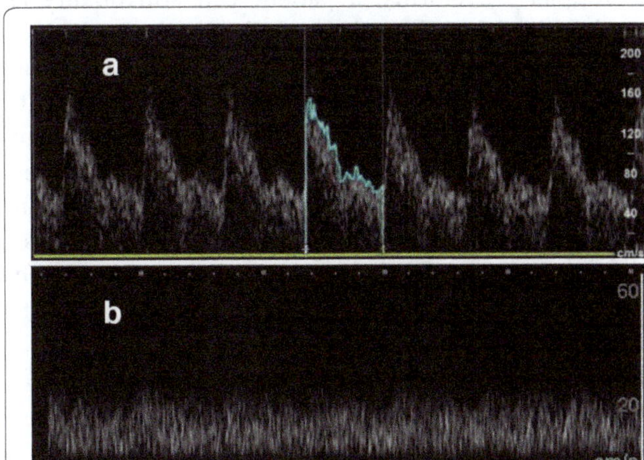


**Fig. 7** Disadvantage to transcranial Doppler when interpreting MCA flows for patient with non-pulsatile flow states (i.e., V–A ECMO, LVAD). **a** Normal pulsatile flow: systolic upstroke with normal step-down of diastolic flow. **b** Non-pulsatile flow: Loss of sharp systolic peak flows, with overall lowering of means flows—which would make interpretation of pulsatility index for ICP as well as mean flows for vasospasm more difficult

**Table 2 Cerebral circulatory arrest criteria by transcranial Doppler**

| |
|---|
| Oscillating wave form (equal systolic forward flow and diastolic reversed flow) |
| Small systolic spikes of < 200 ms duration and < 50 cm/s pulse systolic velocity spike |
| Disappearance of all intra-cranial flow (loss of systolic and diastolic flow, where flow had been present previously intra-cranially, and still present extra-cranially) |

Determination of brain death is typically a clinical diagnosis with parameters like brainstem reflex testing and an apnea test. Certain situations (i.e., presence of spinal reflexes, drug ingestions, and profound hypothermia/shock) may lead to confounding with brain death determination if relying on clinical testing alone. If TCD rules in cerebral circulatory arrest by non-reassuring MCA flows, ancillary testing (4-vessel cerebral angiography, nuclear medicine radionuclide brain perfusion scan, CT or MR cerebral blood flow angiography) could be sought to formally confirm the diagnosis. However, if TCD shows reassuring cerebral blood flows not meeting aforementioned criteria, this would possibly save premature, unnecessary serial ancillary tests, until the diagnosis can be first confirmed on TCD. This helps optimizing the ideal time to obtain ancillary testing when clinical determination of brain death has confounders [65–70].

#### Cerebral circulatory arrest: limitations

In addition to previously discussed limitations in other sections, there are specific limitations to TCD diagnosis of brain death. Despite the presence of reassuring spectral Doppler waveforms, a patient can still qualify as brain dead by other clinical means (brainstem and apnea testing in the absence of confounders). This means cerebral blood flow maybe inadequate to sustain life despite reassuring waveforms. The opposite is also true, as the absence of reassuring spectral Doppler waveforms (meeting above criteria) does not automatically mean brain death, as TCD evaluates cerebral circulatory arrest, not brainstem function. Furthermore, most medical jurisdictions will not accept a TCD as its own ancillary test to confirm brain death [67].

## Conclusions

The advent of intensivist-performed ultrasound and availability of ultrasound machines now provides a unique climate where point-of-care TCD is a reality. Intensivists with this skill are able to provide immediate, 24/7 bedside assessment for midline shift, elevated ICP, vasospasm and intra-cranial hypertension progression. Barriers to training do still exist, but despite these pitfalls and limitations, intensivists performing limited point-of-care TCD as a screening tool to rule-in certain indications is feasible. Reaching competence is attainable, without extensive formal radiology training for diagnostic TCD. Much like many other POC modalities, to rule in various pathologies where prompt bedside diagnosis could be invaluable to the expedition of patient care. We support the use of TCD as a complementary adjunct to routine investigations (formal TCD, CT/MRI, ICP monitors).

## Additional files

**Additional file 1: Video 1.** Vasospasm on TCD. Demonstration of vasospasm pulse wave Doppler of the MCA during TCD interrogation.

**Additional file 2: Video 2.** Raised ICP on TCD. Pulse wave Doppler of the MCA during TCD interrogation demonstrating raised ICP.

#### Abbreviations

TCD: transcranial Doppler; CT: computerized tomography; CT-A: computerized tomography-angiogram; MRI: magnetic resonance imaging; MCA: middle cerebral artery; ICP: intra-cranial pressure; ICA: internal carotid artery; SAH: subarachnoid hemorrhage; IVH: intra-ventricular hemorrhage; ICH: intracranial hemorrhage; EVD: extra-ventricular drain; POC: point-of-care; GCS: Glasgow Coma Scale; TBI: traumatic brain injury; ICU: intensive care unit; $PaCO_2$: pressure in arterial blood of carbon dioxide; PEA: pulseless electrical activity; CPR: cardio-pulmonary resuscitation; ROSC: return of spontaneous circulation; DNR: do not resuscitate; PPV: positive predictive value; MLS: midline shift; CPP: cerebral perfusion pressure; PI: pulsatility index; PSV: peak systolic velocity; ESV: end-diastolic velocity; MV: mean velocity; ABP: arterial blood pressure; MAP: mean arterial pressure; ONSD: optic nerve sheath diameter; V-A ECMO: venous-arterial extracorporeal membrane oxygenation; LVAD: left ventricular assist device.

#### Authors' contributions

VL carried out the conception and design of the review article, the review of the literature, collection of the majority of the cases, image acquisition and drafting/revisions of the manuscript. RA help conceived of the study, and participated in image acquisition of several cases and helped to draft the manuscript while revising the manuscript for important intellectual content. Both authors read and approved the final manuscript.

#### Author details

[1] Department of Medicine, Division of Critical Care, Schulich School of Medicine and Dentistry, Western University, London, ON, Canada. [2] London Health Sciences Centre, Victoria Hospital Rm, D2-528, 800 Commissioners Road East, London, ON N6A 5W9, Canada.

#### Acknowledgements

We would like to acknowledge Dr. Lauren Zarnett (neurosurgery resident at Western University) for her contribution to the cases and her continued support for the TCD modality.

#### References

1. Andrews PJD, Piper IR, Dearden NM, Miller JD (1990) Secondary insults during intrahospital transport of head-injured patients. Lancet 335(8685):327–330
2. Kaups KL, Davis JW, Parks SN (2004) Routinely repeated computed tomography after blunt head trauma: does it benefit patients? J Trauma Acute Care Surg 56(3):475–481
3. Lieben MA (2000) Indications for intracranial pressure monitoring. J Neurotrauma [Internet].17(6/7) http://online.liebertpub.com/doi/pdf/10.1089/neu.2000.17.479. Cited 16 Jan 2017
4. Savers S (2000) Guidelines for cerebral perfusion pressure. J Neurotrauma 17(6–7):507–511

5. Becker DP, Miller JD, Ward JD, Greenberg RP, Young HF, Sakalas R (1977) The outcome from severe head injury with early diagnosis and intensive management. J Neurosurg 47(4):491–502
6. Aaslid R, Markwalder T-M, Nornes H (1982) Noninvasive transcranial Doppler ultrasound recording of flow velocity in basal cerebral arteries. J Neurosurg 57(6):769–774
7. Radiology AC of, others (2012) AIUM practice guideline for the performance of a transcranial Doppler ultrasound examination for adults and children. J Ultrasound Med Off J Am Inst Ultrasound Med 31(9):1489
8. Macdonald RL, Schweizer TA(2016) Spontaneous subarachnoid haemorrhage. Lancet [Internet]. 2016; http://www.sciencedirect.com/science/article/pii/S0140673616306687. Cited 16 Jan 2016
9. Simm RF, de Aguiar PHP, de Oliveira Lima M, Paiva BL (2013) Transcranial Doppler as a routine in the treatment of vasospasm following subarachanoid hemorrhage (SAH). In: Cerebral vasospasm: neurovascular events after subarachnoid hemorrhage [Internet]. Springer;. pp 75–76. http://link.springer.com/chapter/10.1007/978-3-7091-1192-5_16. Cited 16 Jan 2017
10. Bellner J, Romner B, Reinstrup P, Kristiansson K-A, Ryding E, Brandt L (2004) Transcranial Doppler sonography pulsatility index (PI) reflects intracranial pressure (ICP). Surg Neurol 62(1):45–51
11. Rasulo FA, De Peri E, Lavinio A (2008) Transcranial Doppler ultrasonography in intensive care. Eur J Anaesthesiol 25(S42):167–173
12. Rasulo FA, Bertuetti R, Robba C, Lusenti F, Cantoni A, Bernini M et al (2017) The accuracy of transcranial Doppler in excluding intracranial hypertension following acute brain injury: a multicenter prospective pilot study. Crit Care 21(1):44
13. Cardim D, Robba C, Donnelly J, Bohdanowicz M, Schmidt B, Damian M et al (2015) Prospective study on noninvasive assessment of intracranial pressure in traumatic brain-injured patients: comparison of four methods. J Neurotrauma 33(8):792–802
14. O'Brien NF, Maa T, Reuter-Rice K (2015) Noninvasive screening for intracranial hypertension in children with acute, severe traumatic brain injury. J Neurosurg Pediatr 16(4):420–425
15. Hassler W, Steinmetz H, Pirschel J (1989) Transcranial Doppler study of intracranial circulatory arrest. J Neurosurg 71(2):195–201
16. Zweifel C, Czosnyka M, Carrera E, de Riva N, Pickard JD, Smielewski P (2012) Reliability of the blood flow velocity pulsatility index for assessment of intracranial and cerebral perfusion pressures in head-injured patients. Neurosurgery 71(4):853–861
17. Behrens A, Lenfeldt N, Ambarki K, Malm J, Eklund A, Koskinen L-O (2010) Transcranial Doppler pulsatility index: not an accurate method to assess intracranial pressure. Neurosurgery 66(6):1050–1057
18. Moppett IK (2004) Transcranial Doppler ultrasonography in anaesthesia and intensive care. Br J Anaesth 93(5):710–724
19. White H, Venkatesh B (2006) Applications of transcranial Doppler in the ICU: a review. Intensive Care Med 32(7):981–994
20. Seidel G, Gerriets T, Kaps M, Missler U (1996) Dislocation of the third ventricle due to space-occupying stroke evaluated by transcranial duplex sonography. J Neuroimaging 6(4):227–230
21. Gerriets T, Stolz E, Modrau B, Fiss I, Seidel G, Kaps M (1999) Sonographic monitoring of midline shift in hemispheric infarctions. Neurology 52(1):45–49
22. Gerriets T, Stolz E, König S, Babacan S, Fiss I, Jauss M et al (2001) Sonographic monitoring of midline shift in space-occupying stroke. Stroke 32(2):442–447
23. Mayo PH, Beaulieu Y, Doelken P, Feller-Kopman D, Harrod C, Kaplan A et al (2009) American College of Chest Physicians/La Societe de Reanimation de Langue Francaise statement on competence in critical care ultrasonography. Chest J 135(4):1050–1060
24. Kincaid MS (2008) Transcranial Doppler ultrasonography: a diagnostic tool of increasing utility. Curr Opin Anesthesiol. 21(5):552–559
25. Quattrocchi KB, Prasad P, Willits NH, Wagner FC (1991) Quantification of midline shift as a predictor of poor outcome following head injury. Surg Neurol 35(3):183–188
26. Motuel J, Biette I, Srairi M, Mrozek S, Kurrek MM, Chaynes P, et al (2014) Assessment of brain midline shift using sonography in neurosurgical ICU patients. Crit Care [Internet];18(6). http://ccforum.biomedcentral.com/articles/10.1186/s13054-014-0676-9. Cited 16 Jan 2017
27. Kiphuth IC, Huttner HB, Struffert T, Schwab S, Köhrmann M (2011) Sonographic monitoring of ventricle enlargement in posthemorrhagic hydrocephalus. Neurology 76(10):858–862
28. Tsivgoulis G, Alexandrov AV, Sloan MA (2009) Advances in transcranial Doppler ultrasonography. Curr Neurol Neurosci Rep 9(1):46–54
29. Schatlo B, Pluta RM (2007) Clinical applications of transcranial Doppler sonography. Rev Recent Clin Trials 2(1):49–57
30. Naqvi J, Yap KH, Ahmad G, Ghosh J (2013) Transcranial Doppler ultrasound: a review of the physical principles and major applications in critical care. Int J Vasc Med [Internet] http://www.hindawi.com/journals/ijvm/2013/629378/abs/. Cited 16 Jan 2017
31. Saqqur M, Zygun D, Demchuk A (2007) Role of transcranial Doppler in neurocritical care. Crit Care Med 35(5):S216–S223
32. Akif Topcuoglu M (2012) Transcranial Doppler ultrasound in neurovascular diseases: diagnostic and therapeutic aspects. J Neurochem 123(s2):39–51
33. Van Gijn J, Kerr RS, Rinkel GJ (2007) Subarachnoid haemorrhage. Lancet 369(9558):306–318
34. Bleck TP (1997) Rebleeding and vasospasm after SAH: new strategies for improving outcome. J Crit Illn. 12:572–589
35. Rigamonti A, Ackery A, Baker AJ (2008) Transcranial Doppler monitoring in subarachnoid hemorrhage: a critical tool in critical care. Can J Anesth 55(2):112–123
36. Lindegaard K-F, Nornes H, Bakke SJ, Sorteberg W, Nakstad P (1989) Cerebral vasospasm diagnosis by means of angiography and blood velocity measurements. Acta Neurochir (Wien) 100(1–2):12–24
37. Krejza J, Szydlik P, Liebeskind DS, Kochanowicz J, Bronov O, Mariak Z et al (2005) Age and sex variability and normal reference values for the V(MCA)/V(ICA) index. AJNR Am J Neuroradiol 26(4):730–735
38. Mascia L, Fedorko L, terBrugge K, Filippini C, Pizzio M, Ranieri VM et al (2003) The accuracy of transcranial Doppler to detect vasospasm in patients with aneurysmal subarachnoid hemorrhage. Intensive Care Med 29(7):1088–1094
39. Muñoz-Sanchez MA, Murillo-Cabezas F, Egea-Guerrero JJ, Gascón-Castillo ML, Cancela P, Amaya-Villar R et al (2012) Emergency transcranial Doppler ultrasound: predictive value for the development of symptomatic vasospasm in spontaneous subarachnoid hemorrhage in patients in good neurological condition. Med Intensiva 36(9):611–618
40. Wozniak MA, Sloan MA, Rothman MI, Burch CM, Rigamonti D, Permutt T et al (1996) Detection of vasospasm by transcranial Doppler sonography. J Neuroimaging 6(2):87–93
41. Caricato A, Pitoni S, Montini L, Bocci MG, Annetta P, Antonelli M (2014) Echography in brain imaging in intensive care unit: state of the art. World J Radiol 6(9):636
42. Vora YY, Suarez-Almazor M, Steinke DE, Martin ML, Findlay JM (1999) Role of transcranial Doppler monitoring in the diagnosis of cerebral vasospasm after subarachnoid hemorrhage. Neurosurgery 44(6):1237–1247
43. Toi H, Matsumoto N, Yokosuka K, Matsubara S, Hirano K, Uno M (2013) Prediction of cerebral vasospasm using early stage transcranial Doppler. Neurol Med Chir (Tokyo) 53(6):396–402
44. Sloan MA, Alexandrov AV, Tegeler CH, Spencer MP, Caplan LR, Feldmann E et al (2004) Assessment: transcranial Doppler ultrasonography: report of the therapeutics and Technology Assessment Subcommittee of the American Academy of Neurology. Neurology 62(9):1468–1481
45. Alexandrov AV, Sloan MA, Tegeler CH, Newell DN, Lumsden A, Garami Z et al (2012) Practice standards for transcranial Doppler (TCD) ultrasound. part II. clinical indications and expected outcomes. J Neuroimaging Off J Am Soc Neuroimaging 22(3):215–224
46. Connolly ES, Rabinstein AA, Carhuapoma JR, Derdeyn CP, Dion J, Higashida RT et al (2012) Guidelines for the management of aneurysmal subarachnoid hemorrhage: a guideline for healthcare professionals from the American Heart Association/American Stroke Association. Stroke 43(6):1711–1737
47. Marinoni M, Ginanneschi A, Forleo P, Amaducci L (1997) Technical limits in transcranial Doppler recording: inadquate acoustic windows. Ultrasound Med Biol 23(8):1275–1277
48. Baumgartner RW (1999) Transcranial color-coded duplex sonography. J Neurol 246(8):637–647

49. Vollmer DG, Torner JC, Jane JA, Sadovnic B, Charlebois D, Eisenberg HM et al (1991) Age and outcome following traumatic coma: why do older patients fare worse? Spec Suppl 75(1S):S37–S49
50. Graham DI, Adams JH, Gennarelli TA (1993) Pathology of brain damage in head injury. Head Inj.91–113
51. Chan K-H, Miller JD, Dearden NM, Andrews PJ, Midgley S (1992) The effect of changes in cerebral perfusion pressure upon middle cerebral artery blood flow velocity and jugular bulb venous oxygen saturation after severe brain injury. J Neurosurg 77(1):55–61
52. Rosenfeld JV, Maas AI, Bragge P, Morganti-Kossmann MC, Manley GT, Gruen RL (2012) Early management of severe traumatic brain injury. Lancet 380(9847):1088–1098
53. Klingelhöfer J, Conrad B, Benecke R, Sander D (1987) Intracranial flow patterns at increasing intracranial pressure. Klin Wochenschr 65(12):542–545
54. Klingelhöfer J, Conrad B, Benecke R, Sander D, Markakis E (1988) Evaluation of intracranial pressure from transcranial Doppler studies in cerebral disease. J Neurol 235(3):159–162
55. Homburg A-M, Jakobsen M, Enevoldsen E (1993) Transcranial Doppler recordings in raised intracranial pressure. Acta Neurol Scand 87(6):488–493
56. Varsos GV, Richards H, Kasprowicz M, Budohoski KP, Brady KM, Reinhard M et al (2013) Critical closing pressure determined with a model of cerebrovascular impedance. J Cereb Blood Flow Metab 33(2):235–243
57. Czosnyka M, Matta BF, Smielewski P, Kirkpatrick PJ, Pickard JD (1998) Cerebral perfusion pressure in head-injured patients: a noninvasive assessment using transcranial Doppler ultrasonography. J Neurosurg 88(5):802–808
58. Cardim D, Schmidt B, Robba C, Donnelly J, Puppo C, Czosnyka M et al (2017) Transcranial Doppler monitoring of intracranial pressure plateau waves. Neurocrit Care 26(3):330–338
59. de Riva N, Budohoski KP, Smielewski P, Kasprowicz M, Zweifel C, Steiner LA et al (2012) Transcranial Doppler pulsatility index: what it is and what it isn't. Neurocrit Care 17(1):58–66
60. Figaji AA, Zwane E, Fieggen AG, Siesjo P, Peter JC (2009) Transcranial Doppler pulsatility index is not a reliable indicator of intracranial pressure in children with severe traumatic brain injury. Surg Neurol 72(4):389–394
61. Hanlo PW, Gooskens RHJM, Nijhuis IJM, Faber JAJ, Peters RJA, van Huffelen AC et al (1995) Value of transcranial Doppler indices in predicting raised ICP in infantile hydrocephalus. Childs Nerv Syst. 11(10):595–603
62. Rainov NG, Weise JB, Burkert W (2000) Transcranial Doppler sonography in adult hydrocephalic patients. Neurosurg Rev 23(1):34–38
63. Cardim D, Robba C, Bohdanowicz M, Donnelly J, Cabella B, Liu X et al (2016) Non-invasive monitoring of intracranial pressure using transcranial Doppler ultrasonography: is it possible? Neurocrit Care 25(3):473–491
64. Cardim D, Robba C, Donnelly J, Bohdanowicz M, Schmidt B, Damian M et al (2015) Prospective study on noninvasive assessment of intracranial pressure in traumatic brain-injured patients: comparison of four methods. J Neurotrauma 33(8):792–802
65. Monteiro LM, Bollen CW, van Huffelen AC, Ackerstaff RG, Jansen NJ, van Vught AJ (2006) Transcranial Doppler ultrasonography to confirm brain death: a meta-analysis. Intensive Care Med 32(12):1937–1944
66. Kuo JR, Chen CF, Chio CC, Chang CH, Wang CC, Yang CM et al (2006) Time dependent validity in the diagnosis of brain death using transcranial Doppler sonography. J Neurol Neurosurg Psychiatry 77(5):646–649
67. Chassé M, Glen P, Doyle M-A, McIntyre L, English SW, Knoll G et al (2013) Ancillary testing for diagnosis of brain death: a protocol for a systematic review and meta-analysis. Syst Rev 2(1):1
68. Dosemeci L, Dora B, Yilmaz M, Cengiz M, Balkan S, Ramazanoglu A (2004) Utility of transcranial doppler ultrasonography for confirmatory diagnosis of brain death: two sides of the coin. Transplantation 77(1):71–75
69. Poularas J, Karakitsos D, Kouraklis G, Kostakis A, De Groot E, Kalogeromitros A, et al (2006) Comparison between transcranial color Doppler ultrasonography and angiography in the confirmation of brain death. In: Transplantation proceedings [Internet]. Elsevier. pp 1213–1217. http://www.sciencedirect.com/science/article/pii/S004113450600217X Cited 16 Jan 2017
70. De Freitas GR, Andre C (2006) Sensitivity of transcranial Doppler for confirming brain death: a prospective study of 270 cases. Acta Neurol Scand 113(6):426–432

# 13

# Ultrasound assessment of visual loss during severe preeclampsia

Fehmi Ferhi[1,2,3*], Abdeljalil Khlifi[3,4], Feten Hachani[3,4], Khalil Tarmiz[1,2,3] and Khaled Benjazia[1,2,3]

**Abstract**

Bilateral retinal detachments and cortical blindness are rare complications of preeclampsia and the association of the two pathologies is exceptional. We report the case of a preeclamptic patient who presented with an acute bilateral vision loss. Besides, her ocular ultrasound revealed bilateral retinal detachments and an elevated optic nerve sheath diameter. The patient underwent an urgent cesarean section. Subsequently, magnetic resonance imaging and ocular fundus examination confirmed the diagnosis.

**Keywords:** Cortical blindness, Ocular ultrasound, Optic nerve sheath diameter, Preeclampsia, Retinal detachments

## Background

Preeclampsia is a multisystem hypertensive disorder and is mainly responsible for the world's largest maternal morbidity and mortality. Visual symptoms, such as scotomota, amaurosis, blurred vision, diplopia, chromatopsia, or homonymous hemianopsia, may occur in 25% of preeclamptic women [1]. Blindness is usually attributed to retinal abnormalities including edema and vascular changes, such as retinal arteriolar vasospasm, thrombosis of the central retinal artery, or retinal detachment. Transient cortical blindness due to focal cerebral edema is estimated to occur in about 1–15% of eclamptic women [2].

Given the magnitude of the neurological effects of preeclampsia, real-time assessment of the cerebrovascular and ocular changes associated with this condition are challenging with established modalities such as computed tomography, magnetic resonance imaging and ocular fundus examination [3, 4].

We report the case of a preeclamptic patient who presented with acute bilateral vision loss. Bedside ocular ultrasound revealed a bilateral retinal detachment and an elevated optic nerve sheath diameter.

*Correspondence: fehmiferhi@hotmail.fr

[1] Department of Anaesthesiology and Critical Care Medicine, Farhat Hached University Hospital Center, 4002 Sousse, Tunisia

Full list of author information is available at the end of the article

## Case report

A 24-year-old primigravida woman presented to the obstetric emergency department at 35 weeks of gestation complaining of bilateral vision loss. There was nothing abnormal with her previous medical history and she had no history of previous ophthalmologic disorders. The patient reported a mild headache that has been going on for the past 2 days.

Clinical examination showed an important peripheral edema. Vital signs were as follows: pulse rate 105 beats/min, blood pressure 186/115 mmHg, respiratory rate 20 breaths/min, temperature 36.9 °C, and oxygen saturation 98% on air. Visual acuity in the two eyes was finger-counting at less than 1 m. Her pupils were equal and reactive to light. Neurologic examination showed exaggerated deep tendon reflexes.

Proteinuria dipstick was 3+. Laboratory tests revealed anemia at 103 g/L, thrombocytopenia with platelets count at 97 × $10^9$/L and elevated liver enzymes (GOT 82 U/I, GPT 78 U/I, alkaline phosphatase 168 U/I). The remaining laboratory tests, including electrolytes, creatinine, bilirubin, and coagulation tests, were within normal limits.

A bedside ultrasound was performed by an anesthesiologist trained in bedside focused ultrasonography using a 7.5-MHz linear probe (mindray DC 70 Shenzhen, China). Sagittal and transverse planes of the right and left globe were obtained by asking the patient to close her eyelids and then applying ultrasound gel to the inside and outside of a sterile sheath covering the probe as it was gently placed on each eyelid. To measure the optic nerve sheath diameter (ONSD), the placement of the probe was adjusted to view the entry of the optic nerve into the globe. We used an electronic caliper and an axis perpendicular to the optic nerve 3 mm behind the lamina cribosa. The Mechanical Index and Thermal Index were reduced to 0.2 and 1, respectively.

Sonographies detected in the right and left eye a hyper-echoic stripe extending to the optic nerve head, but not across it. The point of fixation of the retina at the optic nerve head was respected. When the patient was also asked to look in various directions with her eyelids closed, the hyper-echoic line undulated with the associated ocular movements, which was suggestive of retinal detachment (RD). The ONSD was measured at 6.9 mm in the right eye (Fig. 1a) and 6.6 mm in the left eye (Fig. 1b), suggesting an elevated intracranial pressure. The patient tolerated the sonogram without pain or complications.

Obstetric ultrasound revealed an intra-uterine fetus with a heart rate of 140 beats/min and a fetal biometry consistent with a 34-week gestation.

Based on these findings, the patient was diagnosed with severe preeclampsia complicated by hemolysis, elevated liver enzymes and low platelets (HELLP) syndrome, bilateral RD and cerebral edema. Therefore, the patient underwent an urgent cesarean section delivery under spinal anesthesia and was immediately administrated an intravenous Magnesium Sulfate and Nicardipine infusion which were maintained 24 h after delivery. Blood pressure was then controlled with Methyldopa 500 mg 6 hourly and Amlodipine 10 mg 12 hourly.

Magnetic resonance imaging (MRI) performed 24 h after delivery showed T2 hyperintensities on flair indicating parieto-occipital and temporal distribution of vasogenic edema. A dilated fundoscopic examination using an ophthalmoscope performed by an ophthalmologist subsequently confirmed the diagnosis of bilateral exudative retinal detachments.

During 1 week, a daily ocular sonogram was performed. The ONSD was back to a normal range after arterial blood pressure control. The RD regressed but it was difficult to objectify it.

Within 3 weeks of delivery, her visual acuity had returned to normal without any further treatment. At that time, the slit lamp examination was normal.

## Discussion

This case highlights a possible association between two etiologies of vision loss during severe preeclampsia and the interest of bedside ocular sonography for reliable assessing.

The most frequent ophthalmologic manifestation of preeclampsia is the vasoconstriction of the retinal arterioles. The prevalence of this disorder increases with severity [5]. It is mostly asymptomatic and regresses without sequelae after delivery. Other clinically noisier manifestations are very rare, and we can mention among them cortical blindness and retinal serous detachment. The association of the two pathologies is exceptional [6].

Computed tomography (CT) and MRI brain imaging are mandatory to make the diagnosis of cerebral edema, but they are expensive and cannot be carried out in real-time assessing [3]. Retinal examination for papilledema or RD seems sometimes difficult. Actually most anesthesiologists and emergency physicians are more comfortable using an ultrasound machine than an ophthalmoscope. In addition, ultrasound is bedside available, reproducible and non-invasive [4].

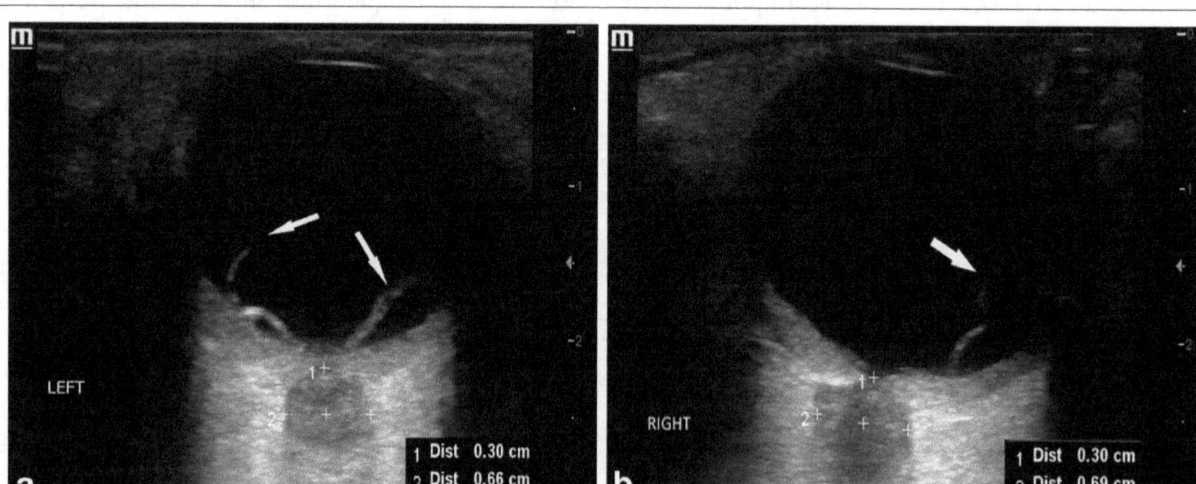


**Fig. 1** **a** Ocular ultrasound of the left eye demonstrating retinal detachment (white arrows) and optic nerve sheath diameter enlargement. **b** Ocular ultrasound of the right eye demonstrating retinal detachment (white arrow) and optic nerve sheath diameter enlargement

Preeclampsia can be associated with brain edema and raised intracranial pressure (ICP) [6]. Increases in ICP are transmitted by the cerebrospinal fluid down the perineural subarachnoid space of the optic nerve, causing an expansion of the nerve sheath [7]. ONSD measured by ultrasound has proved to be highly predictive of intracranial pressure in the settings of traumatic brain injury and neurological pathology [8]. Dubost et al. [9] measured ONSD in patients with preeclampsia and compared the findings with those obtained in healthy pregnant women. They found that median ONSD values were significantly higher in preeclamptic patients at delivery and that in about 20% of preeclamptic patients ONSD values were above 5.8 mm. This threshold diameter was associated with 95% risk of raised ICP (above 20 mmHg) [8]. This technique is rapidly acquired by non-radiologist physicians [10, 11].

RD is a well-documented complication of preeclampsia affecting 0.1–2% of patients [12]. Women who have HELLP syndrome are 7 times more likely to develop RD than those who do not have HELLP syndrome. RD is more frequent in primiparous women. It is usually bilateral and tends to be diagnosed during the last trimester or shortly after delivery [13]. The main pathogenesis of this disease includes generalized vasoconstriction and choroidal ischemia affecting the retinal pigment epithelium, leading to a breakdown of the blood–retinal barrier and a leakage of proteins and fluid from the choriocapillaries into the subretinal space [14]. Focal ischemia caused by capillary obstruction is even more severe when associated to hemolysis of the red blood cells, such as the case of HELLP syndrome [13]. Patients usually have complete recovery of vision with complete resolution of RD within 2–12 weeks postpartum [14].

Ocular ultrasound has proved to be a useful tool for diagnosing most ophthalmic pathologies including retinal detachments, vitreous hemorrhage, papilledema, lens dislocation and globe rupture. The sensitivity and specificity of ultrasound for the diagnosis of retinal detachments were reported to be high [15].

Regarding the mechanical and biological risks of exposing the eye to high-frequency probes, sonography side effects have not been reported up to now. In animal studies, rabbit corneas and retinas were exposed to ultrasound ranging from 10 to 60 MHz for up to 30 min with no deleterious effects [16]. Nevertheless, mechanical energy is transmitted into the eye and more than $4–10 \times 10^6$ oscillations may warm the intraocular fluid. Therefore, it is important to limit the examination time and gain according to the ALARA ("as low as reasonably applicable") principle and reduce Mechanical Index and Thermal Index less than 0.23 and 1, respectively.

Actually preeclampsia especially when severe is associated with an increased risk of maternal retinal disease in the decades following pregnancy [17]. Ocular ultrasound may have a useful role in the assessment strategy of neurological and retinal events in preeclampsia, potentially allowing for more appropriately targeted therapy and survey [3].

In this case, ocular ultrasound was performed by an anesthesiologist using a 7.5-MHz linear probe placed gently over the closed eyelid. This rapid bedside examination quickly helped us to refine our diagnosis in a preeclamptic patient with a life-threatening condition and allowed us to make a rapid decision.

#### Abbreviations

RD: retinal detachments; ONSD: the optic nerve sheath diameter; HELLP syndrome: hemolysis, elevated liver enzymes, and low platelets syndrome; MRI: magnetic resonance imaging; CT: computed tomography; ICP: intracranial pressure.

#### Authors' contributions

FF realized POCUS, AK and FH helped in case-report redaction, KT and KB revised the manuscript. All authors read and approved the final manuscript.

#### Author details

[1] Department of Anaesthesiology and Critical Care Medicine, Farhat Hached University Hospital Center, 4002 Sousse, Tunisia. [2] The Research Unit on Maternal Morbidity and Mortality UR17SP08, Sousse, Tunisia. [3] Ibn Jazzar Medical School Sousse, Avenue Mohamed El Karoui, 4002 Sousse, Tunisia. [4] Department of Obstetrics and Gynaecology, Farhat Hached University Hospital Center, 4002 Sousse, Tunisia.

#### Acknowledgements

None.

#### References

1. Roos NM, Wiegman MJ, Jansonius NM, Zeeman GG (2012) Visual disturbances in (pre)eclampsia. Obstet Gynecol Surv 67(4):242–250. https://doi.org/10.1097/ogx.0b013e318250a457
2. Cunningham FG, Fernandez CO, Hernandez C (1995) Blindness associated with preeclampsia and eclampsia. Am J Obstet Gynecol 172:1291–1298. https://doi.org/10.1016/0002-9378(95)91495-1
3. Kane SC, Brennecke SP, Da Silva Costa F (2017) Ophthalmic artery doppler analysis: a window into the cerebrovasculature of women with preeclampsia. Ultrasound Obstet Gynecol 49(1):15–21. https://doi.org/10.1002/uog.17209
4. Rollins M, Flood P (2012) Imaging intracranial pressure: an introduction to ultrasonography of the optic nerve sheath. Anesthesiology 116:983–984. https://doi.org/10.1097/aln.0b013e31824c16e4
5. Jaffe G, Schatz H (1987) Ocular manifestations of preeclampsia. Am J Ophthalmol 103(3 Pt 1):309–315
6. Zeeman GG (2009) Neurologic complications of pre-eclampsia. Semin Perinatol 33(3):166–172. https://doi.org/10.1053/j.semperi.2009.02.003
7. Hansen H, Helmke K (1996) The subarachnoid space surrounding the optic nerves. An ultrasound study of the optic nerve sheath. Surg Radiol Anat 18(4):323–328. https://doi.org/10.1007/BF01627611
8. Dubourg J, Javouhey E, Geeraerts T, Messerer M, Kassai B (2011) Ultrasonography of optic nerve sheath diameter for detection of raised intracranial pressure: a systematic review and meta-analysis. Intensive Care Med 37(7):1059–1068. https://doi.org/10.1007/s00134-011-2224-2

9. Dubost C, Le Gouez A, Jouffroy V, Roger-Christoph S, Benhamou D, Mercier FJ, Geeraerts T (2012) Optic nerve sheath diameter used as ultrasonographic assessment of the incidence of raised intracranial pressure in preeclampsia: a pilot study. Anesthesiology 116:1066–1071. https://doi.org/10.1097/aln.0b013e318246ea1a
10. Potgieter DW, Kippin A, Ngu F, McKean C (2011) Can accurate ultrasonographic measurement of the optic nerve sheath diameter (a non-invasive measure of intracranial pressure) be taught to novice operators in a single training session? Anaesth Intensive Care 39:95–100
11. Lochner P, Coppo L, Cantello R, Nardone R, Naldi A, Leone MA, Brigo F (2016) Intra- and interobserver reliability of transorbital sonographic assessment of the optic nerve sheath diameter and optic nerve diameter in healthy adults. J Ultrasound 19(1):41–45. https://doi.org/10.1007/s40477-014-0144-z
12. Schultz KL, Birnbaum AD, Goldstein DA (2005) Ocular disease in pregnancy. Curr Opin Ophthalmol 16(5):308–314. https://doi.org/10.1097/01.icu.0000179803.42218.cc
13. Vigil-De Gracia P, Ortega-Paz L (2011) Retinal detachment in association with pre eclampsia, eclampsia and HELLP syndrome. Int J Gynecol Obstet 114:223–225. https://doi.org/10.1016/j.ijgo.2011.04.003
14. Amer R, Nalcı H, Yalçındağ N (2017) Exudative retinal detachment. Surv Ophthalmol 62(6):723–769. https://doi.org/10.1016/j.survophthal.2017.05.001
15. Vrablik ME, Snead GR, Minnigan HJ, Kirschner JM, Emmett TW, Seupaul RA (2015) The diagnostic accuracy of bedside ocular ultrasonography for the diagnosis of retinal detachment: a systematic review and meta-analysis. Ann Emerg Med 65(2):199–203. https://doi.org/10.1016/j.annemergmed.2014.02.020
16. Torloni MR, Vedmedovska N, Merialdi M, Betrán AP, Allen T, ISUOG-WHO Fetal Growth Study Group et al (2009) Safety of ultrasonography in pregnancy: WHO systematic review of the literature and meta-analysis. Ultrasound Obstet Gynecol 33:599–608. https://doi.org/10.1002/uog.6328
17. Auger N, Fraser WD, Paradis G, Healy-Profitós J, Hsieh A, Rhéaume MA (2017) Preeclampsia and long-term risk of maternal retinal disorders. Obstet Gynecol 129(1):42–49. https://doi.org/10.1097/aog.0000000000001758

# 14

# Combined lung and brain ultrasonography for an individualized "brain-protective ventilation strategy" in neurocritical care patients with challenging ventilation needs

Francesco Corradi[1], Chiara Robba[2,3], Guido Tavazzi[4,5] and Gabriele Via[6*]

**Abstract**

When intracranial hypertension and severe lung damage coexist in the same clinical scenario, their management poses a difficult challenge, especially as concerns mechanical ventilation management. The needs of combined lung and brain protection from secondary damage may conflict, as ventilation strategies commonly used in patients with ARDS are potentially associated with an increased risk of intracranial hypertension. In particular, the use of positive end-expiratory pressure, recruitment maneuvers, prone positioning, and protective lung ventilation can have undesirable effects on cerebral physiology: they may positively or negatively affect intracranial pressure, based on the final repercussions on $PaO_2$ and cerebral perfusion pressure (through changes in cardiac output, mean arterial pressure, venous return, $PaO_2$ and $PaCO_2$), also according to the baseline conditions of cerebral autoregulation. Lung ultrasound (LUS) and brain ultrasound (BUS, as a combination of optic nerve sheath diameter assessment and cerebrovascular Doppler ultrasound) have independently proven their potential in respectively monitoring lung aeration and brain physiology at the bedside. In this narrative review, we describe how the combined use of LUS and BUS on neurocritical patients with demanding mechanical ventilation needs can contribute to ventilation management, with the aim of a tailored "brain-protective ventilation strategy."

**Keywords:** ARDS, Brain injury, Lung ultrasound, Brain ultrasound, Neuro-critical care, Respiratory monitoring, Intracranial hypertension, Mechanical ventilation

## Brain injury and severe lung disease: a challenging combination with conflicting therapeutical needs

Intracranial hypertension and severe lung damage may coexist in a variety of clinical settings and pose a difficult challenge, especially in mechanical ventilation management. The two conditions may be caused by the same pathological insult, one be the cause of the other, negatively affect each other in several ways, and in any case may present conflicting therapeutical needs (Fig. 1). This occurs mainly in the context of multiple trauma with severe traumatic brain injury (TBI) [1], but also in patients with subarachnoid hemorrhage [2] and acute liver failure [3]. Acute respiratory syndrome (ARDS) represents altogether a common in-hospital complication after admission for TBI, reaching more than 20% in the adult population [1]. Many ventilation strategies commonly used in patients with ARDS are potentially associated with an increased risk of intracranial hypertension. In particular, the use of positive end-expiratory pressure (PEEP), recruitment maneuvers (RM) and prone positioning (PP) can have undesirable effects on cerebral physiology, by impeding cerebral venous return and decreasing mean arterial pressure (MAP);

*Correspondence: Gabriele.via@gmail.com
[6] Cardiac Anesthesia and Intensive Care, Cardiocentro Ticino, Via Tesserete, 48, Lugano, Switzerland
Full list of author information is available at the end of the article

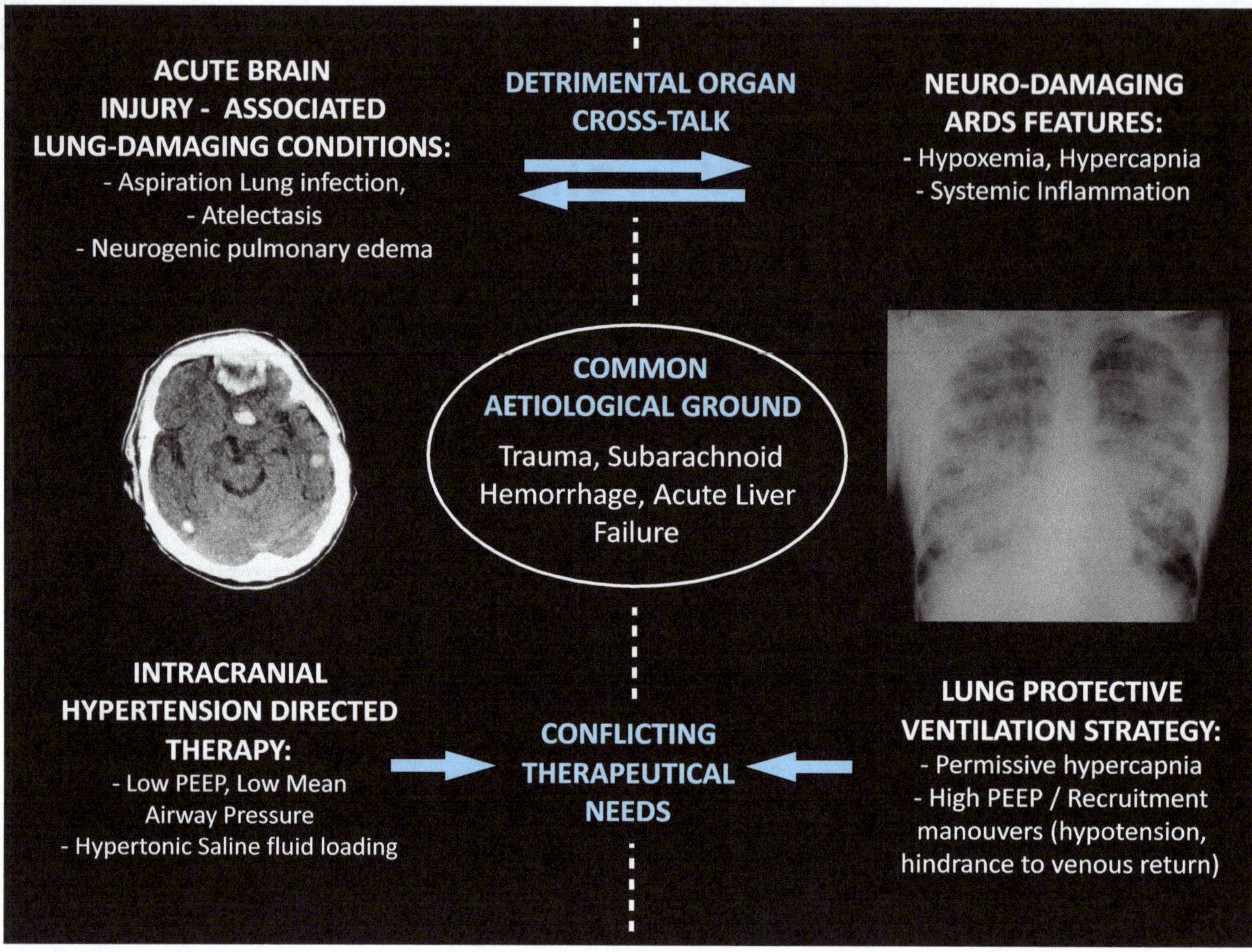


**Fig. 1** Potential pathophysiological interactions between severe brain injury and severe lung injury, and their conflicting therapeutical needs. Severe brain injury and severe lung damage may ensue as consequence of the same noxious agent (for example in severe multiple trauma or severe liver failure), but also one be the cause of the other (e.g., neurogenic pulmonary edema in subarachnoid hemorrhage, or lung aspiration and infection in a comatous patient). Indeed, once coexisting, disease of one organ can negatively affect the other, in a harmful organ cross-talk (e.g., hypoxemia can worsen brain damage). Finally, some therapeutical interventions directed at protecting one organ may have detrimental effects on the other (e.g., mechanical ventilation strategies can either reduce systemic mean arterial pressure, decrease cerebral venous return, or cause cerebral vasodilation, thus inducing a worsening of intracranial hypertension and reducing the cerebral perfusion pressure)

furthermore, lung protective ventilation (aiming at airway plateau pressures < 28–30 $cmH_2O$, driving pressures < 14 $cmH_2O$ or delta transpulmonary pressures < 10–12 $cmH_2O$) may cause hypercarbia, that may result in intracranial pressure (ICP) increases by aggravating a preexisting alteration of cerebral autoregulation [4]. These ARDS ventilation strategies therefore carry a high potential risk for iatrogenic secondary brain damage [5, 6]. Other clinical conditions, even without reaching the severity of ARDS, may pose cerebral protection in conflict with the need of moderate-high PEEP levels. Neurogenic pulmonary edema is a well-known complication of subarachnoid hemorrhage [7], that may represent such a circumstance. Even ventilating an obese neurocritical patient will inevitably raise the conflict between the need to keep the lung open with higher-than-usual PEEP levels [8] and to minimize any hindrance to cerebral venous return. Continuous positive airway pressure has in fact shown to carry the risk of decreasing cerebral perfusion pressure (CPP) and cerebral blood flow (CBF) in both healthy volunteers [9] and brain-injured patients [10].

However, existing data on this phenomenon are conflicting, and must be interpreted with caution. In a first study [9], the drop in CPP and CBF was due to hypocapnic vasoconstriction and not directly related to PEEP. Moreover, the PEEP applied was higher than commonly used in clinical practice and not titrated according to respiratory mechanics. Finally, population studied was composed of spontaneously breathing patients, and the results cannot be assumed to be applicable to deeply sedated patients on invasive mechanical ventilation. In another study [10], alterations of CPP were secondary to MAP reduction and not directly related to PEEP application, but lack of PEEP titration makes the interpretation of data difficult.

Indeed, while properly titrated PEEP can improve cardiac output, especially when left ventricular failure coexists with brain injury, excessive PEEP exposes to lung over-distention and right ventricular impairment [11]. Some authors demonstrated that if PEEP values are below ICP values, then the associated augmentation of intrathoracic pressure does not result in increased ICP [12]. Also, when increased PEEP is applied to brain-injured patients with ARDS, there is a substantial difference in the effects on ICP, depending on whether the application of PEEP causes alveolar hyperinflation or alveolar recruitment and therefore on lung stiffness [13]. Consequently, it is currently unknown which is the optimal level of PEEP in acutely brain-injured patients [14]. Similarly, prone positioning and recruitment maneuvers can increase ICP [6] and their use in brain-injured patients must be weighed in light of the beneficial improvements in oxygenation and gas exchange, which could by far exceed the negative effect of increases of ICP.

In essence, whatever ventilatory adjustment/manouvre may positively or negatively affect ICP in the neurocritical patient, based on its final repercussions on $PaO_2$ and on CPP, according to the baseline conditions of cerebral autoregulation.

Recent advances in critical care ultrasound have shown the wide use and clinical impact of point-of-care ultrasonography in critical care units [15] as well as the utility of a multimodal, integrated approach [16].

## Lung ultrasound (LUS) monitoring in the mechanically ventilated patient

International evidence-based consensus on point-of-care lung ultrasound (LUS) [17] recommends its use to track changes in aeration of lung parenchyma, by providing a semi-quantification [18, 19] of these changes and hence monitor lung disease evolution. Several are its applications. LUS can easily *characterize morphologic features of ARDS* [20], *discriminate between focal and diffuse ARDS,* and provide a picture of the heterogeneity of aeration distribution [21]: focal ARDS is characterized by a normal LUS pattern in upper anterior and lateral lung regions and consolidation or B-lines in lower posterior and lateral ones (dependent lung regions in supine position); in diffuse ARDS, which is present in a minority of patients, aeration loss is homogeneously distributed among lung regions, with a diffuse ubiquitous LUS B-pattern. Overdistention cannot be directly measured by LUS and this represents its greatest limitation, although a reduction of physiological lung sliding in anterior regions may be observed when airway pressure is too high [22].

A simple qualitative LUS evaluation has the potential to predict the occurrence of ARDS in blunt trauma patients [23], and *predict the response to PEEP-induced lung recruitment* and PEEP-induced increase in $PaO_2$ in ARDS patients [24]. Although the same LUS global reareation score applied to ARDS patients failed to predict the response to pronation in terms of oxygenation improvement, basal ARDS morphology described by means of LUS before pronation (focal vs. diffuse morphology) was predictive of effective reareation of dorsal areas, of immediate $PaO_2/FiO_2$ improvement and $pCO_2$ decrease [25, 26]. LUS has also proven utility in *discerning different degrees of disease severity at a very early stage of ARDS* [27]. Finally, it has been demonstrated to accurately *track changes in EVLW,* through a bedside quantitative approach [17, 19, 28, 29].

## Brain ultrasonography (BUS) as bedside monitor of cerebral physiology

Brain ultrasonography, including transcranial Doppler (TCD) and the measurement of optic nerve sheath diameter (ONSD), is an evolving technique that has shown promising results in adult [30, 31] and pediatric populations [32] for the non-invasive assessment of ICP (nICP), cerebral perfusion pressure (CPP), as well as for the calculation of advanced parameters such as critical closing pressure and cerebral compliance [33]. Although the invasive intracranial catheter remains the gold standard for ICP measurement, these methods could be helpful when invasive tools are not indicated (i.e., milder than severe degrees of traumatic brain injury) [34], contraindicated (patients with hemostatic disorders) or unavailable (such as in general intensive care) [30].

Increased intrathoracic pressure and consequent ICP elevation produces specific changes in *cerebral arterial blood flow velocity* (FV) waveform that can be assessed by *decreases in the diastolic FV* and *increases in the pulsatility index* (PI = systolic FV − diastolic FV)/mean FV). In mild to moderate TBI, values of $PI > 1.25$ or a diastolic $FV < 25$ cm/s are considered pathological, and associated to secondary neurological deterioration [34, 35]. *Increases of ONSD* above a cut-off of 6 mm strongly suggest an increased ICP > 20 mmHg [36, 37]. Venous TCD provides further information. A *reduction of venous FV at the level of the straight sinus* (with a cut-off of 38.50 cm/s) has proven to be a good predictor of ICP above 20 mmHg [36]. Therefore, it is intuitive how this index could be useful in neurocritical care patients with challenging mechanical ventilation conditions, where an important pathophysiological mechanism for ICP increase is related to venous return impairment caused by increased intrathoracic pressures.

In a recent study, *TCD and ONSD were tested as surrogate non-invasive measures of ICP changes during prone position and/or PEEP* in non-brain-injured patients undergoing spine surgery [38]: mean ONSD increased significantly upon prone positioning and upon a PEEP application of 8 $cmH_2O$, suggesting that these methods may be applicable in the clinical practice to non-invasively monitor cerebrovascular changes during prone position and PEEP increase during mechanical ventilation. ONSD measurement in the prone position can be easily performed by one operator while an assistant holds the head rotated 30 degrees rightward (to measure the right ONSD) and then 30 degrees leftward (to measure the left ONSD) [38].

Similarly, *BUS can detect relevant changes in cerebrovascular dynamics associated to ICP increases upon recruitment maneuvers* (Fig. 2). In particular, transcranial Doppler has a primarily role in the evaluation of alteration of cerebral blood flow associated with changes in

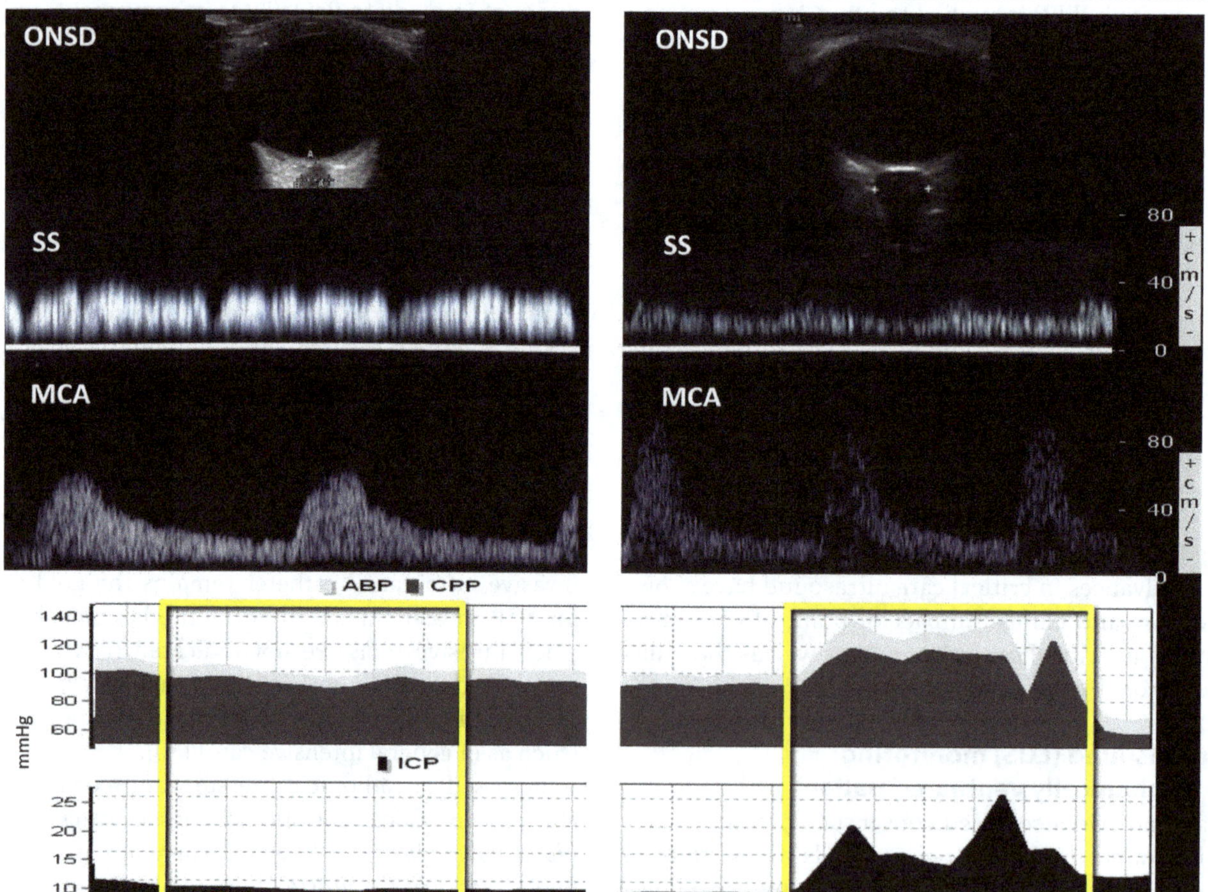


**Fig. 2** Invasive and non-invasive intracranial pressure monitoring, respectively, through ICP Bolt and through brain ultrasound (BUS, optic nerve sheath diameter and cerebrovascular Doppler sampling) in a patient with traumatic brain injury and ARDS. A 26-year-old lady was admitted to the intensive care unit after a road traffic accident. She presented with severe traumatic brain injury (TBI) and chest trauma with lung contusions. She was monitored with invasive ICP, intubated and mechanically ventilated. On day 2, she developed hypoxic respiratory failure with bilateral atelectasia. We therefore performed recruitment maneuvers with ABP, CPP, and ICP monitoring and concomitant ONSD and TCD measurements (venous TCD on the SS and arterious TCD on the MCA). Recordings and scanning were performed at baseline (left panels) and during a recruitment maneuver and subsequent increase in PEEP level (right panels). Initially, ICP was below 20 mmHg (mean ONSD = 5.2), with PEEP = 8, with stable arterial blood pressure (ABP) and cerebral perfusion pressure (CPP). After recruitment maneuvers and setting PEEP at 16, ICP spiked up > 20 mmHg, with reflex mean systemic arterial blood pressure (ABP) and cerebral perfusion pressure (CPP) increase. BUS showed consistent increase in middle cerebral artery (MCA) pulsatility index (decrease in diastolic flow, increase in systolic flow), reduction in straight sinus (SS) flow, and increase in optic nerve sheath diameter (ONSD = 7 mm). $PaCO_2$ remained constant during the procedure and the patients experienced no hypotension nor cardiac output decrease. We therefore reduced PEEP levels and noticed that ICP immediately decreased as well as PI, ONSD and the venous flow on the straight sinus. *MCA* middle cerebral artery, *SS* straight sinus, *ONSD* optic nerve sheath diameter, *ABP* mean systemic arterial blood pressure, *ICP* intracranial pressure, *CPP* cerebral perfusion pressure

(See figure on next page.)

**Fig. 3** Lung ultrasound–Brain ultrasound (LUS–BUS) combined respiratory and neurological monitoring in patients with traumatic brain injury (TBI) and acute respiratory distress syndrome (ARDS). A four-tiered approach is suggested, in order to decide the best ventilatory strategy and simultaneously monitor the effects on intracranial pressure (ICP) and on cerebrovascular dynamics. The goal is to set the ventilation consistently with a lung-protective strategy without negatively affecting the injured brain. Step 1—scanning of ventral and dorsal chest areas allows to differentiate ARDS with focal/patchy morphology (with less recruitment potential and greater risk of anterior lung overdistention) from ARDS with diffuse, more homogenous, morphology (amenable to successful recruitment at higher PEEP levels). Step 2—once this has been established, the kind of recruitment maneuver suitable for the detected ARDS morphology is preceded by BUS. The detection of signs of intracranial hypertension allows the preemptive institution of medical ICP-directed treatment to reduce the negative impact of the ventilatory maneuvers on the brain. Step 3—the recruiting maneuver is performed [under the guide of driving pressure ($\Delta P$) and static respiratory system compliance ($C_{RS}$), Volumetric Capnometry, $SpO_2$] while monitoring changes in lung aeration (LUS) and signs of their potential negative impact on ICP and cerebrovascular dynamics and (BUS). Step 4—the final effect of the recruitment maneuver and the chosen PEEP is finally assessed, both in terms of gas exchanges, lung mechanics, and of net effect on the ICP and cerebrovascular dynamics. Should the ventilation target not be reachable nor compatible with brain protection, other respiratory support strategies/ICP treatments should be considered. *ARDS* acute respiratory distress syndrome, *LUS* lung ultrasound, *BUS* brain ultrasound, *PEEP* positive end expiratory pressure, *PI* middle cerebral artery pulsatility index, $V_d$ middle cerebral artery diastolic arterial flow velocity, *FV* flow velocity; *ONSD* optic nerve sheath diameter, *MAP* mean systemic arterial pressure, *ICP* intracranial pressure, *BGA* blood gas analysis, *TBI* traumatic brain injury, *ECCOR* extracorporeal $CO_2$ removal, *vvECMO* veno-venous extracorporeal membrane oxygenation, *EEG* electroencephalography, $C_{RS}$ respiratory system compliance, $\Delta P$ driving pressure, $Cap_{Vol}$ volumetric capnometry, $SpO_2$ arterial oxygen saturation

intracranial pressure. However, although data about venous TCD and ONSD are limited in this group of patients, we believe that the use of these complementary techniques should be included in a thorough multimodal brain investigation, but not substitute for it, as they enable to assess cerebral haemodynamics from different perspectives.

Therefore, especially in circumstances when invasive ICP pressure may carry excessive risk, be unavailable or contraindicated, BUS has the potential to provide understanding on whether PEEP, recruitment maneuvers or prone positioning are causing pathological changes in cerebral hemodynamics.

## Ultrasound-guided "brain protective ventilation strategy"

Whenever a patient presents brain injury and requires mechanical ventilation, particular care is recommended in the setting and monitoring of airway pressures and of minute ventilation [39]. The combined use of Lung ultrasonography (LUS) and Brain ultrasonography (BUS) could potentially be used to guide mechanical ventilation and at the same time monitor concurrent relevant cerebrovascular physiology, addressing relevant clinical targets: recruitment maneuvers tolerance, choice of the appropriate PEEP level, minimum tolerable minute ventilation.

To tackle the challenging issue of *combined lung and brain protection from secondary damage* in the brain-injured patient under demanding mechanical ventilation, a pragmatic approach to orient mechanical ventilation settings based on LUS and BUS can be proposed, as part of the multimodal, multi-organ monitoring of such complex patients. This approach is based on the concept of noninvasively screening for the potential of a reduced tolerance to ventilatory maneuvers (BUS signs of high ICP/reduced cerebral flow), and of monitoring the cerebral effect itself of the ventilator maneuvers once performed. Where ICP invasive monitoring, that should be considered the gold standard, and other brain monitoring tools are already in place, this approach would represent a complimentary simultaneous assessment of lung recruitability/effective recruitment, screening for the potential of a reduced tolerance to ventilatory maneuvers (BUS signs of high ICP/reduced cerebral flow) and brain response to ventilatory manipulations. When ICP invasive monitoring is not indicated, contraindicated or not available, the combined LUS–BUS approach may represent a non-invasive monitoring tool instrumental to tackle the double challenge of concomitant lung- and neuro-protection in mechanically ventilated patients. A four-tiered LUS–BUS approach to the most severe setting of ARDS in TBI is here presented as example of this concept (Fig. 3).

Essentially, a tailored PEEP-trial is performed under guidance of respiratory mechanics/monitoring parameters [driving pressure ($\Delta P$), Respiratory System Compliance, $SpO_2$, Volumetric Capnometry], and its effects are then monitored with LUS [40] and BUS [38]. The first step is *the evaluation of lung morphology* at a PEEP of 5 $cmH_2O$. This can be done by examination of anterior and dorsal chest areas: the presence of a prevailing normal A pattern [17] or scarce B-lines in the anterior areas, and consolidations in the dorsal ones characterizes focal aeration loss; conversely, if diffuse multiple well-separated or coalescent B-lines (B pattern) [17] are found in anterior areas of the chest, a diffuse, more homogeneous loss of aeration is demonstrated.

The second step focuses on the *screening for BUS signs of intracranial hypertension*: should these be detected

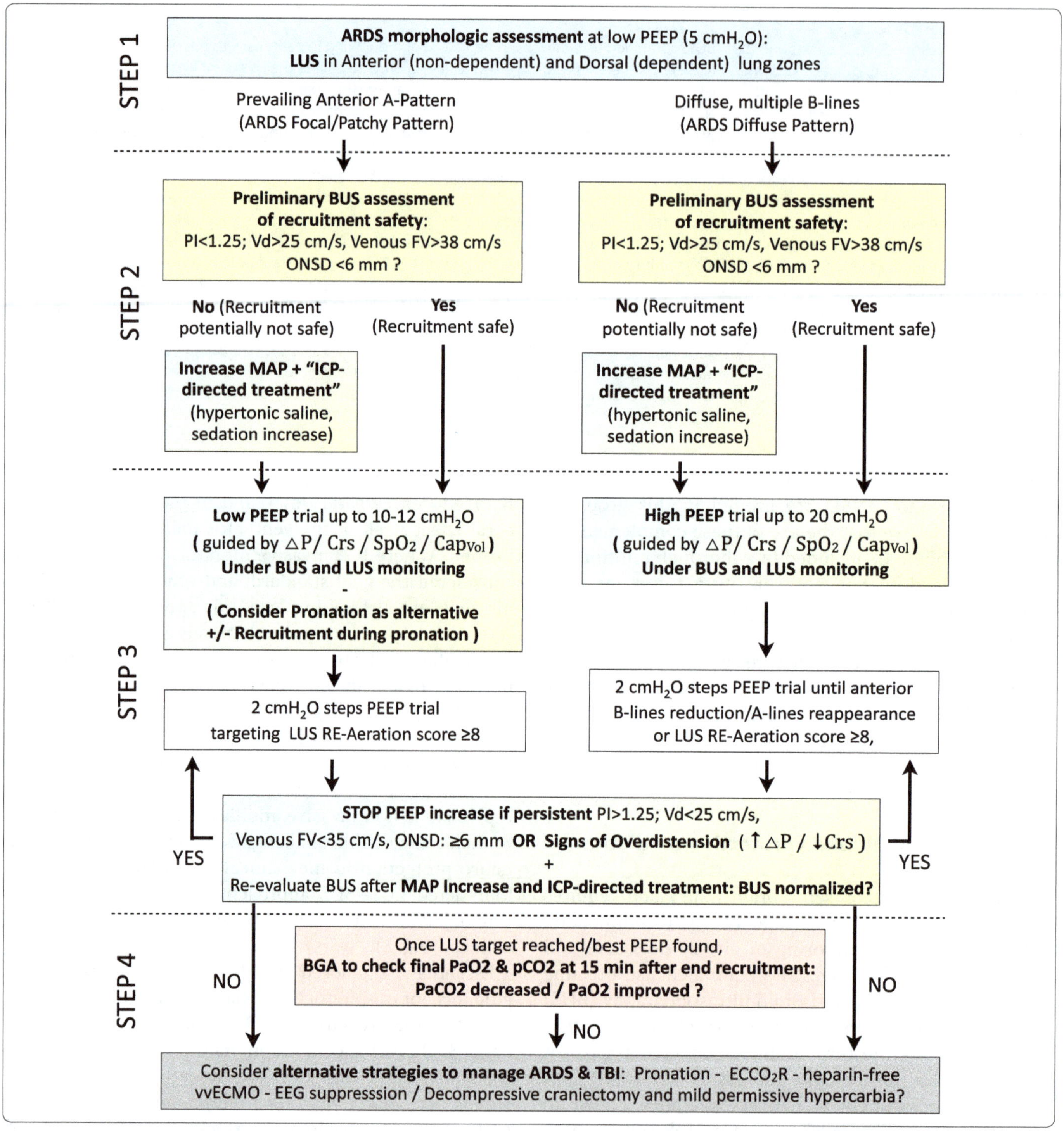


(thus making the PEEP-trial more likely to adversely affect brain vascular dynamics), the expected improvement in oxygenation and hypercarbia upon reduction of alveolar dead space may still be worth the transient side effects of the recruiting PEEP-trial (in terms of cerebral venous return reduction and $pCO_2$ increase). This should though be performed only after ICP-reducing treatments are delivered (sedation, hypertonic saline boluses).

As third step, the *PEEP trial is performed monitoring respiratory mechanics as reference.* For patients with focal loss of aeration, low levels of PEEP ($\leq 10$ $cmH_2O$) can be tested, under BUS monitoring to promptly detect cerebral hemodynamics disturbances (higher levels of PEEP rarely result in recruitment of consolidations in these patients, and expose normally aerated lung zones to over-distension, with no benefit on gas exchanges at the useless price of increasing ICP). For patients with diffuse loss of aeration (diffuse ARDS), higher levels of PEEP (from 12 $cmH_2O$ up) can be tested, still under BUS monitoring. At each increase of PEEP, responsiveness can be monitored by LUS examination of anterior zones [40]; PEEP is increased by 2–4 $cmH_2O$ until anterior zones with moderate or severe aeration loss (respectively separated and coalescent B-lines) become normal (A-lines). Increasing PEEP further to obtain a complete disappearance of B-lines (in lateral zones) or consolidation (in posterior zones) theoretically exposes previously recruited anterior lung zones to over-distension. A semi-quantitative re-aeration score can also be applied in a more exhaustive approach: each intercostal space is examined within each of the 12 regions in both hemi-thoraxes [17]. To apply this scoring method, the most pathological pattern in each region is considered as characterizing the pattern of the entire region. A LUS score of re-aeration would be then calculated, based on the changes of the ultrasound pattern in each region of interest from baseline to end to the recruiting PEEP-trial (a re-aeration score of $\geq 8$ has been associated to a CT-scan measured recruitment greater than 600 ml) [24]. The appearance of BUS signs of worsening intracranial hypertension or respiratory mechanics signs of overdistension warrants cessation of the maneuver and ICP-directed medical treatment.

The final step consists in the *evaluation of the final result of the PEEP-trial.* At the chosen PEEP level and after sufficient time for gas exchanges to stabilize, BGA assessment will describe the $PaO_2$ and $PaCO_2$ obtained. Should the new ventilation setting yield no improvement in arterial blood gases, or should this improvement have occurred at the expenses of excessive ICP (persistent BUS signs of elevated ICP), alternative respiratory support strategies [41, 42] or TBI treatments [43] could be considered.

## Conclusion

Respiratory and cerebral monitoring are complex parts of critical care. We herewith presented the concept of a combined bedside ultrasound respiratory and neurological monitoring of the neurocritical patient on mechanical ventilation, based on recent evidence suggesting the added value that both techniques represent for bedside monitoring. At present, the use of PEEP to treat ARDS in TBI patients may be appropriate; but the decision to increase PEEP in a neurocritical patient should be accompanied by maintenance of systemic arterial pressure and gas-exchange stability, and a close monitoring of cerebral parameters (mainly ICP and CPP). The concomitant combined use of ultrasound for lung and brain monitoring in the challenging setting of co-existing TBI and ARDS could serve the purpose of guiding the ventilator strategy (PEEP setting, recruitment vs. pronation) and of promptly screening for signs of increased/worsening intracranial hypertension (i.e., screening for tolerance to PEEP, to sub-optimal $PaCO_2$). However, LUS–BUS monitoring should be integrated into the well established diagnostic-monitoring workup, including the evaluation of respiratory mechanics, gas-exchange, computer tomography scan and multi-modal brain monitoring. Further research is advocated to validate this ultrasound-aided approach.

**Authors' contributions**

FC and GV conceived and reviewed the manuscript, CR and GT reviewed the manuscript. All authors read and approved the final manuscript.

**Author details**

[1] Servizio di Anestesia e Rianimazione, Ente ospedaliero Ospedali Galliera, Genoa, Italy. [2] Anaesthesia and Intensive Care, IRCSS S. Martino Hospital, Genoa, Italy. [3] Neurocritical Care Unit, Addenbrookes Hospital Cambridge, Cambridge, UK. [4] Emergency Department, Anaesthesia and Intensive Care Unit, Fondazione IRCCS Policlinico S. Matteo, Pavia, Italy. [5] Department of Clinical, Surgical, Diagnostic and Paediatric Sciences, Anaesthesia, Intensive Care and Pain Therapy Unit, University of Pavia, Pavia, Italy. [6] Cardiac Anesthesia and Intensive Care, Cardiocentro Ticino, Via Tesserete, 48, Lugano, Switzerland.

**Acknowledgements**

None.

**References**

1. Rincon F, Ghosh S, Dey S, Maltenfort M, Vibbert M, Urtecho J, McBride W, Moussouttas M, Bell R, Ratliff JK, Jallo J (2012) Impact of acute lung injury and acute respiratory distress syndrome after traumatic brain injury in the United States. Neurosurgery 71(4):795–803
2. Veeravagu A, Chen YR, Ludwig C, Rincon F, Maltenfort M, Jallo J, Choudhri O, Steinberg GK, Ratliff JK (2014) Acute lung injury in patients with subarachnoid hemorrhage: a nationwide inpatient sample study. World Neurosurg 82(1–2):e235–e241
3. Damm TW, Kramer DJ (2016) The liver in critical illness. Crit Care Clin 32(3):425–438
4. Meng L, Gelb AW (2015) Regulation of cerebral autoregulation by carbon dioxide. Anesthesiology 122(1):196–205
5. Beuret P, Carton MJ, Nourdine K, Kaaki M, Tramoni G, Ducreux JC (2002) Prone position as prevention of lung injury in comatose patients: a prospective, randomized, controlled study. Intensive Care Med 28(5):564–569
6. Roth C, Ferbert A, Deinsberger W, Kleffmann J, Kastner S, Godau J, Schuler M, Tryba M, Gehling M (2014) Does prone positioning increase intracranial pressure? A retrospective analysis of patients with acute brain injury and acute respiratory failure. Neurocrit Care 21(2):186–191
7. Bruder N, Rabinstein A, Participants in the International Multi-Disciplinary Consensus Conference on the Critical Care Management of Subarachnoid H (2011) Cardiovascular and pulmonary complications of aneurysmal subarachnoid hemorrhage. Neurocrit Care 15(2):257–269
8. Wang C, Zhao N, Wang W, Guo L, Guo L, Chi C, Wang X, Pi X, Cui Y, Li E (2015) Intraoperative mechanical ventilation strategies for obese patients: a systematic review and network meta-analysis. Obes Rev 16(6):508–517
9. Yiallourou TI, Odier C, Heinzer R, Hirt L, Martin BA, Stergiopulos N, Haba-Rubio J (2013) The effect of continuous positive airway pressure on total cerebral blood flow in healthy awake volunteers. Sleep Breath 17(1):289–296
10. Shapiro HM, Marshall LF (1978) Intracranial pressure responses to PEEP in head-injured patients. J Trauma 18(4):254–256
11. Mekontso Dessap A, Boissier F, Charron C, Begot E, Repesse X, Legras A, Brun-Buisson C, Vignon P, Vieillard-Baron A (2016) Acute cor pulmonale during protective ventilation for acute respiratory distress syndrome: prevalence, predictors, and clinical impact. Intensive Care Med 42(5):862–870

12. McGuire G, Crossley D, Richards J, Wong D (1997) Effects of varying levels of positive end-expiratory pressure on intracranial pressure and cerebral perfusion pressure. Crit Care Med 25(6):1059–1062
13. Mascia L, Grasso S, Fiore T, Bruno F, Berardino M, Ducati A (2005) Cerebro-pulmonary interactions during the application of low levels of positive end-expiratory pressure. Intensive Care Med 31(3):373–379
14. Young N, Rhodes JK, Mascia L, Andrews PJ (2010) Ventilatory strategies for patients with acute brain injury. Curr Opin Crit Care 16(1):45–52
15. Zieleskiewicz L, Muller L, Lakhal K, Meresse Z, Arbelot C, Bertrand PM, Bouhemad B, Cholley B, Demory D, Duperret S, Duranteau J, Guervilly C, Hammad E, Ichai C, Jaber S, Langeron O, Lefrant JY, Mahjoub Y, Maury E, Meaudre E, Michel F, Muller M, Nafati C, Perbet S, Quintard H, Riu B, Vigne C, Chaumoitre K, Antonini F, Allaouchiche B, Martin C, Constantin JM, De Backer D, Leone M, Car'Echo, AzuRea Collaborative N (2015) Point-of-care ultrasound in intensive care units: assessment of 1073 procedures in a multicentric, prospective, observational study. Intensive Care Med 41(9):1638–1647
16. Bataille B, Riu B, Ferre F, Moussot PE, Mari A, Brunel E, Ruiz J, Mora M, Fourcade O, Genestal M, Silva S (2014) Integrated use of bedside lung ultrasound and echocardiography in acute respiratory failure: a prospective observational study in ICU. Chest 146(6):1586–1593
17. Volpicelli G, Elbarbary M, Blaivas M, Lichtenstein DA, Mathis G, Kirkpatrick AW, Melniker L, Gargani L, Noble VE, Via G, Dean A, Tsung JW, Soldati G, Copetti R, Bouhemad B, Reissig A, Agricola E, Rouby JJ, Arbelot C, Liteplo A, Sargsyan A, Silva F, Hoppmann R, Breitkreutz R, Seibel A, Neri L, Storti E, Petrovic T, International Liaison Committee on Lung Ultrasound for International Consensus Conference on Lung U (2012) International evidence-based recommendations for point-of-care lung ultrasound. Intensive Care Med 38(4):577–591
18. Corradi F, Ball L, Brusasco C, Riccio AM, Baroffio M, Bovio G, Pelosi P, Brusasco V (2013) Assessment of extravascular lung water by quantitative ultrasound and CT in isolated bovine lung. Respir Physiol Neurobiol 187(3):244–249
19. Corradi F, Brusasco C, Vezzani A, Santori G, Manca T, Ball L, Nicolini F, Gherli T, Brusasco V (2016) Computer-aided quantitative ultrasonography for detection of pulmonary edema in mechanically ventilated cardiac surgery patients. Chest 150(3):640–651
20. Lichtenstein D, Goldstein I, Mourgeon E, Cluzel P, Grenier P, Rouby JJ (2004) Comparative diagnostic performances of auscultation, chest radiography, and lung ultrasonography in acute respiratory distress syndrome. Anesthesiology 100(1):9–15
21. Corradi F, Brusasco C, Pelosi P (2014) Chest ultrasound in acute respiratory distress syndrome. Curr Opin Crit Care 20(1):98–103
22. Markota A, Golub J, Stozer A, Fluher J, Prosen G, Bergauer A, Svensek F, Sinkovic A (2016) Absence of lung sliding is not a reliable sign of pneumothorax in patients with high positive end-expiratory pressure. Am J Emerg Med 34(10):2034–2036
23. Leblanc D, Bouvet C, Degiovanni F, Nedelcu C, Bouhours G, Rineau E, Ridereau-Zins C, Beydon L, Lasocki S (2014) Early lung ultrasonography predicts the occurrence of acute respiratory distress syndrome in blunt trauma patients. Intensive Care Med 40(10):1468–1474
24. Bouhemad B, Brisson H, Le-Guen M, Arbelot C, Lu Q, Rouby JJ (2011) Bedside ultrasound assessment of positive end-expiratory pressure-induced lung recruitment. Am J Respir Crit Care Med 183(3):341–347
25. Haddam M, Zieleskiewicz L, Perbet S, Baldovini A, Guervilly C, Arbelot C, Noel A, Vigne C, Hammad E, Antonini F, Lehingue S, Peytel E, Lu Q, Bouhemad B, Golmard JL, Langeron O, Martin C, Muller L, Rouby JJ, Constantin JM, Papazian L, Leone M, Network CAEC, AzuRea Collaborative N (2016) Lung ultrasonography for assessment of oxygenation response to prone position ventilation in ARDS. Intensive Care Med 42(10):1546–1556
26. Guerin C, Gattinoni L (2016) Assessment of oxygenation response to prone position ventilation in ARDS by lung ultrasonography. Intensive Care Med 42(10):1601–1603
27. Zhao Z, Jiang L, Xi X, Jiang Q, Zhu B, Wang M, Xing J, Zhang D (2015) Prognostic value of extravascular lung water assessed with lung ultrasound score by chest sonography in patients with acute respiratory distress syndrome. BMC Pulm Med 15:98
28. Volpicelli G, Skurzak S, Boero E, Carpinteri G, Tengattini M, Stefanone V, Luberto L, Anile A, Cerutti E, Radeschi G, Frascisco MF (2014) Lung ultrasound predicts well extravascular lung water but is of limited usefulness in the prediction of wedge pressure. Anesthesiology 121(2):320–327
29. Agricola E, Bove T, Oppizzi M, Marino G, Zangrillo A, Margonato A, Picano E (2005) "Ultrasound comet-tail images": a marker of pulmonary edema: a comparative study with wedge pressure and extravascular lung water. Chest 127(5):1690–1695
30. Moretti R, Pizzi B (2009) Optic nerve ultrasound for detection of intracranial hypertension in intracranial hemorrhage patients: confirmation of previous findings in a different patient population. J Neurosurg Anesthesiol 21(1):16–20
31. Whiteley JR, Taylor J, Henry M, Epperson TI, Hand WR (2015) Detection of elevated intracranial pressure in robot-assisted laparoscopic radical prostatectomy using ultrasonography of optic nerve sheath diameter. J Neurosurg Anesthesiol 27(2):155–159
32. Albin MS (2014) Measuring the ICP in neonates and infants noninvasively is also important. J Neurosurg Anesthesiol 26(4):407
33. Robba C, Cardim D, Sekhon M, Budohoski K, Czosnyka M (2018) Transcranial Doppler: a stethoscope for the brain-neurocritical care use. J Neurosci Res 96(4):720–730
34. Bouzat P, Francony G, Declety P, Genty C, Kaddour A, Bessou P, Brun J, Jacquot C, Chabardes S, Bosson JL, Payen JF (2011) Transcranial Doppler to screen on admission patients with mild to moderate traumatic brain injury. Neurosurgery 68(6):1603–1609 **(discussion 1609–1610)**
35. Bouzat P, Almeras L, Manhes P, Sanders L, Levrat A, David JS, Cinotti R, Chabanne R, Gloaguen A, Bobbia X, Thoret S, Oujamaa L, Bosson JL, Payen JF, Asehnoune K, Pes P, Lefrant JY, Mirek S, Albasini F, Scrimgeour C, Thouret JM, Chartier F, Ginet M, Investigators T-TS (2016) Transcranial Doppler to predict neurologic outcome after mild to moderate traumatic brain injury. Anesthesiology 125(2):346–354
36. Robba C, Cardim D, Tajsic T, Pietersen J, Bulman M, Donnelly J, Lavinio A, Gupta A, Menon DK, Hutchinson PJA, Czosnyka M (2017) Ultrasound non-invasive measurement of intracranial pressure in neurointensive care: a prospective observational study. PLoS Med 14(7):e1002356
37. Ohle R, McIsaac SM, Woo MY, Perry JJ (2015) Sonography of the optic nerve sheath diameter for detection of raised intracranial pressure compared to computed tomography: a systematic review and meta-analysis. J Ultrasound Med 34(7):1285–1294
38. Robba C, Bragazzi NL, Bertuccio A, Cardim D, Donnelly J, Sekhon M, Lavinio A, Duane D, Burnstein R, Matta B, Bacigaluppi S, Lattuada M, Czosnyka M (2017) Effects of prone position and positive end-expiratory pressure on noninvasive estimators of ICP: a pilot study. J Neurosurg Anesthesiol 29(3):243–250
39. Rajajee V, Riggs B, Seder DB (2017) Emergency neurological life support: airway, ventilation, and sedation. Neurocrit Care 27(Suppl 1):4–28
40. Bouhemad B, Mongodi S, Via G, Rouquette I (2015) Ultrasound for "lung monitoring" of ventilated patients. Anesthesiology 122(2):437–447
41. Munoz-Bendix C, Beseoglu K, Kram R (2015) Extracorporeal decarboxylation in patients with severe traumatic brain injury and ARDS enables effective control of intracranial pressure. Crit Care 19:381
42. Wu SC, Chen WT, Lin HH, Fu CY, Wang YC, Lo HC, Cheng HT, Tzeng CW (2015) Use of extracorporeal membrane oxygenation in severe traumatic lung injury with respiratory failure. Am J Emerg Med 33(5):658–662
43. Stocchetti N, Maas AI (2014) Traumatic intracranial hypertension. N Engl J Med 370(22):2121–2130

# 15

# Ultrasound evaluation of the airway in the ED

Elizabeth A. Hall[1,2*], Ibrahim Showaihi[3], Frances S. Shofer[4], Nova L. Panebianco[1] and Anthony J. Dean[5]

**Abstract**

**Background:** Recognition of the difficult airway is a critical element of emergency practice. Mallampati score and body mass index (BMI) are not always predictive and they may be unavailable in critically ill patients. Ultrasonography provides high-resolution images that are rapidly obtainable, mobile, and non-invasive. Studies have shown correlation of ultrasound measurements with difficult laryngoscopy; however, none have been performed in the Emergency Department (ED) using a consistent scanning protocol.

**Objectives:** This study seeks to determine the feasibility of ultrasound measurements of the upper airway performed in the ED by emergency physicians, the inter-rater reliability of such measurements, and their relationship with Mallampati score and BMI.

**Methods:** A convenience sample of volunteer ED patients and healthy volunteers with no known airway issues, aged > 18 years, had images taken of their airway using a standardized ultrasound scanning protocol by two EM ultrasound fellowship trained physicians. Measurements consisted of tongue base, tongue base-to-skin, epiglottic width and thickness, and pre-epiglottic space. Mean and standard deviation (SD) were used to summarize measurements. Inter-rater reliability was assessed by intraclass correlation coefficients (ICCs). Analysis of variance with linear contrasts was used to compare measurements with Mallampati scores and linear regression with BMI.

**Results:** Of 39 participants, 50% were female, 50% white, 42% black, with median age 32.5 years (range 19–90), and BMI 26.0 (range 19–47). Mean ± SD for each measurement (mm) was as follows: tongue base (44.6 ± 5.1), tongue base-to-skin (60.9 ± 5.3), epiglottic width (15.0 ± 2.8) and thickness (2.0 ± 0.37), and pre-epiglottic space (11.4 ± 2.4). ICCs ranged from 0.76 to 0.88 for all measurements except epiglottis thickness (ICC = 0.57). Tongue base and tongue base-to-skin thickness were found to increase with increasing Mallampati score ($p = .04, .01$), whereas only tongue-to-skin thickness was loosely correlated with BMI ($r = .38$).

**Conclusions:** A standardized ultrasound scanning protocol demonstrates that the airway can be measured by emergency sonologists with good inter-operator reliability in all but epiglottic thickness. The measurements correlate with Mallampati score but not with BMI. Future investigation might focus on ultrasound evaluation of the airway in patients receiving airway management to determine whether ultrasound can predict challenging or abnormal airway anatomy prior to laryngoscopy.

**Keywords:** Point-of-care ultrasound, Upper airway ultrasound, Airway management

## Background

Recognizing difficult airways in the Emergency Department (ED) is an important skill anatomic variations in airway structures cannot be fully assessed prior to intubation. Identification of a difficult airway prior to intubation allows for optimal preparation, equipment selection, and participation of experienced personnel.

Pre-intubation evaluation of the airway has traditionally depended on clinical parameters such as body mass index, neck circumference, and the Mallampati scoring method [1]. None of these parameters is reliably

*Correspondence: Elizabeth.Hall1@gmail.com
[1] Department of Emergency Ultrasound, Emergency Medicine, Hospital at the University of Pennsylvania, Philadelphia, PA, USA
Full list of author information is available at the end of the article

predictive [2–5]. A meta-analysis of 55 studies identified that only 35% of difficult intubations had a Mallampati score of III or IV [6]. Thus, it is clear that airway evaluation prior to laryngoscopy might benefit from improved methods of assessment.

Ultrasound is a mobile, non-ionizing, non-invasive tool that readily provides images of airway anatomy. Research in the anesthesiology literature has demonstrated that ultrasound can visualize key anatomical structures through transcutaneous views of the neck [7–10].

Studies examining the ability of ultrasound to predict difficult airways have been performed in adult patients in the pre-operative surgical setting using variable patient positioning and scanning protocols. Ultrasound measurements at the level of tongue, pharynx, larynx, and trachea have been compared to Cormack–Lehane Grades (CLG) determined during direct laryngoscopy [11]. Difficult laryngoscopy was found to correlate with ultrasound measurements taken at the hyoid bone, thyrohyoid membranes, and hyomental distance with patients in the sniffing position [12–14]. A South Korean study used ultrasound to examine the epiglottis in normal patients and those diagnosed with acute epiglottis and found a significant difference in the anteroposterior diameter, promoting ultrasound as a possible tool for diagnosing acute epiglottis [15]. Despite these results, several studies have had contradictory findings, and all were limited by small sample size, marked differences in population characteristics, and an absence of a specified ultrasound scanning protocol [16].

The current study investigates the feasibility of soft tissue measurements performed by clinician sonologists in the ED environment using a defined scanning protocol. The goal of this study was (1) to determine the inter-rater reliability of airway measurements obtained by emergency sonologists using a standardized scanning protocol and (2) to compare these measurements to widely used clinical predictors of difficult airway, specifically the Mallampati score and BMI.

## Methods

### Study design

This was a prospective study, using a convenience sample of ED patients and volunteer members of the ED staff. Airway ultrasound measurements were obtained by two emergency medicine (EM) physicians using a standardized scanning protocol. Both physicians were currently enrolled in an emergency ultrasound fellowship program. Mean and standard deviation (SD) were used to summarize measurements. The results obtained by the two sonologists were compared. Inter-rater reliability between the two sonologists was assessed by intraclass correlation coefficients (ICCs). Analysis of variance with linear contrasts was used to compare measurements with Mallampati scores and linear regression with body mass index (BMI).

### Study setting and population

The study was performed in a metropolitan tertiary care center with an annual ED census of 72,000 patients. The ED supports an Emergency Medicine Residency Program and an Emergency Ultrasound Fellowship. Subjects were ED patients presenting for complaints unrelated to the airway. They were asked to enroll voluntarily with the understanding that the ultrasound would likely have no impact on their clinical care. The study was approved by the institutional review board of the Hospital at the University of Pennsylvania.

### Selection of participants

We enrolled a convenience sample of patients and volunteers between March 2016 and September 2016. Patient inclusion criteria included age older than 17 years and ability to provide written consent in English. Volunteers were excluded if they had a history of congenital or acquired airway abnormalities.

### Study protocol

Any ED patient or ED staff volunteer that met inclusion criteria was approached by the research physicians for enrollment in the study and a written informed consent was obtained. Subjects had ultrasound measurements and images of their tongue base, tongue base-to-skin, epiglottic width and thickness, and pre-epiglottic space recorded separately by both physicians. The data were collected at bedside and each research physician was blinded to the other's assessment. Demographic information including sex, age, race, BMI, and Mallampati scores were collected.

### Ultrasound technique

A standardized scanning protocol was used for subject positioning and measurement. Subjects were placed in the supine position without a pillow, with head and neck in extension, and tongue in resting position and touching the lower incisors. A Mindray M9 ultrasound machine (Mindray Bio-Medical Electronics Co, Shenzhen, China) with a curved linear 5- to 3-MHZ probe was used to obtain the tongue base and tongue base-to-skin thickness. A linear 10- to 5-MHZ probe was used to obtain the epiglottic width and thickness, and pre-epiglottic space measurements. All ultrasound images were obtained using the minimal transducer pressure necessary to obtain good skin contact. Subjects were asked to rest the tip of their tongue against their lower incisors while the measurements were being made. The curvilinear probe was placed in the longitudinal position or long axis along the submental space and the maximum thickness of the tongue was recorded as well as the maximum thickness of the tongue to the skin surface at the neck (Fig. 1a). The linear probe in a transverse plane was used to measure the epiglottic width and thickness at the level of the thyrohyoid membrane midway between the hyoid bone and the thyroid cartilage (Fig. 1b). The epiglottis was identified at the thyrohyoid membrane by making slight cranial or caudal angulated movements with the transducer and observing the bright air–mucosa interface at the posterior edge of the epiglottis. The epiglottis thickness was measured at the point of greatest visible thickness determined by the sonologist. At the same level, the pre-epiglottic space was measured from the anterior surface of the epiglottis to the anterior surface of the strap muscles (Fig. 1b). Demographic variables and Mallampati scores were collected by the same co-investigators after ultrasound measurements had been completed.

## Results

Forty subjects were enrolled, of which one subject was excluded because epiglottic views were unobtainable, and in this patient, all other measurements were excluded for reasons of consistency. Of the 39 subjects with complete data, 31 were ED patients and 8 were volunteers: 50% were female, 50% white, 42% black, with median age 32.5 years (range 19–90) and BMI 26.0 (range 19–47). Mean ± SD for each measurement (mm) were as follows: tongue base (44.6 ± 5.1), tongue base-to-skin (60.9 ± 5.3), epiglottic width (15.0 ± 2.8) and thickness (2.0 ± 0.37), and pre-epiglottic space (11.4 ± 2.4). Intraclass correlation coefficients (ICCs) ranged from 0.76 to 0.88 for all measurements except epiglottis thickness (ICC = 0.57) and Bland–Altman plots demonstrated consistency over the range of values between the two physicians (Figs. 2, 3). Tongue base and tongue base-to-skin thickness were found to linearly increase with Mallampati score ($p$ = .04, .01) (Fig. 4), whereas only tongue-to-skin thickness was loosely correlated with BMI ($r$ = .38).

## Discussion

The study found that the airways of a randomly chosen population of ED patients with a range of BMI and Mallampati scores can be measured by emergency sonologists with good inter-operator reliability. This study, to our knowledge, is the first that documents the feasibility of these measurements made by clinician-performed ultrasonography in the emergency department environment. Only one subject in 40 had an airway parameter that could not be obtained by ultrasound. Almost all of the measurements used including tongue base, tongue base-to-skin, epiglottic width, and pre-epiglottic space had fair to good ICCs ranging from 0.76 to 0.88. Epiglottic thickness, however, had a poor ICC at 0.57 which is related to the inherently small values of this structure, making standard errors in ultrasound measurements (often in the 1–2 mm range) mathematically much more impactful. This explanation is consistent with the finding that the ICC for epiglottic width (a larger distance) was similar to that of other parameters. Possibly using the 'zoom' mode on the ultrasound machine to enlarge the image might have improved the ICC for epiglottic

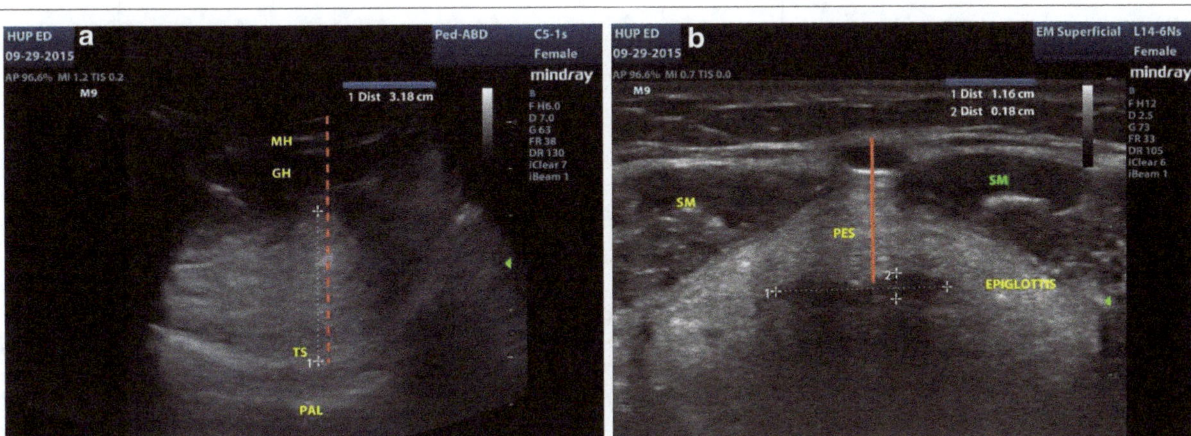


**Fig. 1** **a** Sagittal paramedian view of the tongue from the submental area with the white dotted line representing the tongue base measurement and the red dotted line as tongue base-to-skin thickness. The patient's face would be in the direction of the right of the screen. *MH* mylohyoid muscle, *GH* geniohyoid muscle, *TS* tongue surface, *PAL* palette. **b** Transverse ultrasound image at the level of the thyrohyoid membrane. The pre-epiglottic space (red line, PES) is measured from the anterior surface of the epiglottis to the anterior margin of the strap muscles (SM) midway between the hyoid bone and the thyroid cartilage. The epiglottis is indicated by the two white caliper lines showing width (dotted line #1) and thickness (dotted line #2)

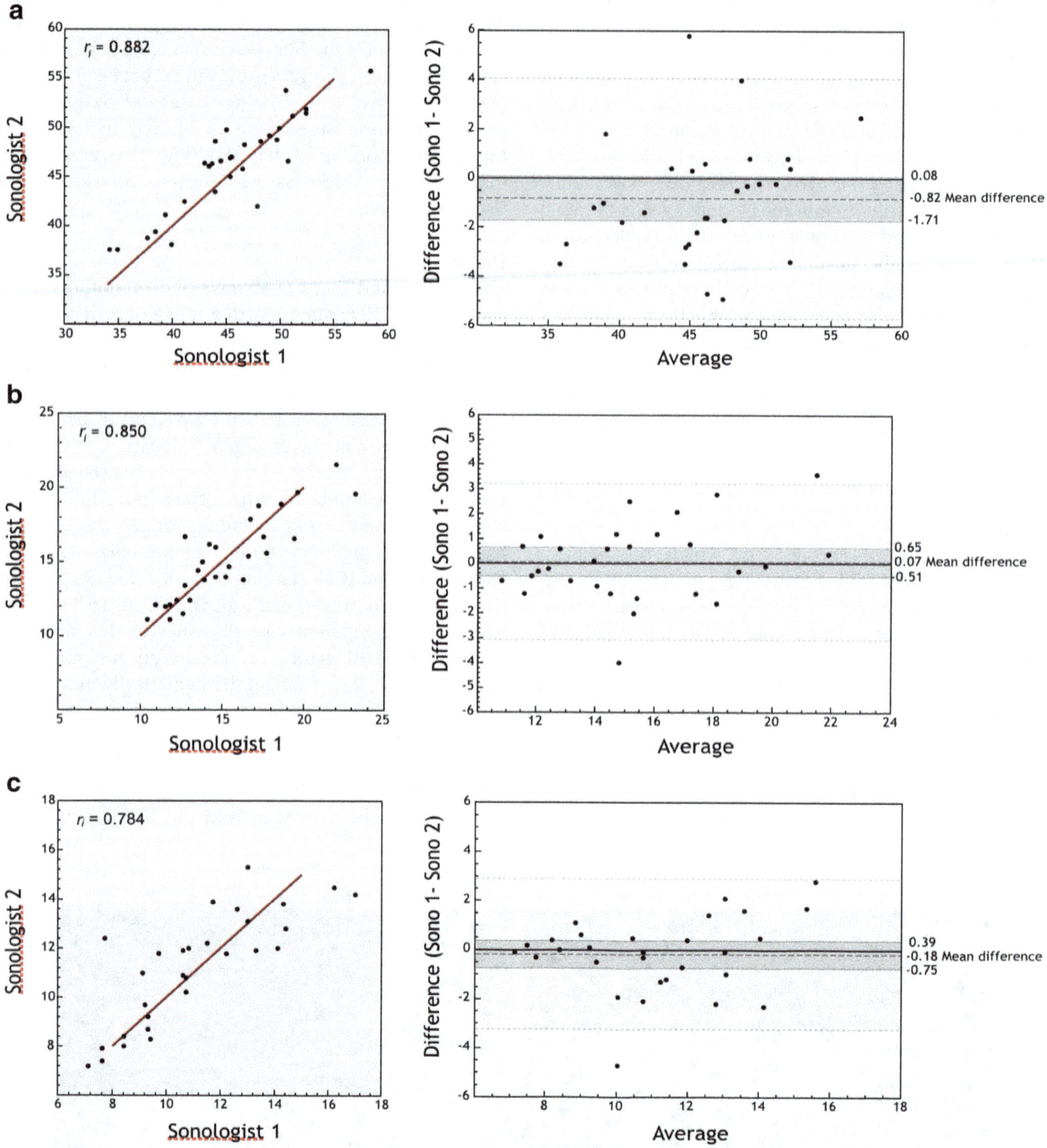


**Fig. 2** ICC graphs and Bland–Altman plots: agreement between sonologists in measurements. *Y* axis for Bland–Altman plots represents average of sonologists measurements. Mean difference between sonologists with 95% confidence intervals on the means shown (darker gray). Lighter gray bands represent the 95% confidence bands. **a** Tongue base thickness (mm). **b** Epiglottis LA (mm). **c** Pre-epiglotic space (mm)

thickness measurement; however, such maneuvers increase the complexity and time required for the task, both of which can be disadvantageous in the context of the time constraints inherent in emergency airway management [17].

Future studies comparing soft tissue measurements to metrics of airway difficulty such as the Cormack–Lehane

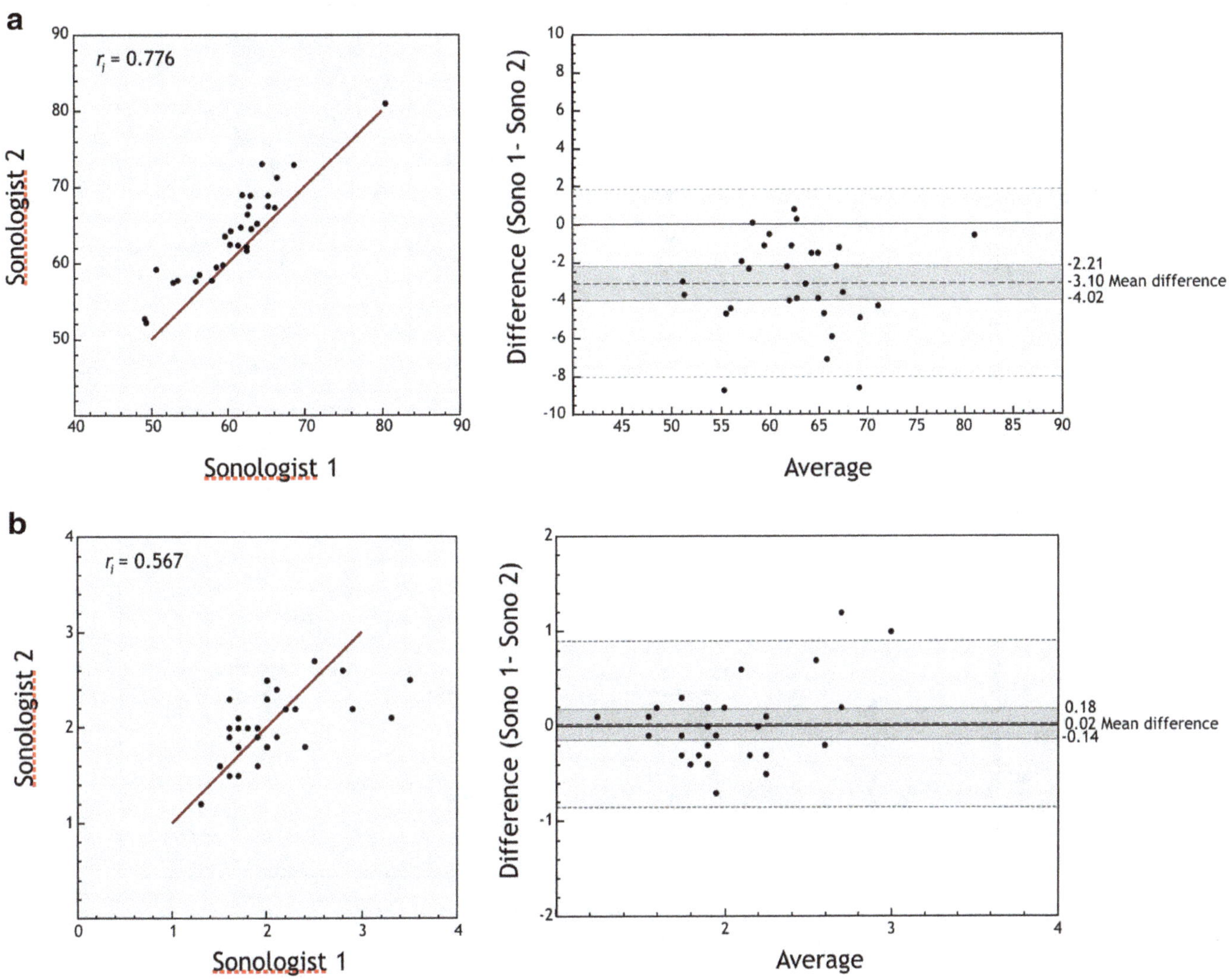


**Fig. 3** ICC graphs and Bland–Altman plots: agreement between sonologists in measurements. *Y* axis for Bland–Altman plots represents average of sonologists measurements. Mean difference between sonologists with 95% confidence intervals on the means shown (darker gray). Lighter gray bands represent the 95% confidence bands. **a** Skin tongue thickness (mm). **b** Epiglottis SA (mm)

grading system will reveal whether epiglottic thickness is necessary or even helpful in this setting. Our study also suggests that epiglottic thickness has little variation in the general population, which also makes it less likely to be a discriminatory metric. Of course such reasoning would not have any place in situations where acute epiglottic inflammation or edema are of concern, such as in cases of smoke inhalation, angioedema, or epiglottitis. Similarly, the absence of thickening might give some assurance in cases where epiglottic enlargement or obstruction is a concern.

There are several limitations in this study. Experienced airway sonologists are aware that differences in probe pressure applied while scanning the neck can significantly alter measurements of these superficial neck structures. It was thus emphasized during the ultrasound airway training that the sonologist place the probe against the neck with the least pressure needed to maintain skin contact. The goal of minimal probe pressure also coheres with the principle of avoiding anything that might narrow the upper airway in a dyspneic patient receiving preoxygenation.

The tongue is a dynamic muscle and its position within the mouth can significantly change its size and shape, and also possibly the thickness of the soft tissues of the hypopharynx [18, 19]. Patients were therefore asked to rest their tongue with the anterior tip touching the lower incisors. In unconscious, hypoxic, or altered patients, this would not be possible limiting the generalizability of the findings of the current study to the real clinical

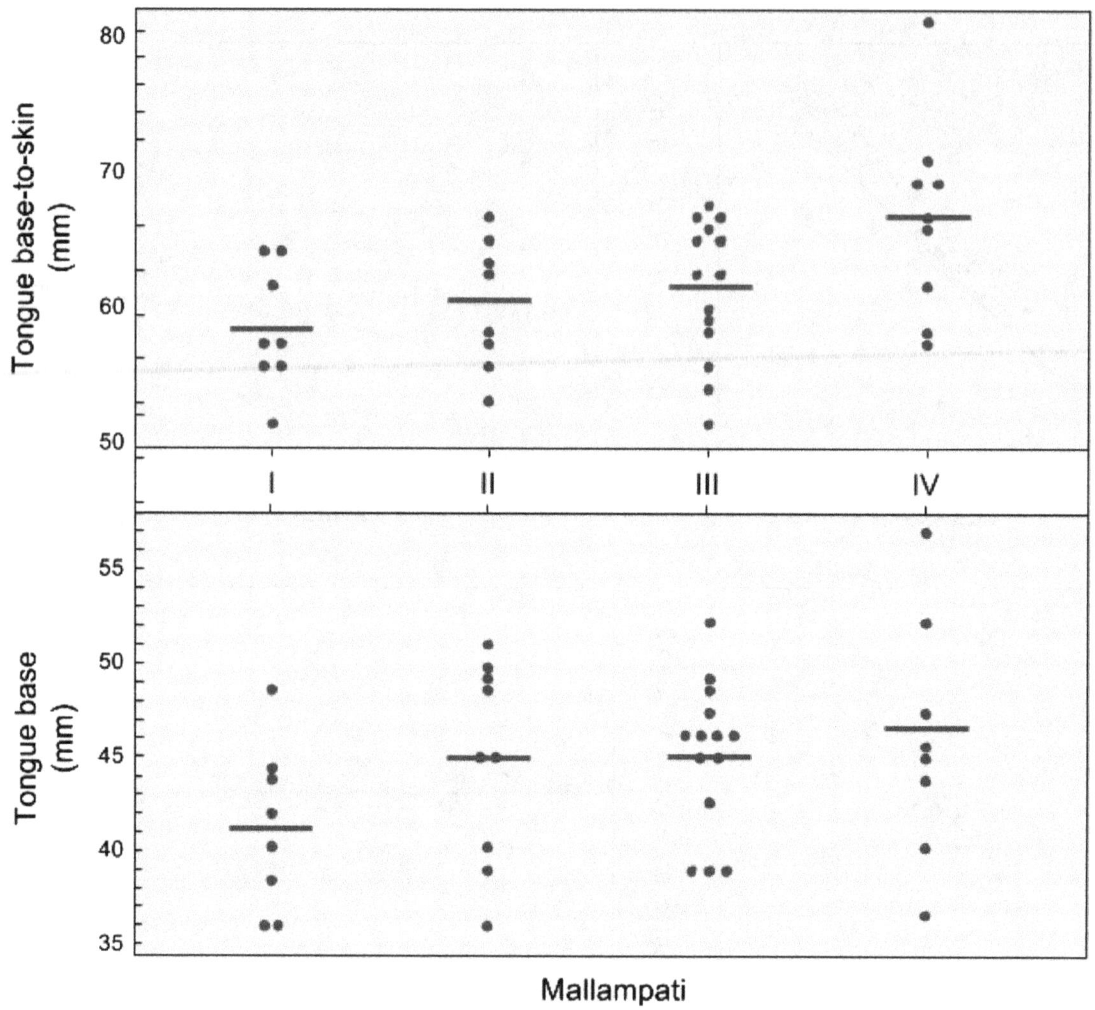


**Fig. 4** Tongue US measurements demonstrate linear increase as compared to Mallampati

environment. We also chose to position patients' supine with the neck extended, to ensure rigorous standardization. Since the "sniffing position" (neck flexed with the external auditory meatus level with the sternum and some head extension) is currently recommended for laryngoscopy, this also limits the generalizability of our study in the clinical environment. We believe that future studies might want to use the "sniffing position" for purposes of standardization, with the additional advantage that it would allow the ultrasound to be performed while the patient is being set up for intubation. Another limitation of the study is its failure to obtain data regarding the time needed to perform the ultrasound exam. In the context of emergent airway management, any ultrasound requiring much more than 30–60 s would be unlikely to see widespread acceptance by clinicians unless the information it provided was of critical importance. The time taken to perform ultrasound assessment will need to be the subject of future inquiry, but in the current feasibility paper the time required for ultrasound assessment was not recorded because it was felt that any information obtained would not be valid in a real clinical context. Along these lines, it would be ideal if a single measurement was found to be predictive of difficult laryngoscopy, thereby obviating the need for the multiple measurements made in the current study. The study tried to correlate the ultrasound findings with established metrics used in pre-intubation airway assessment, but for reasons of patient comfort and practicability, some metrics were not included, such as hyoid-mental distance. This metric was not included because it was thought that it would likely be used in a pre-intubation airway evaluation regardless of whether or not an ultrasound was performed because it can be obtained without an ultrasound machine. Future studies might investigate this issue.

Finally, the ultrasound exams performed in the current study were done by advanced emergency sonologists receiving fellowship training. This will limit the generalizability of the study among emergency physicians, although it should be generalizable among anesthesiologists and critical care physicians with ultrasound experience and interest in the airway.

The tongue base and tongue base-to-skin measurements were found to correlate with increasing Mallampati score. This finding is not surprising given that Mallampati score is based on oropharyngeal anatomy, and it makes these ultrasound measurements less valuable, since the Mallampati can be obtained rapidly by visual inspection. Furthermore, the wide range of measured mean soft tissue thickness within each Mallampati grade makes it unlikely that ultrasound will be a useful substitute for the Mallampati score. In fact, one study found that combining Mallampati score with sonographic assessment of the skin to epiglottis distance was a stronger predictor of difficult airway compared to individual parameters [20]. Tongue base-to-skin thickness was the only measurement to loosely correlate with BMI [3, 5]. We expected this measurement to have a stronger relationship with BMI. Regardless, with respect to airway management previous research has demonstrated that large neck circumference is a more reliable predictor of difficult laryngoscopy than Mallampati, although also not without limitations [2, 21–23]. One study demonstrated that ratio of tongue thickness to thyromental distance was an independent predictor of difficult airway in patients undergoing anesthesia [24]. Since Cormack–Lehane grading can only be performed after intubation is under way, it would be of interest in future studies to determine whether pre-intubation ultrasound measurements of the pre-epiglottic space are predictive of CLG. Future studies would also need to assess whether the allocation of time and resources for ultrasonography during the fraught period prior to an emergency intubation are warranted by the additional information it generates. For purposes of expediency a single parameter would be ideal. In this context, pre-epiglottic distance appeared to be a potentially useful metric since it was measured with high ICC. It also has the advantage that the normal range of values that we measured was relatively wide: a standard deviation of 2.4 mm from the mean value of 11.4 mm gives an SD of 21% of the mean value. This means that standard errors of measurement are likely to have less impact and that real differences are likely to be detected. Additional investigation using a defined and standardized scanning method in pre-operative patients undergoing intubation is needed to determine whether ultrasound can serve as a non-invasive real-time predictor of difficult intubation.

## Conclusions

The current study demonstrates that emergency sonologists are able to obtain ultrasound measurements of the upper airway with a high degree of inter-operator reliability in a cross-section of undifferentiated patients and volunteers in the ED. Future studies are needed to determine whether similar accuracy is possible among patients receiving acute airway management in the ED; whether they are predictive of a difficult airway, and whether ultrasound measurements are sufficiently valuable to warrant the expenditure of time and resources needed to obtain them.

### Abbreviations

MS: Mallampati score; BMI: body mass index; ED: Emergency Department; EM: Emergency Medicine; SD: standard deviation; ICC: intraclass correlation coefficient; CLG: Cormack–Lehane Grade.

### Authors' contributions

EAH: study design, data collection, and manuscript preparation. IS: study design and data collection. FSS: study design, data analysis, and manuscript preparation. NLP: study design and manuscript review. AJD: manuscript review. All authors read and approved the final manuscript.

### Author details

[1] Department of Emergency Ultrasound, Emergency Medicine, Hospital at the University of Pennsylvania, Philadelphia, PA, USA. [2] Ashtabula, OH 44004, USA. [3] Department of Emergency Ultrasound, Hospital at the University of Pennsylvania, Philadelphia, PA, USA. [4] Epidemiology & Biostatistics, Department of Emergency Medicine, Hospital at the University of Pennsylvania, Philadelphia, PA, USA. [5] Division of Emergency Ultrasonography, Hospital at the University of Pennsylvania, Philadelphia, PA, USA.

### Acknowledgements

None.

### References

1. Mallampati SR, Gatt SP, Gugino LD, Desai SP, Waraksa B, Freiberger D, Liu PL (1985) A clinical sign to predict difficult tracheal intubation: a prospective study. Can Anaesth Soc J 32(4):429–434
2. Brodsky JB, Lemmens HJ, Brock-Utne JG, Vierra M, Saidman LJ (2002) Morbid obesity and tracheal intubation. Anesth Analg 94(3):732–736
3. Ezri T, Gewurtz G, Sessler DI, Medalioin B, Smuk P, Hagberg C, Susmalian S (2003) Prediction of difficult laryngoscopy in obese patients by ultrasound quantification of anterior neck soft tissue. Anesthesia 58:1111–1114
4. Lundstrom LH, Moller AM, Rosenstock C, Astrup G, Wetterslev J (2009) High body mass index is a weak predictor for difficult and failed tracheal-intubation. Anesthesiology 110(2):266–274
5. Ezri T, Medalion B, Weisenberg M, Szmuk P, Warters RD, Charuzi I (2003) Increased body mass index per se is not a predictor of difficult laryngoscopy. Can J Anaesth 50:179–183
6. Lundstrom LH, Vester-Andersen M, Moller AM, Charuluxananan S, L'Hermite J, Wetterslev J (2011) Poor prognostic value of the modified Mallampati score: a meta-analysis involving 177,088 patients. Br J Anaesth 107(5):659–667
7. Kristensen MS (2011) Ultrasonography in the management of the airway. Acta Anaesthesiol Scaninavica 55(10):1155–1173
8. Singh M, Chin KJ, Chan VWS, Wong DT, Prasad GA, Yu E (2010) Use of sonography for airway assessment: an observational study. J Ultrasound Med 29(1):79–85
9. Green JS, Tsui BCS (2010) Applications of ultrasonography in ENT: airway assessment and nerve blockage. Anesthesiol Clin 28(3):541–553
10. Lakha K, Delplace X, Cottier JP, Tranquart F, Sauvagnac X, Mercier C, Fusciardi J, Laffon M (2007) The feasibility of ultrasound to assess subglottic diameter. Anesth Analg 104(3):611–614
11. Cook TM (2000) A new practical classification of laryngeal view. Anaesthesia 55(3):274–279

12. Adhikari S, Zeger W, Schmier C, Crum T, Craven A, Frrokaj I, Pang H, Shostrom V (2011) Pilot study to determine the utility of point-of-care ultrasound in the assessment of difficult laryngoscopy. Acad Emerg Med 18(7):754–758
13. Wu J, Dong J, Ding Y, Zheng J (2014) Role of anterior neck soft tissue quantifications by ultrasound in predicting difficult laryngoscopy. Med Sci Monit Int Med J Exp Clin Res 20:2343
14. Pinto J, Cordeiro L, Pereira C, Gama R, Fernandes HL, Assuncao J (2016) Predicting difficult laryngoscopy using ultrasound measurement of distance from skin to epiglottis. J Crit Care 33:26–31
15. Ko DR, Chung YE, Park I, Lee HJ, Park JW, You JS, Chung TN, Park YS, Chung SP, Kim S (2012) Use of bedside sonography for diagnosing acute epiglottitis in the emergency department. J Ultrasound Med 31(1):19–22
16. Fulkerson JS, Moore HM, Anderson TS, Lowe JRJ (2017) Ultrasonography in the perioperative difficult airway assessment. J Clin Monit Comput 31(3):513–530
17. Werner SL, Jones RA, Emerman CL (2004) Sonographic assessment of the epiglottis. Acad Emerg Med 11(12):1358–1360
18. Wojtczak JA (2012) Submandibular sonography: assessment of hyomental distances and ratio, tongue size, and floor of the mouth musculature using portable sonography. J Ultrasound Med 31(4):523–528
19. Hui CM, Tsui BC (2014) Sublingual ultrasound as an assessment method for predicting difficult intubation: a pilot study. Anaesthesia 69(4):314–319
20. Parameswari A, Govind M, Vakamudi M (2017) Correlation between preoperative ultrasonographic airway assessment and laryngoscopic view in adult patients: a prospective study. J Anaesthesiol Clin Pharmacol 33(3):353–358
21. Koay CK (1998) Difficult tracheal intubation—analysis and management in 37 case. Singap Med J 39:112–114
22. Gupta S, Sharma R, Jain D (2005) Airway assessment: predictors of difficult airway. Indian J Anaesth 49(4):257–262
23. Fox W, Harris S, Kennedy N (2008) Prevalence of difficult intubation in a bariatric population, using the beach chair position. Anaesthesia 63(12):1339–1342
24. Yao W, Wang B (2017) Can tongue thickness measured by ultrasonography predict difficult intubation? Br J Anaesth 118(4):601–609

# 16

# Lung and diaphragm ultrasound as predictors of success in weaning from mechanical ventilation

Eva Tenza-Lozano[1*], Ana Llamas-Alvarez[1], Enrique Jaimez-Navarro[1] and Javier Fernández-Sánchez[2]

**Abstract**

**Background:** Lung and diaphragm ultrasound methods have recently been introduced to predict the outcome of weaning from mechanical ventilation (MV). The aim of this study is to assess the reliability and accuracy of these techniques for predicting successful weaning in critically ill adults.

**Methods:** We conducted two studies: a cross-sectional interobserver agreement study between two sonographers and a prospective cohort study to assess the accuracy of lung and diaphragm ultrasound for predicting weaning and extubation outcome. For the interobserver agreement study, we included 50 general critical care patients who were consecutively admitted to the ICU. For the predictive accuracy study, we included consecutively 69 patients on MV who were ready for weaning. We assessed interobserver agreement of ultrasound measurements, using the weighted kappa coefficient for LUSm score (modified lung ultrasound score) and the intraclass correlation coefficient (ICC) and Bland–Altman method for TI (diaphragm thickening index). We assessed the predictive value of LUSm and TI in weaning outcome by plotting the corresponding ROC curves.

**Results:** We found adequate interobserver agreement for both LUSm (weighted kappa 0.95) and TI (ICC 0.78, difference according to Bland–Altman analysis ± 12.5%). LUSm showed good-moderate discriminative power for successful weaning and extubation (area under the ROC curve (AUC) for successful weaning 0.80, and sensitivity and specificity at optimal cut-off point 0.76 and 0.73, respectively; AUC for successful extubation 0.78, and optimal sensitivity and specificity 0.76 and 0.47, respectively. TI was more sensitive but less specific for predicting successful weaning (AUC 0.71, optimal sensitivity and specificity 0.93 and 0.48) and successful extubation (AUC 0.76, optimal sensitivity and specificity 0.93 and 0.58). The area under the ROC curve for predicting weaning success was 0.83 for both ultrasound measurements together.

**Conclusions:** Interobserver agreement was excellent for LUSm and moderate-good for TI. A low TI value or high LUSm value indicates high risk of weaning failure.

**Keywords:** Lung ultrasound, Diaphragm ultrasound, Weaning, Withdrawal of mechanical ventilation

## Background

Although widespread use of MV in the intensive care unit (ICU) saves hundreds of lives daily, prolonged MV can lead to increased mortality and morbidity [1–3]. On the one hand, therefore, weaning should be considered as early as possible. On the other hand, however, premature withdrawal can result in extubation failure, which is also associated with increased morbidity and mortality [1, 4, 5].

Several ventilatory indices have been developed for identifying the right time to extubate the patient who has required endotracheal intubation and MV, but none met the criteria required to provide suitably accurate success rates [6]. More recently, lung and diaphragm ultrasound methods have been introduced, assessing pulmonary airway patterns and diaphragm function. Bouhemad [7] was the first author to propose the LUS score for calculating

*Correspondence: evitatl@hotmail.com
[1] Intensive Care Unit, Department of Intensive Care Medicine, Elche General University Hospital, Camino de la Almazara 11, 03203 Elche, Spain
Full list of author information is available at the end of the article

lung aeration patterns in patients with ventilator-associated pneumonia. In later articles, this score was used to predict weaning outcome [8–11], with promising results. Several parameters measured through diaphragm ultrasound have been proposed for the same purpose [11–21]. These include diaphragm thickness, diaphragm movement or excursion during the respiratory cycle [22], and diaphragm thickening or thickening fraction (TI). Although some studies have shown diaphragm excursion and thickness to be of low predictive value in the assessment of diaphragm function [18, 19, 23], a recent meta-analysis corroborates this and the best use of TI to weaning outcome [24].

The data suggest that TI and LUS are good non-invasive indicators of weaning outcome. However, the reliability and accuracy of these studies is limited, mainly due to small sample sizes, inadequate spectra of patients and study heterogeneity [24]. The aim of this study is to assess the reliability and accuracy of lung and diaphragm ultrasound for predicting successful weaning in general critical care patients on mechanical ventilation.

## Methods

### Design

We performed two independent studies: a cross-sectional concordance study between two sonographers (interobserver agreement study) and a prospective cohort study to assess the accuracy of lung and diaphragm ultrasound for predicting weaning and extubation outcome (predictive accuracy study).

### Population

For the interobserver agreement study, we included 50 patients (with or without MV), who were consecutively admitted to the ICU of our hospital from December 2016 to February 2017, and who required a thoracic ultrasound examination for clinical reasons.

For the predictive accuracy study, we included consecutively all patients on MV admitted to the ICU from 15 January 2016 to 15 April 2017 who have signed the informed consent (Additional file 1) and met the following inclusion criteria (1) over 18 years of age; (2) more than 24 h on MV; (3) ready for weaning.

We applied the same exclusion criteria for both studies: (1) spinal cord injury higher than T8; (2) arrhythmias and haemodynamic instability; (3) terminal extubation; (4) pregnancy; (5) pneumothorax, pneumomediastinum, thoracostomy, chest tube or chest injuries that prevent ultrasound; (6) pleural lesions or pleurodesis.

### Measurements/procedures

#### *Ultrasound technique*

Two sonographers trained in lung and diaphragm ultrasound, according to international recommendations [25] (Additional files 1, 2 and 3), performed the ultrasound measurements. They used a 2–4 MHz convex probe in B mode, as described in other studies [7, 8]. The scoring system adopted distinguishes four ventilation patterns as follows: normal aeration (N; presence of lung sliding with A lines and fewer than two isolated B lines), moderate loss of pulmonary ventilation (B1; more than two well-defined B lines), severe loss of pulmonary ventilation (B2; multiple coalescing B lines) and pulmonary consolidation (C; presence of a tissue pattern). Scores of 0–3 were respectively attributed to the four categories (0 point for N, 1 point for B1, 2 points for B2 and 3 points for C), and for each region the worst visible pattern was recorded. Rather than using the original LUS score, in our study, we applied a modified procedure (LUSm), evaluating four lung regions on each side instead of the standard six. Our intention in making this modification was to avoid having to move the critical patient, thus preventing the associated complications and facilitating the examination process for the operators. We assessed four areas: anterior–superior, anterior-inferior, lateral and postero-basal. The postero-basal area is where most of the pathology of the critical patient according to Lichtenstein [26] occurs. The total LUSm score for all areas ranged from 0 to 24 points.

In the diaphragm ultrasound examination, the sonographers measured diaphragm thickness using a 7–10 MHz linear probe in B mode (Micromax® Sonosite) following the technique described in other studies [11–18, 20, 27]. The right hemidiaphragm was visualised in the zone of apposition, on the midaxillary line between the 8th and 10th intercostal spaces, with the patient in a semi-decubitus position (20°–40°). The diaphragm was viewed in M-mode as a hypoechoic structure between two echoic lines (the diaphragmatic pleura and the peritoneal membrane). The sonographers captured almost three images in M-mode during spontaneous patient breathing, measuring diaphragm thickness at the end of expiration and at the end of inspiration. We made the average of three TI measurements using the following formula: (end inspiratory diaphragm thickness − end expiratory diaphragm thickness)/end inspiratorydiaphragm thickness.

#### *Interobserver agreement study*

Both sonographers took TI and LUSm measurements in the same sample of 50 stable patients, with a time difference of less than 5 h between the two operators. This sample was different from the predictive accuracy study.

#### *Predictive accuracy study*

In the predictive accuracy study, the patients who were ready to start weaning, according to the international consensus conference criteria [28], the respirator was selected with 8 cm $H_2O$ pressure support (PS) and 5 cm $H_2O$ positive end-expiratory pressure (PEEP) and ultrasound and ventilatory measurements were made. The ventilatory measurements are made automatically by the respirator (model: GE DATEX- OHMEDA Engström Carestation). Afterwards, SBT was continued with a T-tube or with 8 cm $H_2O$ PS and 5 PEEP, depending on the decision of the responsible physician, who evaluated which of the patients successfully passed the SBT, and those who did were extubated. The medical team was blinded to the ultrasound results, and the research team played no role in the patient's weaning. Weaning failure according to the 2007 international consensus conference [28] is defined as either failure of SBT or failure of extubation. Extubation failure is defined as the occurrence of reintubation, non-invasive ventilatory support or death within 48 h following extubation.

### Statistical analysis

Data were expressed as medians and interquartile ranges (IQR) or percentages. To compare continuous variables, we used the unpaired Student's *t* test, Mann–Whitney *U* test and Wilcoxon test. For categorical variables, we applied the Chi-square or Fisher's exact test.

To evaluate interobserver agreement for LUSm, we calculated the quadratic-weighted kappa coefficient (which is comparable to ICC) and for the TI variable we used ICC and the Bland–Altman method.

In the predictive accuracy study, we calculated the AUCs and their corresponding sensitivities, specificities and likelihood ratios (LR+and LR−) at the optimal cut-off points, to determine the predictive value of TI and LUSm for weaning and extubation success. We developed a predictive model using binary logistic regression, with the ultrasound measures (LUSm and TI) as independent variables to predict successful weaning.

We used the StatsDirect v3.0.194 package to perform the statistical analysis.

### Ethical aspects

The research ethics committee of Elche General University Hospital approved the study and all enrolled patients gave their informed consent.

## Results

In the interobserver agreement study, the quadratic-weighted kappa value for LUSm was 0.95 (95% CI 0.92, 0.98), which shows almost perfect interobserver agreement. For the TI variable, we calculated an ICC value of 0.78 (95% CI 0.65, 0.87), showing moderate to good interobserver agreement, and a difference in measurements according to the Bland–Altman method of ±12.5% (Fig. 1).

Over the study period, 139 patients underwent MV, of whom 52 did not meet the inclusion criteria (48 deaths before attempted weaning, 2 self-extubations, 2 on MV for less than 24 h) and 17 were not included for reasons beyond the research team's control (eight withdrawn more gradually from MV, two with no informed consent, two transferred to another hospital, four eligible patients of whom the investigator was not notified, one case of a non-functioning ultrasound scanner). The baseline

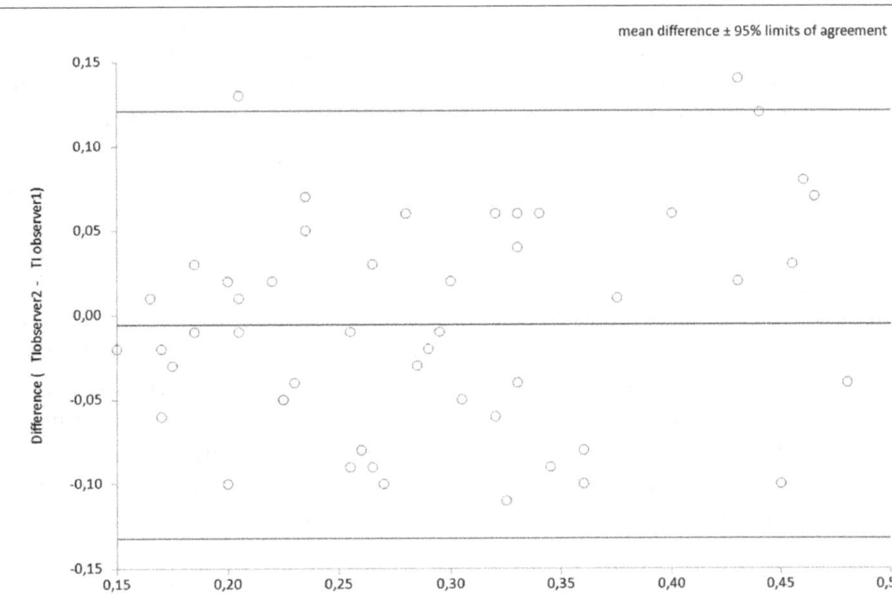


**Fig. 1** Bland–Altman method for interobserver difference in TI measurement

characteristics of the 69 patients recruited are shown in Table 1. Pressure support was used in 49% of SBTs, a T-tube in 42% and both methods in 9%. Eight patients failed SBT and 61 were extubated, of whom 17 failed extubation. This means that a total of 25 patients failed weaning. Most patients who failed extubation recovered with non-invasive-ventilation (NIV) and high-flow nasal cannula (HFNC); only five patients (8.2%) were reintubated (Fig. 2).

If we compare the group that was successfully weaned (SW) with those who failed weaning (FW) (Table 1), we observe that the FW group was associated with more time on MV, more cases of chronic obstructive pulmonary disease (COPD), higher LUSm and mortality, and lower TI and $SpO_2$. The median difference in TI and LUSm between the SW and FW groups was 11% and 3 points, respectively.

The area under the ROC curve for predicting weaning success was 0.80 for LUSm (95% CI 0.69, 0.91), 0.71 for TI (95% CI 0.58, 0.84) (Fig. 3) and 0.83 for both (Fig. 4). Table 2 shows the sensitivity, specificity and likelihood ratios at the optimal cut-off points for successful weaning. The area under the ROC curve for predicting extubation success was 0.78 for LUSm (95% CI 0.64, 0.91) and 0.76 for TI (95% CI, 0.61–0.9) (Fig. 3). Table 3 shows the sensitivity, specificity and likelihood ratios at the same cut-off points as those shown in the previous two tables.

## Discussion

According to our data, the reproducibility of lung ultrasound is excellent for the variable LUSm and moderate to good for TI. Regarding the prognostic accuracy of ultrasound for weaning outcome, we found that if TI is below 24% or LUSm is greater than 7 points, the patient has a high risk of weaning failure, with an AUC of 0.8 for LUSm and 0.71 for TI. We found similar values for extubation outcome.

Mean time on MV [29, 30], mortality of the patients included in the study (16%) [4], and SBT failure rate (11.6%) [31] was consistent with previously published results. Extubation failure occurred in 24.6% of the patients, a slightly higher proportion than the 10% to 20% reported in a number of other studies [1, 5, 32–35]. Of the 17 patients who failed extubation, only five (8.2%) required reintubation, a lower rate than reported in other studies [36, 37]. This shows that NIV plays a decisive role in reducing the need for reintubation without increasing morbidity or mortality [37, 38]. As such, through conceptually defined as a criteria of weaning failure [28], we consider that recovery with NIV in fact constitutes a success for the patient's clinical situation. We observed that FW patients were more likely to have COPD. This is a logical finding, as COPD is a risk factor for extubation failure [39, 40]. Of the standard predictors of weaning assessed in our study ($PI_{Max}$, RSBI, P0.1), we found none to be useful. In a study with the largest number of patients performed for the study of weaning predictors [6], about 500 patients, to assess the predictability of many indices as possible weaning predictors (minute volume, respiratory rate, $PaO_2$, RSBI, $PI_{Max}$, Maximum expiratory pressure, dynamic respiratory compliance, CROP index), it is observed that none of them has value as a predictor of weaning.

The results obtained for LUSm are consistent with previously reported data [8–11]. Our cut-off point is lower (7 LUSm points) because we assessed eight lung areas, whereas the other studies assessed 12. Our aim was to assess all the areas normally affected in critical patients [26], while simplifying the technique so that the patient did not have to be moved, and the associated complications could be avoided. We therefore consider LUSm to constitute a useful new proposal that is beneficial for both the patient and the operator. For TI, we found a cut-off point of 24% for predicting successful weaning, within the range of values reported in other studies (20–36%) [11–20]. The LUS and TI variables tested in those studies showed a higher predictive value for weaning success (Table 2), but a number of factors may have influenced this result. In those studies, patient selection was in some cases very strict, resulting in a homogeneous sample with specific characteristics (patients with COPD [15], tracheotomised patients with prior weaning failure [13], patients with ICU-acquired weakness [17]). Since these samples already had a higher probability of weaning failure, their results cannot be generalised to the whole population of critical care patients. Other limitations in the reviewed studies included elimination of deceased patients [20], diaphragm ultrasound when the patient was on MV rather than during SBT [20], use of a non-validated probe for diaphragm measurement [18], periods of up to 36 h between the ultrasound scan and extubation [12], and using STB failure rather than extubation failure as an endpoint [13]. Only one of the reviewed studies included a reproducibility study comparing TI measurement by two observers, with results very similar to ours (ICC 0.81) [14].

In our study, we chose not to select specific populations of patients for our study, to obtain a heterogeneous sample and produce generalizable results. The ultrasound measurements were taken within the first minutes of pressure support ventilation, the physicians were blinded to the ultrasound data, no patients were lost to follow-up, and the median time between SBT and extubation was 120 min.

One limitation of our study is the small sample size, which led to imprecise results with broad confidence intervals, especially for TI. Further studies with larger

**Table 1 Characteristics of patients included in the study**

| Variables | All patients (69) | SW (44) | FW (25) | *P* value |
|---|---|---|---|---|
| Sex (men)[a] | 43 (62.3) | 26 (63.4) | 15 (62.5) | 0.8 |
| Age (years)[b] | 66 (53, 78) | 65 (53, 78) | 69 (64, 78) | 0.37 |
| Time on MV (days)[b] | *4 (3, 7)* | *4 (2, 6)* | *5 (3, 9)* | *0.04* |
| Time SBT-extubation (minutes)[b] | 120 (30, 120) | 120 (30, 120) | 60 (30, 120) | 0.15 |
| Mode of STB | | | | |
| T–T | 29 (42%) | 17 (38.6%) | 12 (48%) | 0.14 |
| PS 8 and PEEP 5 | 34 (49%) | 21 (47.7%) | 13 (52%) | |
| T–T + PS 8 PEEP 5 | 6(9%) | 6 (13.6%) | 0 | |
| Comorbidity[a] | | | | |
| Chronic heart disease | 18 (26) | 14 (31.8) | 4 (16) | 0.25 |
| Neurological disease | 18 (26) | 12 (27.3) | 6 (24) | 0.99 |
| COPD | *13 (18.8)* | *5 (11.4)* | *8 (32)* | *0.05* |
| Diabetes mellitus | 19 (27.5) | 12 (27.3) | 7 (28) | 0.99 |
| Cancer | 8 (11.6) | 4 (9.1) | 4 (16) | 0.45 |
| Chronic kidney failure | 12 (17.4) | 6 (13.6) | 6 (24) | 0.33 |
| Liver disease | 8 (11.6) | 3 (6.8) | 5 (20) | 0.36 |
| Pathology at ICU admission[a] | | | | |
| Neurological disease | 29 (42) | 18 (41) | 11 (44) | |
| Respiratory disease | 24 (34, 8) | 16 (36.4) | 8 (32) | |
| Cardiovascular disease | 10 (14.5) | 8 (18.2) | 2 (8) | 0.7 |
| Sepsis | 7 (10.1) | 5 (11.4) | 2 (8) | |
| Digestive pathology | 4 (5.8) | 1 (2.3) | 3 (12) | |
| Polytrauma | 1 (1.4) | 1 (2.3) | 0 | 0.7 |
| LUSm[b] | *6 (4, 8)* | *5 (3, 7)* | *8 (7, 11)* | *0.0001* |
| TI (%)[b] | *36 (27, 41)* | *38 (31, 45)* | *27 (20, 40)* | *0.003* |
| APACHE II on SBT day[b] | 4 (2, 6) | 4 (2, 6) | 5 (3, 9) | 0.07 |
| VE (L/min)[b] | 8.6 (7.5, 10) | 8.25 (7.3, 9.8) | 9 (8.1, 11.6) | 0.13 |
| Compliance (mL/cm $H_2O$)[b] | 56 (41, 67) | 55.5 (43, 69) | 59 (40.5, 67) | 0.86 |
| $PI_{Max}$ (cm $H_2O$)[b] | − 25 (− 23, − 25) | − 25 (− 25, − 18) | − 25 (− 26, − 24) | 0.28 |
| P0.1 (cm $H_2O$)[b] | 1 (1, 3) | 1 (1, 3) | 1.5 (1, 2.5) | 0.47 |
| RSBI (breaths/min/L)[b] | 35 (20, 50) | 31 (20, 43) | 37 (30, 54) | 0.16 |
| RR (breaths/min)[b] | 17 (15, 20) | 17 (14, 19) | 19 (16, 22) | 0.09 |
| Tidal volume (ml)[b] | 400 (450, 585) | 508 (452, 572) | 500 (440, 600) | 0.71 |
| $FiO_2$ (%)[b] | 30 (28, 35) | 30 (28, 35) | 30 (28, 35) | 0.83 |
| $SpO_2$ (%)[b] | 98 (97, 100) | 99 (97, 100) | 97 (96, 99) | 0.027 |
| $PaCO_2$ (mm Hg)[b] | 40 (36, 46) | 41 (36, 45.6) | 39.6 (37, 45) | 0.63 |
| $PaO_2$, (mm Hg)[b] | 93 (79, 115) | 96.5 (83, 117) | 92 (74, 115) | 0.61 |
| pH[b] | 7.42 (7.32, 7.47) | 7.4 (7.3, 7.5) | 7.4 (7.4, 7.4) | 0.93 |
| Lactate (mmol/L)[b] | 1.2 (1, 1.7) | 1.2 (1, 1.5) | 1.3 (1.1, 2) | 0.2 |
| ICU mortality[a] | *7 (14)* | *1 (2.3)* | *6 (24)* | *0.005* |
| Hospital mortality[a] | *11 (16)* | *3 (6.8)* | *8 (32)* | *0.003* |
| ICU stay (days)[b] | *11 (7, 19)* | *8 (6, 15)* | *18 (11, 21)* | *0.002* |
| Hospital stay (days)[b] | 19 (14, 30) | 17 (13.5, 31) | 23 (17, 30) | 0.08 |

SW, successful weaning; FW, failed weaning; MV, mechanical ventilation; T–T, disconnection with T-tube with oxygen; PS 8 and PEEP, 5 disconnection with pressure support and 5 cm $H_2O$ positive end-expiratory pressure; ICU, intensive care unit; LUSm, modified lung ultrasound score; TI, diaphragm thickness index; APACHE II, acute physiology and chronic health evaluation II; SBT, spontaneous breathing trial; VE, minute ventilation; $PI_{Max}$, maximal inspiratory pressure; P0.1, airway occlusion pressure; RR, respiratory rate; RSBI, rapid shallow breathing index; $FiO_2$, fraction of inspired oxygen; $SpO_2$, oxygen saturation; $PaCO_2$, partial pressure of carbon dioxide; $PaO_2$, partial pressure of oxygen; ICU, intensive care unit

[a] n (%), [b]Median (IQR)

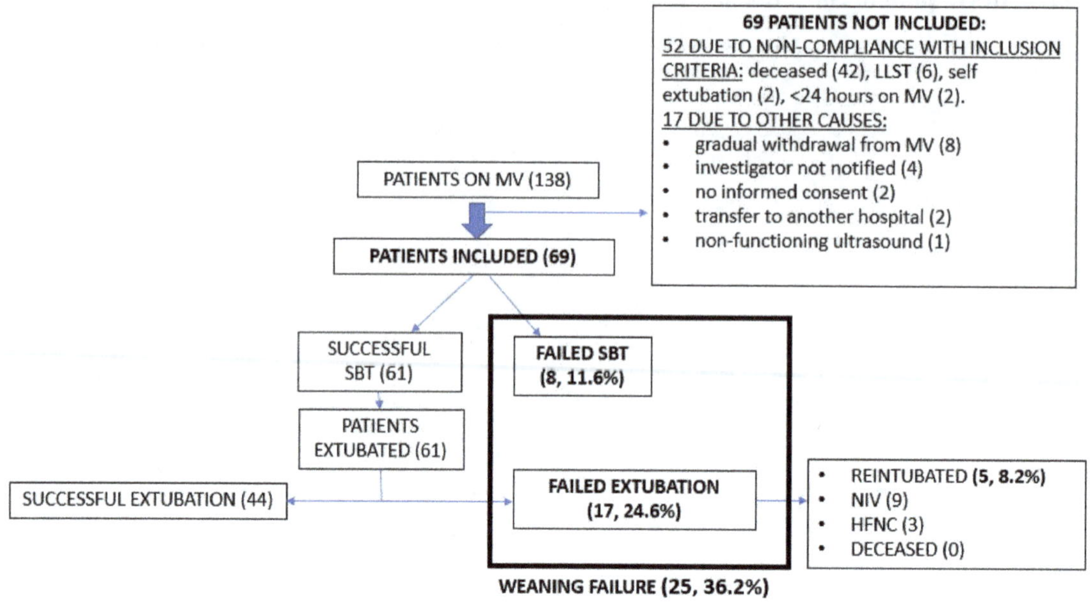


**Fig. 2** Flowchart of patients

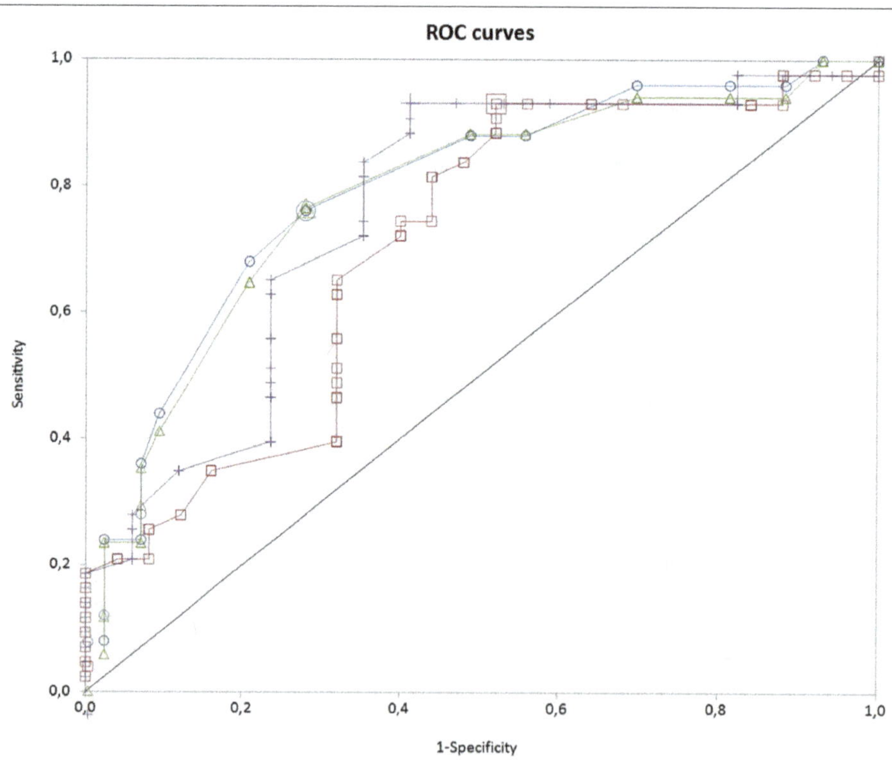


**Fig. 3** ROC curves for predictive value of TI in successful weaning (SW) (+), in successful extubation (SE) (White square) and LUSm in SW (White circle) and SE (Increment). In SW: LUSm AUC 0.8; TI AUC 0.71. In SE: LUSm AUC 0.78; TI AUC 0.76

samples of patients are required to establish the true predictive power of these ultrasound techniques.

It should be noted that the interobserver difference in TI measurement (±12.5%) was greater than the median difference in TI between the SW/FW groups (11%). In our sample, therefore, a degree of uncertainty was associated with this parameter. This is probably because the formula for calculating TI is such that a difference of a

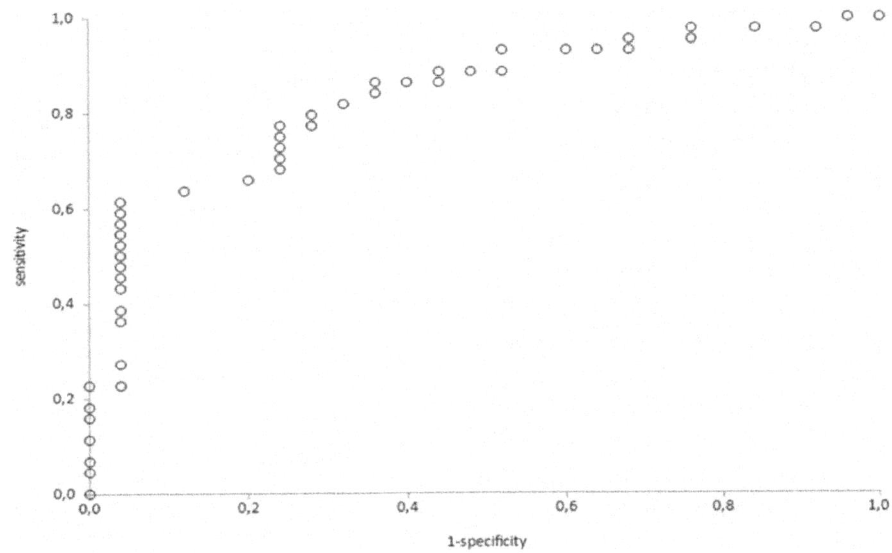


**Fig. 4** ROC curve for predictive value of TI plus LUSm in successful weaning (SW). AUC 0.83

**Table 2 Comparison with other studies of predictive value of TI and LUS for successful weaning**

| Study (ref)—variable | n | AUC | Sensitivity | Specificity | LR+ | LR− | Cut-off point (%) |
|---|---|---|---|---|---|---|---|
| Binet [9]—LUS | 48 | 0.89 | 1 | 0.44 | 1.80 | 0 | 14 |
| Osman [11]—LUS | 68 | 0.94 | 1 | 0.94 | 18 | 0 | 12 |
| Shoaeir [10]—LUS | 50 | 0.95 | 0.83 | 1 | | 0.17 | 10 |
| Soummer [8]—LUS | 86 | 0.87 | 0.68 | 0.86 | 4.96 | 0.37 | 13 |
| Tenza—LUSm | 69 | 0.80 | 0.76 | 0.73 | 2.8 | 0.44 | 7 |
| Ali [16]—TI | 54 | – | 0.96 | 0.85 | 6.27 | 0.04 | 30[a] |
| Baess [18]—TI | 30 | 0.65 | 0.70 | 0.71 | 2.43 | 0.42 | 30[a] |
| Blumhof(14)—TI | 33 | 0.86 | 0.85 | 0.77 | 3.67 | 0.20 | 20[a] |
| DiNino [12]—TI | 63 | 0.79 | 0.88 | 0.71 | 3.07 | 0.17 | 30[a] |
| Farghaly [16]—TI | 54 | 0.71 | 0.9 | 0.64 | 2.52 | 0.16 | 34.5[a] |
| Fayed [15]—TI | 112 | 0.93 | 0.98 | 0.73 | 3.66 | 0.04 | 29[a]; 24[b] |
| Ferrari [13]—TI | 46 | 0.95 | 0.83 | 0.88 | 7.03 | 0.20 | 36[a] |
| Jung [17]—TI | 33 | – | 0.61 | 0.93 | 9.17 | 0.42 | 20[a] |
| Osman [11]—TI | 68 | 0.89 | 0.88 | 1 | – | 0.12 | 28[a] |
| Tenza—TI | 69 | 0.71 | 0.93 | 0.48 | 1.8 | 0.14 | 24[a] |

AUC, area under the ROC curve; LR+, positive likelihood ratio; LR−, negative likelihood ratio; LUS, lung ultrasound score; LUSm, modified lung ultrasound score; TI, diaphragm thickness index

[a] Right hemidiaphragm; [b] Left hemidiaphragm

**Table 3 Predictive value of LUSm and TI for successful extubation**

| Variable | AUC | Sensitivity | Specificity | LR+ | LR− | Cut-off point (%) |
|---|---|---|---|---|---|---|
| LUSm | 0.78 | 0.76 | 0.72 | 2.74 | 0.33 | 7 |
| TI | 0.76 | 0.93 | 0.58 | 2.26 | 0.12 | 24 |
| LUSm + TI | 0.83 | 0.86 | 0.56 | 1.97 | 0.24 | |

AUC, area under the ROC curve; LR+, positive likelihood ratio; LR−, negative likelihood ratio; LUSm, modified lung ultrasound score; TI, diaphragm thickness index tenth of a millimeter in the measurement of inspiratory or expiratory diaphragm thickness has a considerable effect on the result. None of the studies reviewed considers this possibility. We believe the problem can be overcome with better ultrasound equipment and a more effective TI measuring technique, so that the true value of this parameter can be reported.

In the future, in order that results can be compared across studies, we believe a number of items should be standardised: the ultrasound technique, the definitions of weaning failure and extubation failure, the time between ultrasound and extubation, blinding of ultrasound findings, and the protocol. If results are to be applied to the whole population of general critical care patients on MV, a heterogeneous sample should be used. Studies in this domain should also assess reproducibility by measuring interobserver agreement in ultrasound measurements. In addition, it may be useful to consider other parameters, such as time on MV, disease severity, comorbidities, etc., alongside lung and diaphragm ultrasound measurements, to better predict weaning success.

## Conclusions

In our study, interobserver agreement was excellent in LUSm measurements and moderate to good in TI measurements. The TI variable showed a degree of uncertainty for predicting weaning outcome, but overall its predictive value was found to be acceptable. LUSm produced stronger results in this regard. Lung and diaphragm ultrasound are promising techniques for predicting weaning outcome, but more studies are required to verify their reproducibility. These studies should have a standardised design and should assess interobserver agreement of ultrasound techniques. Using a non-specific sample would ensure that results can be generalised to all patients on MV.

## Additional files

**Additional file 1.** Lung ultrasound video.

**Additional file 2.** Diaphragm ultrasound video.

**Additional file 3.** Diaphragm ultrasound video.

### Abbreviations

MV: mechanical ventilation; ICU: intensive care unit; LUS: lung ultrasound score; LUSm: modified lung ultrasound score; TI: diaphragm thickening index; ROC curves: receiver operating characteristic curves; ICC: intraclass correlation coefficient; AUC: area under the ROC curve; SBT: spontaneous breathing; PEEP: positive end-expiratory pressure; IQR: interquartile ranges; LR+: positive likelihood ratio; LR-: negative likelihood ratio; CI: confidence interval; NIV: non-invasive ventilation; HFNC: high-flow nasal cannula; SW: successfully weaned; FW: failed weaning; COPD: chronic obstructive pulmonary disease; VE: minute ventilation; $PI_{Max}$: maximal inspiratory pressure; P0.1: airway occlusion pressure; RR: respiratory rate; RSBI: rapid shallow breathing index; $FiO_2$: fraction of inspired oxygen; $SpO_2$: oxygen saturation; $PaCO_2$: partial pressure of carbon dioxide; $PaO_2$: partial pressure of oxygen; APACHE II: acute physiology and chronic health evaluation II.

### Authors' contributions

ET-L is guarantor for the entire manuscript. ET-L had full access to all the data in the study; takes responsibility for the integrity of the data and the accuracy of the data analysis; contributed to the study concept and design, data analysis and drafting of the manuscript; and served as principal author. AML-A contributed to the literature search. ET-L and EJ-N contributed to the ultrasound measurements. JF-S contributed to the study design and revision of the manuscript. All authors read and approved the final manuscript.

### Author details

[1] Intensive Care Unit, Department of Intensive Care Medicine, Elche General University Hospital, Camino de la Almazara 11, 03203 Elche, Spain. [2] Department of Clinical Medicine, Miguel Hernandez University, Sant Joan d'Alacant, Spain.

### Acknowledgements

The authors appreciate the assistance of Jaime Latour-Pérez, PhD, for his contribution to the study design, drafting of the manuscript and statistical analysis, and Julia Turner, MSc, for her help with the language editing and review of the manuscript.

### References

1. Peñuelas O, Frutos-Vivar F, Fernández C, Anzueto A, Epstein SK, Apezteguía C et al (2011) Characteristics and outcomes of ventilated patients according to time to liberation from mechanical ventilation. Am J Respir Crit Care Med 184(4):430–437
2. Powers SK, Kavazis ANLS (2009) Prolonged mechanical ventilation alters diaphragmatic structure and function. Crit Care Med 37(10 suppl):S347–S353
3. Levine S, Nguyen T, Taylor N, Friscia ME, Budak MT, Rothenberg P, Zhu J, Sachdeva R, Sonnad S, Kaiser LR, Rubinstein NA, Powers SKSJ (2008) Rapid disuse atrophy of diaphragm fibers in mechanically ventilated humans. N Engl J Med 358(13):1327–1335
4. Béduneau G, Pham T, Schortgen F, Piquilloud L, Zogheib E, Jonas M, Grelon F, Runge I, Terzi N, Grangé S, Barberet G, Guitard PG, Frat JP, Constan A, Chretien JM, Mancebo J, Mer BL (2016) Epidemiology of weaning outcome according to a new definition. The WIND study. Am J Respir Crit Care Med 195(6):772–783
5. Funk GC, Anders S, Breyer MK, Burghuber OC, Edelmann G, Heindl W et al (2010) Incidence and outcome of weaning from mechanical ventilation according to new categories. Eur Respir J 35(1):88–94
6. Savi A, Teixeira C, Silva JM, Borges LG, Pereira PA, Pinto KB et al (2012) Weaning predictors do not predict extubation failure in simple-to-wean patients. J Crit Care 27(2):221-e1–221-e8. https://doi.org/10.1016/j.jcrc.2011.07.079
7. Bouhemad B, Liu ZH, Arbelot C, Zhang M, Ferarri F, Le-Guen M, Girard M, Lu QRJ (2010) Ultrasound assessment of antibiotic-induced pulmonary reaeration in ventilator-associated pneumonia. Crit Care Med 38(1):84–92
8. Soummer A, Perbet S, Brisson H, Arbelot C, Constantin J-M, Lu Q et al (2012) Ultrasound assessment of lung aeration loss during a successful weaning trial predicts postextubation distress. Crit Care Med 40(7):2064–2072
9. Binet C, Neron L, Rochart N, Cousson J, Floch T, Charbit B et al (2014) Validation d'un indice échographique prédictif d'échec de sevrage de la ventilation mécanique. Ann Fr Anesth Reanim 33:A383
10. Shoaeir M, Noeam KMA (2016) Lung aeration loss as a predictor of reintubation using lung ultrasound in mechanically ventilated patients. Biolife 4(3):514–520
11. Osman AM, Hashim RM (2017) Diaphragmatic and lung ultrasound application as new predictive indices for the weaning process in ICU patients. Egypt J Radiol Nucl Med 48:61–66
12. DiNino E, Gartman EJEJ, Sethi JMJM, McCool FDD (2014) Diaphragm ultrasound as a predictor of successful extubation from mechanical ventilation. Thorax 69(5):423–427. https://doi.org/10.1136/thoraxjnl-2013-204111

13. Ferrari G, De Filippi G, Elia F, Panero F, Volpicelli GAF (2014) Diaphragm ultrasound as a new index of discontinuation from mechanical ventilation. Crit Ultrasound J. 6(1):8
14. Blumhof S, Wheeler D, Thomas K, McCool FD, Mora J (2016) Change in diaphragmatic thickness during the respiratory cycle predicts extubation success at various levels of pressure support ventilation. Lung 194(4):519–525
15. Fayed AM, Abd El Hady MA, Shaaban MSFD (2016) Use of ultrasound to assess diaphragmatic thickness as a weaning parameter in invasively ventilated chronic obstructive pulmonary disease patients. J Am Sci. 12(6):96–105
16. Farghaly S, Hasan AA (2015) Diaphragm ultrasound as a new method to predict extubation outcome in mechanically ventilated patients. Aust Crit Care. https://doi.org/10.1016/j.aucc.2016.03.004
17. Jung B, Moury PH, Mahul M, de Jong A, Galia F, Prades A et al (2016) Diaphragmatic dysfunction in patients with ICU-acquired weakness and its impact on extubation failure. Intensive Care Med 42(5):853–861
18. Baess AI, Abdallah TH, Emara DM, Hassan M (2016) Diaphragmatic ultrasound as a predictor of successful extubation from mechanical ventilation: thickness, displacement, or both? Egypt J Bronchiol 10(2):162–166
19. Umbrello M, Formenti P (2016) Ultrasonographic assessment of diaphragm function in critically ill subjects. Respir Care 61(4):542–555
20. Ali ER, Mohamad AM (2016) Diaphragm ultrasound as a new functional and morphological index of outcome, prognosis and discontinuation from mechanical ventilation in critically ill patients and evaluating the possible protective indices against VIDD. Egypt J Chest Dis Tuberc. https://doi.org/10.1016/j.ejcdt.2016.10.006
21. Zambon M, Greco M, Bocchino S, Cabrini L, Beccaria PF, Zangrillo A (2016) Assessment of diaphragmatic dysfunction in the critically ill patient with ultrasound: a systematic review. Intensive Care Med 43(1):29–38
22. Palkar A, Narasimhan M, Greenberg H, Singh K, Koenig S, Mayo P et al (2018) Diaphragm excursion-time index: a new parameter using ultrasonography to predict extubation outcome. Chest 153(5):1213–1220. https://doi.org/10.1016/j.chest.2018.01.007
23. Dubé B-P, Dres M, Mayaux J, Demiri S, Similowski T, Demoule A (2017) Ultrasound evaluation of diaphragm function in mechanically ventilated patients: comparison to phrenic stimulation and prognostic implications. Thorax. https://doi.org/10.1136/thoraxjnl-2016-209459
24. Llamas-Alvarez AM, Tenza-Lozano EM, Latour-Perez J (2017) Diaphragm and lung ultrasound to predict weaning outcome: systematic review and meta-analysis. Chest 152(6):1140–1150
25. Bouhemad B, Zhang M, Lu QRJ (2007) Clinical review: bedside lung ultrasound in critical care practice. Crit Care 11(1):205. https://doi.org/10.1186/cc5668
26. Lichtenstein DAMG (2008) Relevance of lung ultrasound in the diagnosis of acute respiratory failure: the BLUE protocol. Chest 134(1):117–125
27. Matamis D, Soilemezi E, Tsagourias M, Akoumianaki E, Dimassi S, Boroli F et al (2013) Sonographic evaluation of the diaphragm in critically ill patients. Technique and clinical applications. Intensive Care Med 39(5):801–810. https://doi.org/10.1007/s00134-013-2823-1
28. Boles J-M, Bion J, Connors A, Herridge M, Marsh B, Melot C et al (2007) Weaning from mechanical ventilation. Eur Respir J 29(5):1033–1056. https://doi.org/10.1183/09031936.00010206
29. Esteban A, Anzueto A, Frutos F, Alía I, Brochard L, Stewart TE, Benito S, Epstein SK, Apezteguía C, Nightingale P, Arroliga AC, Tobin MJ (2002) Characteristics and outcomes in adult patients receiving mechanical ventilation: a 28-day international study. JAMA 287(3):345
30. Esteban A, Frutos-Vivar F, Muriel A, Ferguson ND, Peñuelas O, Abraira V et al (2013) Evolution of mortality over time in patients receiving mechanical ventilation. Am J Respir Crit Care Med 188(2):220–230
31. Figueroa-Casas JB, Broukhim A, Vargas A, Milam L, Montoya R (2014) Interobserver agreement of spontaneous breathing trial outcome. Respir Care 59(9):1324–1328
32. Esteban A, Alía I, Tobin MTA et al (1999) Effect of spontaneous breathing trial duration on outcome of attempts to discontinue mechanical ventilation. Am J Resp Crit Care Med 159:512–518
33. Frutos-Vivar F, Esteban A, Apezteguia C, González M, Arabi Y, Restrepo MI et al (2011) Outcome of reintubated patients after scheduled extubation. J Crit Care 26(5):502–509. https://doi.org/10.1016/j.jcrc.2010.12.015
34. Tonnelier A, Tonnelier JM, Nowak E, Gut-Gobert C, Prat G, Renault A et al (2011) Clinical relevance of classification according to weaning difficulty. Respir Care 56(5):583–590
35. Sellares J, Ferrer M, Cano E, Loureiro H, Valencia M, Torres A (2011) Predictors of prolonged weaning and survival during ventilator weaning in a respiratory ICU. Intensive Care Med 37(5):775–784
36. Thille AW, Boissier F, Ben-Ghezala H, Razazi K, Mekontso-Dessap A, Brun-Buisson C et al (2016) Easily identified at-risk patients for extubation failure may benefit from noninvasive ventilation: a prospective before-after study. Crit Care 20(1):48
37. Ferrer M, Esquinas A, Arancibia F, Thomas Bauer T, Gonzalez G, Carrillo A et al (2003) Noninvasive ventilation during persistent weaning failure: a randomized controlled trial. Am J Respir Crit Care Med 168(1):70–76
38. Nava S, Gregoretti C, Fanfulla F, Squadrone E, Grassi M, Carlucci A, Beltrame FNP (2005) Noninvasive ventilation to prevent respiratory failure after extubation in high-risk patients. Crit Care Med 33(11):2465–2470
39. Esteban A, Alía I, Gordo FFR et al (1997) Extubation outcome after spontaneous breathing trials with T-tube or pressure support ventilation. Am J Respir Crit Care Med 156:459–465
40. Thille AW, Harrois A, Schortgen F, Brun-Buisson C, Brochard L (2011) Outcomes of extubation failure in medical intensive care unit patients. Crit Care Med 39(12):2612–2618

# 17

# Pre-hospital lung ultrasound for cardiac heart failure and COPD: is it worthwhile?

Mirko Zanatta*, Piero Benato, Sigilfredo De Battisti, Concetta Pirozzi, Renato Ippolito and Vito Cianci

**Abstract**

**Background:** Pre-hospital ultrasound is a new challenge and lung ultrasound could be an interesting opportunity in the pre-hospital medical service. The aim of our study was to evaluate the efficacy of lung ultrasound in out-of-hospital non-traumatic respiratory insufficiency.

**Methods:** We planned a case-controlled study in the ULSS 5 ovest vicentino area (Vicenza—Italy) enrolling subjects with severe dyspnea caused by cardiac heart failure or acute exacerbation of chronic obstructive pulmonary disease. We compared drugs administration, oxygen delivery, and laboratory tests between those patients with ultrasound integrated management and those without ultrasound.

**Results:** Pre-hospital lung ultrasound had a high specificity (94.4%) and sensitivity (100%) for the correct identification of alveolar interstitial syndrome using B lines, whereas the percentages obtained with pleural effusion were lower (83.3, 53.3%, respectively). The patients with ultrasound integrated management received a more appropriate pharmacological therapy (*p* 0.01), as well as non-invasive ventilation (CPAP) was used more frequently in those with an acute exacerbation of chronic obstructive pulmonary disease (*p* 0.011). Laboratory tests and blood gases analysis were not significant different between the two study groups. In a sub-analysis of the patients with an A profile, we observed a significant lower concentration of $PCO_2$ in those with an ultrasound integrated management ($PCO_2$: 42.62 vs 52.23 *p* 0.049). According with physicians' opinion, pre-hospital lung ultrasound gave important information or changed the therapy in the 42.3% of cases, whereas it just confirmed physical examination in the 67.7% of cases.

**Conclusions:** Pre-hospital lung ultrasound is easy and feasible, and learning curve is rapid. Our study suggests that cardiac heart failure and acute exacerbation of chronic obstructive pulmonary disease can be considered two indications for pre-hospital ultrasound, and can improve the management of patient with acute respiratory insufficiency.

**Keywords:** Pre-hospital, Lung, Ultrasound, Dyspnea, Heart failure, COPD

## Background

Pre-hospital ultrasound is considered one of the top five research priorities according to the opinion of a consensus meeting of a European expert panel, to identify which ultrasound examinations can be reliably transferred to the pre-hospital setting, how they affect patient management and pathway, and how providers can achieve and maintain specific ultrasound skills [1].

The indications are few and well defined, physicians and operators must be adequately trained, and the examinations must be short, focused, and strictly connected with the patients' symptoms and history. The technical skills are the same of in-hospital critical ultrasound or even simpler [2–8].

The FAST protocol has been used successfully for the management of trauma, both inside and outside the hospital [9, 10].

Ultrasound was included in the latest guidelines for cardiopulmonary resuscitation as a supplementary tool for the identification of reversible causes of cardiac arrest [11].

In the same document, ultrasound was recognized as an additional device for airway management and for

*Correspondence: mirko.zanatta@aulss8.veneto.it
Emergency Department of Arzignano Hospital, AULSS 8 Berica, Via Parco 1, 36071 Arzignano, Vicenza, Italy

post-procedural check of the correct placement of an endo-tracheal tube [11, 12].

The lung ultrasound has changed significantly in-hospital management of non-traumatic respiratory insufficiency, and it could be a new and interesting opportunity also in the pre-hospital setting with a few and clear indications: the determination of the lung profile (A: no signs of increased extravascular lung water—"dry lung"; B: increased extravascular lung water—"wet lung"), the identification of pleural effusions, and the diagnosis of pneumothorax [2, 13].

Lung evaluation is rapid and physicians can reach a reliable diagnosis in a few minutes [13–15].

A rapid two-point technique (upper anterior and basal lateral areas) is usually enough to rule in or rule out an interstitial syndrome, a pneumothorax, or a pleural effusion [13, 15–17].

Nevertheless, there are not many studies evaluating the real effectiveness of the pre-hospital lung ultrasound: Neesse et al. [15] showed that the identification of a pleural effusion is useful for the differentiation between a cardiac heart failure (CHF) and an acute exacerbation of a chronic obstructive pulmonary disease (COPD). Strnad et al. and Ferrari and collaborators suggested that lung ultrasound is reliable to monitor response to pre-hospital treatment with continuous positive airway pressure (CPAP) in patients with CHF [18, 19].

The primary and secondary outcomes of our work evaluated the efficacy of lung ultrasound in out-of-hospital non-traumatic respiratory insufficiency, by analyzing clinical and laboratory parameters after the arrival at the emergency department. In particular, we compared drug administration, ventilation, oxygen delivery, and laboratory tests between those patients with ultrasound integrated management and those without ultrasound.

## Methods

We planned a case-controlled study in the pre-hospital emergency setting of the ULSS 5 ovest vicentino area (Vicenza—Italy) between January 2016 and December 2016.

This area included one major emergency department with 35.000 accesses par year, and a minor emergency department located in the countryside with 6000 accesses par year, each one with an emergency physician-led advanced life support (ALS) ambulance.

The former had an ultrasound portable device (Nanomax Sonosite) in the ambulance; the latter did not. All controlled cases were collected from the second one.

All patients included in the studied were treated in the major emergency department.

Inclusion criteria was severe dyspnea as prevalent symptom most likely caused by CHF or COPD exacerbation and digital pulse oximetry $\leq 90\%$, whereas exclusion criteria were other causes of respiratory insufficiency (for example: trauma, pulmonary embolism, cancer) and subjects less that 18 years old.

The two groups were matched for age, gender, type of respiratory insufficiency, and digital pulse oximetry recorded by the ambulance crew.

All recruited patients underwent a rapid and complete physical examination. Blood pressure, heart frequency, and pulse oximetry were tested.

Oxygen was delivered using an oxymask and inspiratory fraction of oxygen was extrapolated by oxygen flow according with the operating instructions.

Non-invasive ventilation was performed using a Boussignac system that allowed the application of a continuous positive airway pressure (PEEP) from 5 to 10 $cmH_2O$ and the possibility to choose among three different percentages of oxygen: 30, 50, and 100%. The criteria used for using the CPAP were the presence of at least one of the following findings: a persistent oximetry lower than 90% even after oxygen supplementation with the oxymask, respiratory rate higher than 30 per min, mild drowsiness.

Lung ultrasound was performed after the clinical examination with a rapid two-point technique (upper anterior and basal lateral areas). The type of lung profile (A profile: dry lung; B profile: wet lung) and the presence of a pleural effusion were recorded.

An interstitial syndrome was defined by the presence of three or more B lines in a longitudinal plane between two ribs in two or more regions bilaterally with a symmetrical pattern, with or without a pleural effusion.

All ultrasound examinations were performed with the same ultrasound device (Sonosite Nanomax) using a convex probe (3.5–5 MHz). A linear probe was used to improve the accuracy in case of an undefined diagnosis.

Operators were certified emergency physicians who had accomplished a full mentoring program for "UltraSound Life Support".

In-hospital assessment included a physical examination, laboratory tests, blood gases analysis, a chest X-ray, in-hospital lung ultrasound, a focused echocardiography, and a static and dynamic evaluation of the vena cava.

The diagnosis made after discharge from the emergency department or after hospitalization was compared with the one made by the physician in the ambulance.

In-hospital lung ultrasound was blinded with respect to pre-hospital one and performed soon after the arrival at the hospital by the emergency physician of the emergency department.

The study evaluated the feasibility of pre-hospital lung ultrasound and the improvement of both pharmacological and oxygen administration in the ambulance and of the blood gases analysis (pH and $CO_2$) at the arrival at the emergency department.

Finally, we compared hospitalization rate and the time spent in the emergency department between the two study groups.

The study was conducted in accordance with Helsinki Declaration, it had been previously approved by local medical ethics committee and a written informed consent was collected from all the patients.

### Statistical analysis

We expressed as mean and standard deviation all the anthropometric and laboratory parameters of the patients.

Standard *T* test was used for the comparison of parametric variables, whereas Chi-square analysis was chosen for non-parametric data.

Sensitivity, specificity, and positive (PPV) and negative (NPV) predictive values were calculated to test the diagnostic capability of the pre-hospital lung ultrasound.

Finally physician's opinions about the utility of the pre-hospital ultrasound were transformed into percentages.

Results were considered statistically significant for *p* value lower than 0.05.

Statistical analysis was made using SPSS 16.0.

## Results

We recruited 30 patients affected by non-traumatic respiratory insufficiency caused by CHF (12 patients) or acute exacerbation of COPD (18 patients), who underwent an ultrasound integrated management (US group) and were compared with 30 patients managed without ultrasound (NUS group).

The characteristics of the two groups are described in Table 1. The two groups were comparable for age, gender, type of respiratory insufficiency, and pulse oximetry values at the arrival of the ALS ambulance.

Pre-hospital lung ultrasound was accurate for the identification of the correct lung profile, in particular for the diagnosis of an interstitial syndrome.

B lines had both a high sensitivity (100%) and specificity (94.4%), and a high PPV and NPV (92.3 and 100%, respectively) for the diagnosis of cardiac heart failure.

The presence of a pleural effusion was not as accurate as B lines for CHF: sensitivity 83.3%, specificity 58.3%, PPV 75.0%, and NPV 70.0%.

Finally, the same percentages obtained by the combination of B lines with pleural effusion for the diagnosis of CHD were 77.8, 100, 100, and 75.5%, respectively.

The number of patients who received an appropriate pharmacological treatment was significantly higher in US group ($p < 0.001$), especially in those subjects with an A profile (non-cardiogenic respiratory insufficiency—COPD; $p < 0.0001$). In this subgroup, the mean dose of furosemide was significantly lower in the US group than the NUS group (3.33 mg vs 15.29 mg $p = 0.036$). On the contrary, in the subgroup of patients with a B profile (CHF), the mean dosage of furosemide was higher in the US groups (42.50 mg vs 29.41 mg), even though not significantly (Fig. 1).

**Table 1 General characteristics of the two study groups**

| | Mean NUS | SD NUS | Mean US | SD US | *p* |
|---|---|---|---|---|---|
| Age | 83.87 | ±10.08 | 80.30 | ±12.27 | ns |
| Hb | 123.93 | ±18.90 | 125.35 | ±25.72 | ns |
| WBC | 14.33 | ±15.59 | 12.56 | ±5.16 | ns |
| Cr | 1.47 | ±1.35 | 1.29 | ±1.76 | ns |
| CRP | 91.70 | ±92.69 | 75.08 | ±73.46 | ns |
| pH | 7.36 | ±0.09 | 7.38 | ±0.08 | ns |
| $PCO_2$ | 49.32 | ±16.87 | 44.36 | ±11.69 | ns |
| SBP | 144.20 | ±38.27 | 142.58 | ±33.48 | ns |
| DBP | 86.43 | ±16.70 | 79.72 | ±22.73 | ns |
| HR | 102.89 | ±27.83 | 104.72 | ±21.94 | ns |
| $O_2$% | 82.20 | ±7.81 | 79.43 | ±11.83 | ns |

*Hb* haemoglobin (g/L), *WBC* white blood cells (x $10^9$ L), *Cr* creatinine (mg/dL), *CRP* C reactive protein, *$PCO_2$* partial pressure of carbon dioxide, *SBP* systolic blood pressure (mmHg), *DBP* diastolic blood pressure (mmHg), *HR* heart rate, *$O_2$%* pulse oximetry

The corticosteroid administration (methylprednisolone) was comparable both between the two groups with an A profile (34.72 vs 29.00 mg) and with a B profile (9.62 vs 11.36 mg) (Fig. 1).

We did not find any difference in the pre-hospital administration of other medications such us morphine, salbutamol, nitroglycerin, and vasoactive agents.

Comparing the use of CPAP, in those patients with an A profile, it was employed more in the US group than in the NUS one (*p* 0.011), whereas the use was comparable in the two groups with a B profile. Moreover, the $FIO_2$ administered was not significantly different between groups.

Blood gases analysis was not significantly different in the US group than in the NUS group.

Anyway, a sub-analysis of patients with the A profile showed that $PCO_2$ was significantly lower in the US group than NUS group ($PCO_2$: 42.62 vs 52.23 *p* 0.049) (Fig. 2).

We did not found any significant difference in all the other laboratory examinations (Table 1).

Two patients were intubated in the NUS group and one in the US group, without any statistical significance.

The convex probe was always the probe of choice and the linear probe was never used.

Hospitalization rate was comparable between the two study groups, whereas we observed a reduction of the

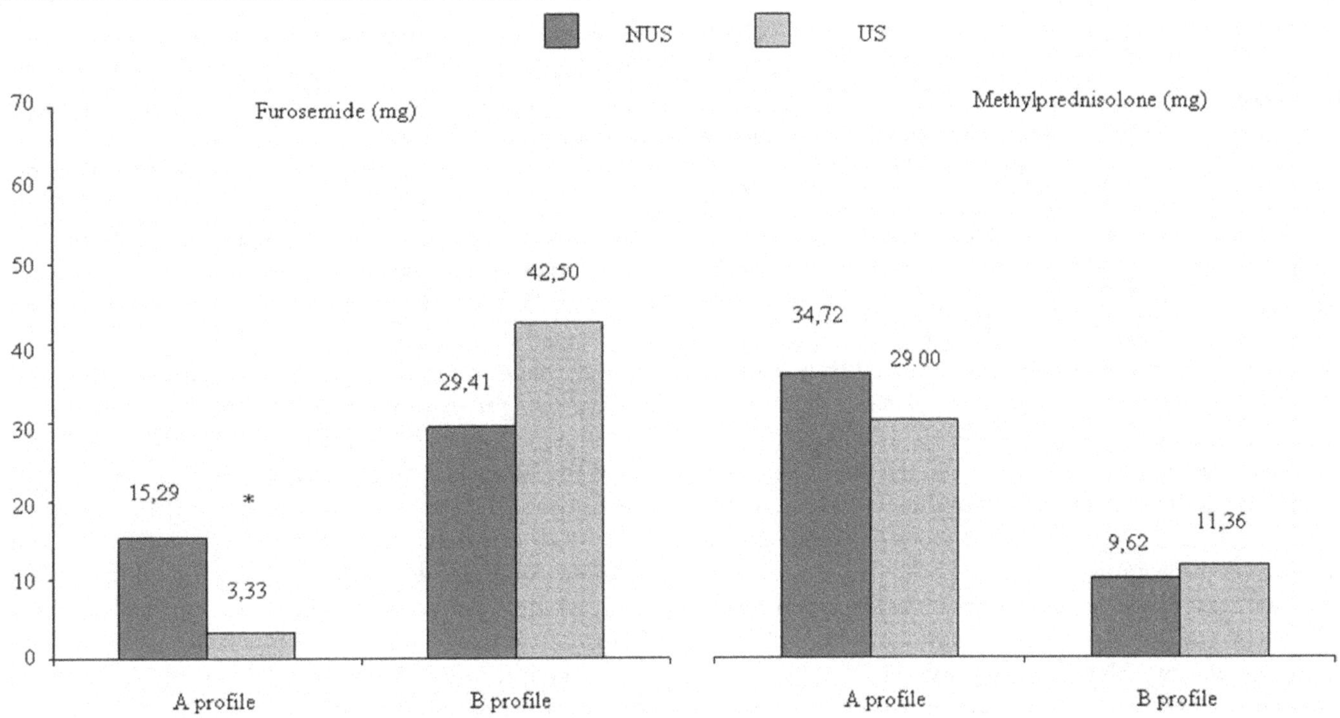


**Fig. 1** Pharmacological therapy in the two study groups splitted by lung profile

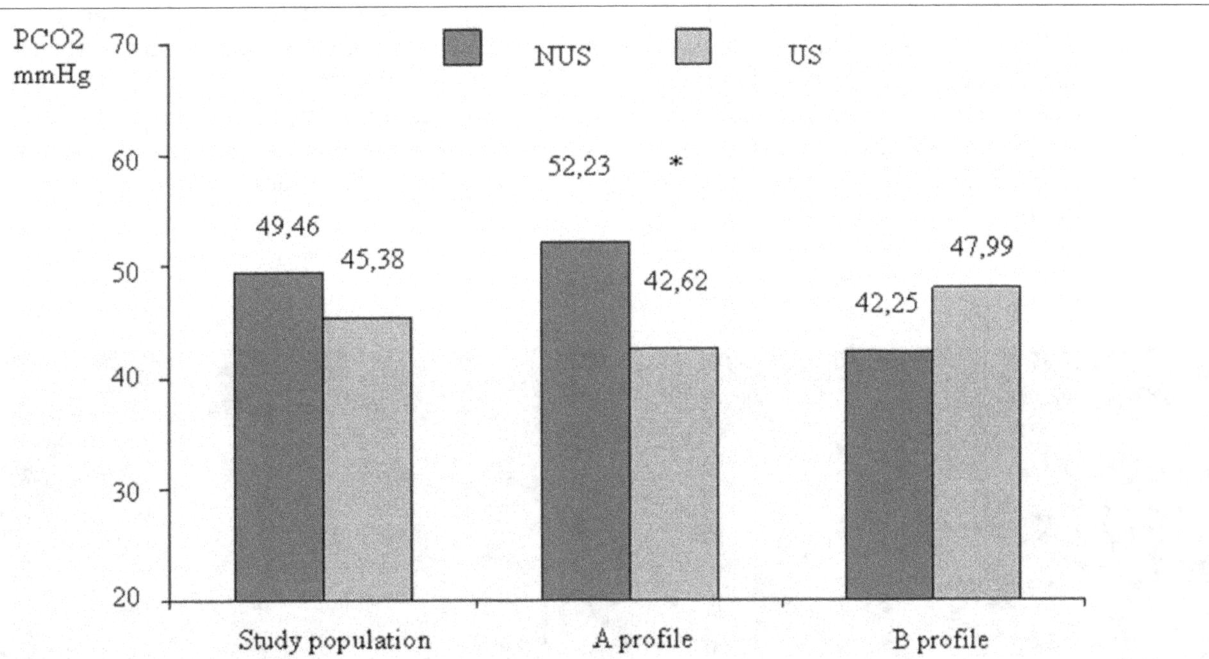


**Fig. 2** $PCO_2$ concentration in the two study groups splitted by lung profile

overall time spent in the emergency department by the US group (267.77 ± 406.15 vs 463.24 ± 521.29 min), but these data did not reach a full statistical significance.

According with physicians' opinion, pre-hospital lung ultrasound either gave important information or changed the therapy in the 42.3% of cases, whereas it just confirmed physical examination and therapy in the remaining 67.7% of cases.

## Discussion

Lung ultrasound is undoubtedly an effective and reliable instrument capable to improve medical care [13].

It has changed in-hospital management of respiratory insufficiency, it has demonstrated remarkable results in patients with trauma of the chest, and both the FAST and the Extended-FAST (EFAST) are two effective protocols that are used worldwide [9, 10, 20–23].

Anyway it is not clear if the same efficacy can be exploited in the pre-hospital medical service for non-traumatic respiratory insufficiency [15–18].

The critical points are three: which are the most remarkable indications? Does it influence the management of respiratory insufficiency? Does it change short- and long-term prognosis?

In our article, we focused our attention on patients affected by cardiac heart failure and acute exacerbation of chronic obstructive pulmonary disease.

We chose CHF and COPD, because their ultrasound patterns are completely different and ultrasound has a high sensitivity and specificity for the identification of the type of lung profile: the former has a B profile (wet lung) and the latter an A profile (dry lung) (Fig. 3) [13, 24].

Our data confirm that pre-hospital ultrasound can differentiate them with a high sensitivity and sensibility.

The examination time was very rapid, all the scans lasted less than 3 min, the two points technique was adequate to examine the chest and the convex probe was always appropriate [2, 13].

The linear probe would have been used if lung profile had not been clear enough, but it never happened.

We tested B lines, the pleural effusion, and the combination between them as ultrasonographic signs for the diagnosis of CHD.

Neesse et al. [15] showed that the identification of a pleural effusion is useful for the diagnosis of CHD in the pre-hospital setting. Nevertheless, our data indicate that B lines had a higher sensitivity and specificity and the combination of the two findings did not improve the diagnostic capability.

Since the identification of B lines is simpler and faster than the diagnosis of pleural effusion, we think that the presence of a bilateral, diffuse, and symmetrical B profile of the lungs is enough for the diagnosis of CHD in a pre-hospital setting.

We did not have any recordings about the time required for the sole identification of the lung profile, but it would have been certainly shorter than the 3 min described above, probably within 1 min.

The second question regards the possibility to influence medical decision-making?

A more accurate diagnosis brought about a more adequate therapy.

In the US group, the patients with CHF received a higher dosage of furosemide, even though not significantly, whereas it was significantly lower in case of COPD. The data are certainly more remarkable in those with an acute exacerbation of COPD, because it reduced inappropriate drug administration preventing hypotension, dehydration, and electrolyte imbalance.

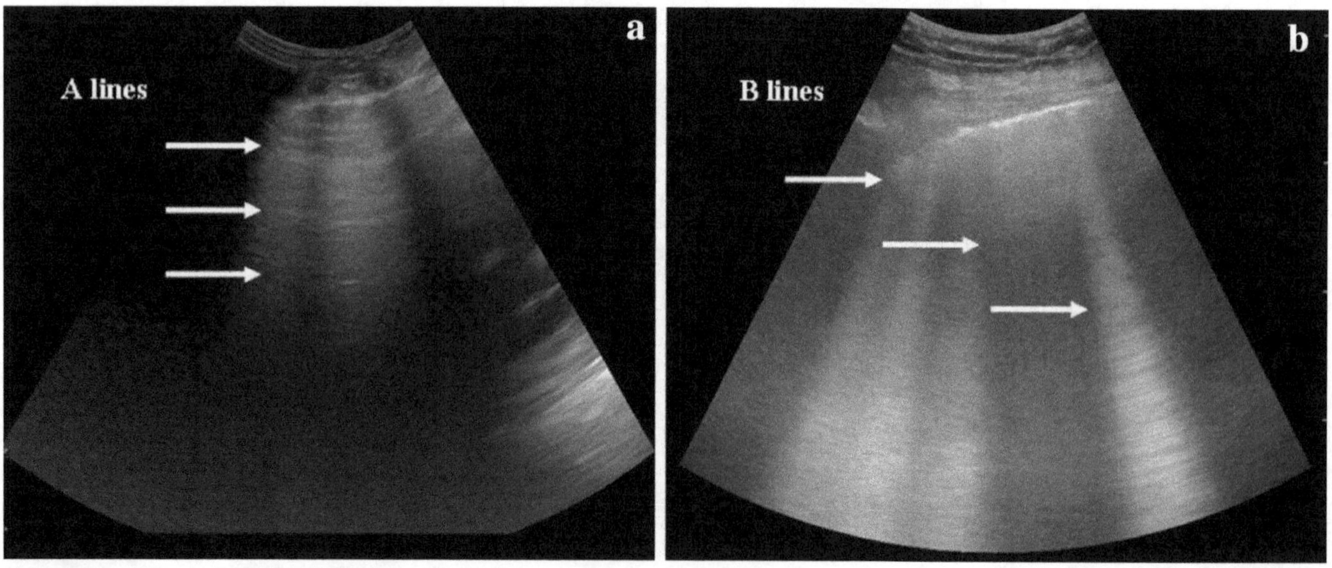


**Fig. 3** **a** A profile—dry lung; **b** B profile—wet lung

Non-invasive ventilation (CPAP) was used thoroughly in patients affected by CHD, whereas, in those with COPD exacerbation, it was applied more often in the US group than in the NUS group. We think that the possibility to identify the correct lung profile made the physicians more confident in choosing the most appropriate type of ventilation and setting for the CPAP.

Eventually in-hospital blood gas analysis showed a lower level of $PCO_2$ in patients affected by COPD when ultrasound was used. The better diagnostic performances given by ultrasound helped the physicians to titrate the oxygen better, reducing the risk of hypercapnia and acidosis.

One of the most remarkable consideration that comes out from these results is that ultrasound made more homogeneous the pre-hospital approach, independently from the medical specialization of the physicians. Indeed, since the physicians who worked in the ambulance with the ultrasound and in the one without were the same, we might assess that the improvement of diagnostic accuracy and medical assistance was determined by the ultrasound integrated approach.

This was possible, because the identification of the lung patter is simple and extremely different between a pulmonary oedema and an acute exacerbation of COPD (Fig. 3). The possibility to "watch the diagnosis on the screen" permitted to choose easily the most appropriate therapy, despite all the confounding elements that are usually caused by the noise and the narrow spaces inside the ambulance or by the patient conditions.

Moreover, the learning curve for the identification of the lung profile is easy and rapid [25]. Consequently, it lets also paramedics, who work in the pre-hospital medical service, to approach lung ultrasound, as it has already been done with FAST, so that the choice of ventilation, oxygen administration, and CPAP setting would become easier and safer for everyone.

Finally, we are not able to answer the third question: we did not collect enough information about the prognosis and the outcome of patients. Anyway, we found a reduction of the time spent in the ED by the patients with the ultrasound integrated approach. We think that the result is interesting even if it was not completely significant and, according to the extent of the reduction, the lack of significance might be caused by the small number of subjects. The possibility to reach the correct diagnosis and to set the right therapy earlier permitted to speed up the in-hospital management of the patients.

## Limitations

The study has certainly several limitations.

First of all, the number of patients is low and should be increased, including other causes of respiratory insufficiency.

Then, it is a case–control study, whereas a randomized-controlled trial could have been more adequate from a statistical point of view.

Most of pre-hospital scans were not re-evaluated by a blinded second operator, because they had not been stored or recorded properly.

The two study groups were matched by comparing digital oxygen values recorded by the ambulance crew, without considering the duration of symptoms and previous history of COPD.

## Conclusions

Pre-hospital lung ultrasound is easy and feasible, and learning curve is very rapid [25].

Pulmonary oedema and COPD should be considered as proven indications for pre-hospital ultrasound, since it can improve both pharmacological therapy and oxygen delivery.

Our study population was small, so that other studies should be planned to support our findings, and to establish the influence of ultrasound on invasive management of airways and on short- and long-term prognosis.

### Abbreviations

ALS: advanced life support; COPD: chronic obstructive pulmonary disease; CHF: cardiac heart failure; CPAP: continuous positive airway pressure; Cr: serum creatinine; CPR: C reactive protein; DBP: diastolic blood pressure; FAST: fast assessment sonography for trauma; EFAST: extended fast assessment sonography for trauma; $FIO_2$: fraction of inspired oxygen; Hb: haemoglobin concentration; HR: heart rate; LUS: lung ultrasound; NUS group: group without an ultrasound integrated management; $PCO_2$: partial pressure of carbon dioxide; PEEP: continuous positive airway pressure; PPV: positive predictive value; NPV: negative predictive value; $O_2$%: pulse oximetry; SBP: systolic blood pressure; US group: ultrasound integrated management group; WBC: white blood cells.

### Authors' contributions

MZ: study conception and design, acquisition of data, analysis and interpretation of data, drafting the manuscript, and critical revision. PB: study conception and design, acquisition of data, and critical revision. SDB: acquisition of data and critical revision. CP: acquisition of data and critical revision. RI: acquisition of data and critical revision. VC: study conception and design, drafting the manuscript, and critical revision. All authors read and approved the final manuscript.

### Acknowledgements

We thank Cristina Dalla Pellegrina, a nurse of our emergency department, for her precious job in filing all the documents.

### References

1. Fevang E, Lockey D, Thompson J, Lossius HM, Torpo Research Collaboration (2011) Top five research priorities in physician-provided pre-hospital critical care: a consensus report from a European research collaboration. Scand J Trauma Resusc Emerg Med 13:19–57
2. Zanatta M, Benato P, Cianci V (2016) Pre-hospital ultrasound: current indications and future perspectives. Int J Crit Care Emerg Med 2:019. https://doi.org/10.23937/2474-3674/1510019

3. Bush M (2006) Portable ultrasound in pre-hospital emergencies: a feasibility study. Acta Anaesthesiol Scand 50:754–758
4. Taylor J, McLaughlin K, McRea A, Lang E, Anton A (2014) Use of prehospital ultrasound in North America: a survey of emergency medical services medical directors. BMC Emerg Med 1:14–16
5. Knudsen L, Sandberg M (2011) Ultrasound in pre-hospital care. Acta Anaesthesiol Scand 55:377–378
6. El Sayed MJ, Zaghrini E (2013) Prehospital emergency ultrasound: a review of current clinical applications, challenges, and future implications. Emerg Med Int 2013:531674. https://doi.org/10.1155/2013/531674
7. Lapostolle F, Petrovic T, Lenoir G, Catineau J, Galinski M, Metzger J, Chanzy E, Adnet F (2006) Usefulness of hand-held ultrasound devices in out-of-hospital diagnosis performed by emergency physicians. Am J Emerg Med 24:237–242
8. O'Dochartaigh D, Douma M, MacKenzie M (2017) Five-year retrospective review of physician and non-physician performed ultrasound in a Canadian critical care helicopter emergency medical service. Prehosp Emerg Care 21:24–31
9. Rozycki GS, Ochsner MG, Schmidt JA, Frankel HL, Davis TP, Wang D, Champion HR (1995) A prospective study of surgeon-performed ultrasound as the primary adjuvant modality for injured patient assessment. J Trauma 39:492–500
10. Scalea TM, Rodriguez A, Chiu WC, Brenneman FD, Fallon WF Jr, Kato K, McKenney MG, Nerlich ML, Ochsner MG, Yoshii H (1999) Focused assessment with sonography for trauma (FAST): results from an international consensus conference. J Trauma 46:466–472
11. Neumar RW, Shuster M, Callaway CW, Gent LM, Atkins DL, Bhanji F, Brooks SC, de Caen AR, Donnino MW, Ferrer JM, Kleinman ME, Kronick SL, Lavonas EJ, Link MS, Mancini ME, Morrison LJ, O'Connor RE, Samson RA, Schexnayder SM, Singletary EM, Sinz EH, Travers AH, Wyckoff MH, Hazinski MF (2015) Part 1: executive summary: 2015 American heart association guidelines update for cardiopulmonary resuscitation and emergency cardiovascular care. Circulation 132(18 Suppl 2):S315–S367. https://doi.org/10.1161/CIR.0000000000000252
12. Brun PM, Besserau J, Cazes N, Querrelou E, Chenaitia H (2012) Lung ultrasound associated to capnography to verify correct endotracheal tube positioning in prehospital. Am J Emerg Med 30(2080):e5–e6
13. Volpicelli G, Elbarbary M, Blaivas M, Lichtenstein DA, Mathis G, Kirkpatrick AW, Melniker L, Gargani L, Noble VE, Via G, Dean A, Tsung JW, Soldati G, Copetti R, Bouhemad B, Reissig A, Agricola E, Rouby JJ, Arbelot C, Liteplo A, Sargsyan F, Hoppmann R, Breitkreutz R, Seibel A, Neri L, Storti E, Petrovic T, International Liaison Committee on Lung Ultrasound (ILC-LUS) for International Consensus Conference on Lung Ultrasound (ICC-LUS) (2012) International evidence-based recommendations for point-of-care lung ultrasound. Intensive Care Med 38:577–591
14. Hoyer HX, Vogl S, Schiemann U, Haug A, Stolpe E, Michalski T (2010) Prehospital ultrasound in emergency medicine: incidence, feasibility, indications and diagnoses. Eur J Emerg Med 17:254–259
15. Neesse A, Jerrentrup A, Hoffman S, Sattler A, Gorg C, Kill C, Gress TM, Kunsch S (2012) Prehospital chest emergency sonography trial in Germany: a prospective study. Eur J Emerg Med 19:161–166
16. Zechner PM, Aichinger G, Riguad M, Wildner G, Prause G (2010) Prehospital lung ultrasound in the distinction between pulmonary edema and exacerbation of chronic obstructive pulmonary disease. Am J Emerg Med 28:389.e1-2
17. Stefanone G, Boero E, Sverzellati N, Cardinale L, Bussi M, Boccuzzi F, Tullio M, Lamorte A, Stefanone V, Ferrari G, Veltri A, Francisco MF (2014) Semi-quiantification of pneumothorax volume by lung ultrasound. Intensive Care Med 40:1460–1467
18. Strnad M, Prosen G, Borovnik Leskjak V (2016) Bedside lung ultrasound for monitoring effectiveness of prehospital ultrasound treatment with continuous positive airway pressure in acute decompensated heart failure. Eur J Emerg Med 23:50–55
19. Ferrari G, Esquinas AM (2015) Lung ultrasound in prehospital acute cardiac pulmonary edema: a new practical toll for CPAP assessment. Eur J Emerg Med 22:146–147
20. Kirkpatrick AW, Sirois M, Laupland KB, Liu D, Rowan K, Ball CG, Hameed SM, Brown R, Simons R, Dulchavsky SA, Hamiilton DR, Nicolaou S (2004) Hand-held thoracic sonography for detecting post-traumatic pneumothoraces: the extended focused assessment with sonography for trauma (EFAST). J Trauma 57:288–295
21. Jorgensen H, Jensen CH, Dirks J (2010) Does pre-hospital ultrasound improve treatment of the trauma patient? A systematic reviews. Eur J Emerg Med 17:249–253
22. Rudolph SS, Sorensen MK, Svane C, Hessefeldt R, Steinmez J (2014) Effect of pre-hospital ultrasound on clinical outcomes of non-trauma patients—a systematic review. Resuscitation 85:21–30
23. O'Dochartaigh D, Douma M (2015) Pre-hospital ultrasound of the abdomen and thorax changes trauma patients management: a systematic review. Injury 11:2093–2102
24. Copetti R, Soldati G, Copetti P (2008) Chest sonography: a useful tool to differentiate acute cardiogenic pulmonary edema from acute respiratory distress syndrome. Cardiovasc Ultrasound 29:6–16
25. Picano E, Frassi F, Agricola E, Gligorova S, Gargani L, Mottola G (2006) Ultrasound lung comets: a clinically useful sign of extravascular lung water. J Am Soc Echocardiogr 19:356–363

18

# Is point-of-care ultrasound disruptive innovation? Formulating why POCUS is different from conventional comprehensive ultrasound

Jesper Weile[1,2*], Jacob Brix[3] and Anders Broens Moellekaer[1,2]

**Abstract**

**Background:** Point-of-care ultrasound (PoCUS) is spreading throughout Emergency Medicine, Critical Care and Prehospital Care. However, there is an underlying inherited conflict with the established specialties performing comprehensive examinations. It has been stated that PoCUS is disruptive innovation. If this is true the definition might open up for a new perspective on differentiating comprehensive ultrasound from PoCUS. PoCUS in the light of disruptive innovation is a different perspective on ultrasound that has not before been academically scrutinized.

**Methods:** In this paper we investigate if PoCUS is in fact disruptive innovation. This is done by comparative analysis with the point of departure in disruptive innovation theory known from the business world.

**Results:** We find that a disruptive innovation process is happening. This new knowledge allows us to put forward advice for the stakeholders in the field of ultrasound. It also allows us to challenge the conventional pyramid of expertise used to describe different types of ultrasound. The perspective of this paper is mutual understanding of similarities and differences between conventional and point-of-care ultrasound. Only with this understanding the stakeholders can collaborate and use the full spectrum of ultrasound for the benefit of the patient.

**Keywords:** Point-of-care ultrasound, Disruptive innovation, Disruption, Ultrasonography

## Background

Point-of-care ultrasound (PoCUS) is different from conventional comprehensive ultrasound examinations—*but what exactly differentiates the two?* Critics would state that PoCUS are merely inferior examinations compared to comprehensive conventional ultrasound examinations performed in an unsuited environment. This standpoint is visualized in the conventional pyramid of expertise, where PoCUS is placed at the bottom [1]. Proponents have stated that PoCUS, "has become a more physiological study than an anatomical one" [2]. These two standpoints represent a disagreement and this conflict does not serve the general purpose of treating every patient to the best of knowledge. Resolving this conflict necessitates a clear theoretical classification between PoCUS and conventional comprehensive ultrasound examinations.

Leaders in ultrasound, such as Resa Lewiss from the University of Colorado School of Medicine, have claimed that PoCUS is disruptive innovation [3]. Clayton Christensen, the father of the disruptive innovation theory, has suggested that healthcare should embrace disruptive innovation [4]. According to Christensen, if a given technology and the business model pertaining to it is undergoing *a process of disruptive innovation*, appreciating this will enable established market players to act and react accordingly [5].

Hence, understanding if PoCUS is undergoing a process of disruptive innovation will aid in a theoretical description of the difference between PoCUS and conventional comprehensive ultrasound examinations and contribute to solving the inherent conflict between conventional comprehensive ultrasound and PoCUS.

*Correspondence: jesper.weile@clin.au.dk
[2] Research Center for Emergency Medicine, Aarhus University Hospital, Aarhus, Denmark
Full list of author information is available at the end of the article

To our knowledge it has not been academically investigated if PoCUS adheres to the definition of being true disruptive innovation. This paper will use a comparative analysis, with the point of departure in disruptive innovation theory, to determine whether PoCUS is in fact true disruptive innovation.

If this assumption is true the paper aims first to challenge the conventional pyramid of expertise and second to provide recommendations for stakeholders on how to act or react to the disruptive innovation that is taking place [5].

### Disruptive innovation

Disruptive innovation is defined as a process in which a new competitor successfully challenges an established market. The disruptive innovation process can have two different strategies: (1) focus on a low-price alternative to existing technology, where the "job of the product" corresponds with the users' minimum requirement for relevancy, or (2) focus on creating a new market (potentially in an existing market) in which there is no competition. Hence, disruptive innovation is both different from and in conflict with traditional business models [5, 6]. In 1997, Christensen presented the difference between sustaining and disruptive innovation as shown in Fig. 1 [7]. According to this model the market region's ability to absorb technology is a developing area ready for increasingly complex technology. Every technology follows a trajectory, which evolves from being below the market, to entering the market, and finally to being developed beyond the customer's demands. A sustaining innovation process focuses on continuingly delivering products that exceed the current level of customer needs. A disruptive innovation process represents the opportunity for a parallel trajectory, entering the market at the low end of customer demands, where the existing technology's sustaining innovation has become over-performing and overpriced.

There are many well-known examples of innovative disrupters introducing new platforms with inferior quality at a lower price. One example is how the compact disc (CD) was rapidly pushed from the market after the introduction of the iPod and iTunes Store. In this example, the improvement of CDs, as well as CD players, is the "sustaining innovation." The compressed files on the iPod were products of inferior sound quality compared to CDs; however, the sound quality was acceptable to meet the minimum requirements of ordinary users listening to music. At the same time, the business model changed from buying a full, physical album to online purchases of either one song or even a full album at a lower price. While the product and the business model changed, despite the inferior quality of the new product, in 2012 there where seven times more purchases of music in iTunes than purchases of physical CDs [8].

### The ultrasound examination as a commodity

The ultrasound examination itself represents value-creation, if regarded as a self-contained commodity. In this case, the patient is a potential customer (e.g.,

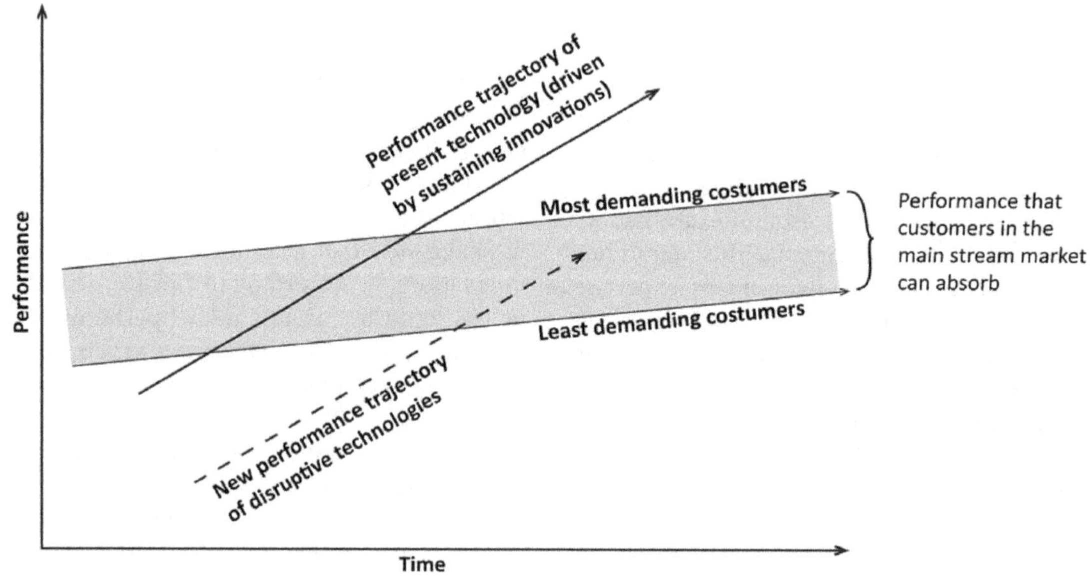


**Fig. 1** Disruptive innovation. The graph outlines how the disruptive innovation enters the market in it's own trajectory to the right of the original technology trajectory. Improvement of the original technology within one trajectory is considered sustaining innovation. From Christensen, Clayton M.: The innovator's dilemma: when new technologies cause great firms to fail (1997)

the patient with a sudden onset of dyspnea who aims to purchase an ultrasound examination to investigate cardiac function or an examination of the lungs). The doctors from different specialties are the service providers of the ultrasound examination. Specialties such as radiology and cardiology can be considered the "established service providers" of comprehensive conventional ultrasound examinations, and the "new suppliers" of ultrasound examinations would be specialties in which the simple PoCUS examination has become relevant such as anesthesiology or emergency medicine. In PoCUS multiple abbreviated protocols have been proposed. The general idea of these is abbreviation of a corresponding comprehensive examination. Examples of this are protocols such as FEEL (Focused Echocardiographic Evaluation in Life Support) [9], FEER (Focused Echocardiographic Evaluation in Resuscitation [10] or FATE (Focus Assessed Transthoracis Echocardiography) [11] vs. the minimum requirements for comprehensive echocardiography protocol put forward by leading medical societies [12, 13]. The abbreviated examination aims to be simpler, but faster and with a much wider indication.

Hence, the PoCUS examination could represent the creation of a new market in an existing market. This is argued because PoCUS can be performed anywhere with any type of ultrasound machine, and consequently, the hardware technology itself is less important. This is a new business model and an opposite approach to ultrasound examination compared to comprehensive conventional echocardiography or a comprehensive conventional radiological ultrasound examination; PoCUS brings the ultrasound to the patient, as opposed to the patient being referred and transported to the ultrasound examination room hence making the examination available at all times.

In summary, the PoCUS examination meets the cri teria of an occurring process of disruptive innovation:

1) The examination is inferior compared to what exists on the market (e.g. eyeballing four cardiac windows in PoCUS protocols vs. extensive views and qualitative measurements on flow and left ventricular ejection fraction in the comprehensive echocardiography protocol).
2) The examination is at a lower cost (time equals cost) compared to existing technology.
3) The PoCUS examination follows the dogma of a different business model (the care giver provides the product instantly at the bedside).

## Challenging the pyramid of expertise

In the conventional perception of ultrasound, the PoCUS examination is placed at the bottom of an expertise pyramid as shown in Fig. 2. In this view, the pyramid is a learning ladder that one climbs from the bottom to the top by acquiring expertise [1].

PoCUS is based on the premise that the examinations are acceptable for their intended purpose but inferior in quality when compared to comprehensive examinations. However, the PoCUS examinations excel in speed and availability for every patient and are as accessible as the stethoscope. The conventional pyramid is static and leaves no room for PoCUS to offer superiority on any parameter compared to comprehensive examinations. If the physician performing PoCUS rises to a higher level of expertise in the pyramid, speed is lost, as the examiner extends the exam toward something more comprehensive and time consuming. Availability is also lost, as only a few doctors (who are not always present in the department) can be expected to perform the examination at the expert level. Hence climbing the pyramid of expertise also weakens the product.

Applying the theory of disruptive innovation to the PoCUS examination can be presented as shown in Fig. 3. Here, the comprehensive ultrasound examination and the PoCUS examination are perceived as two parallel trajectories. The trajectory of the comprehensive examination

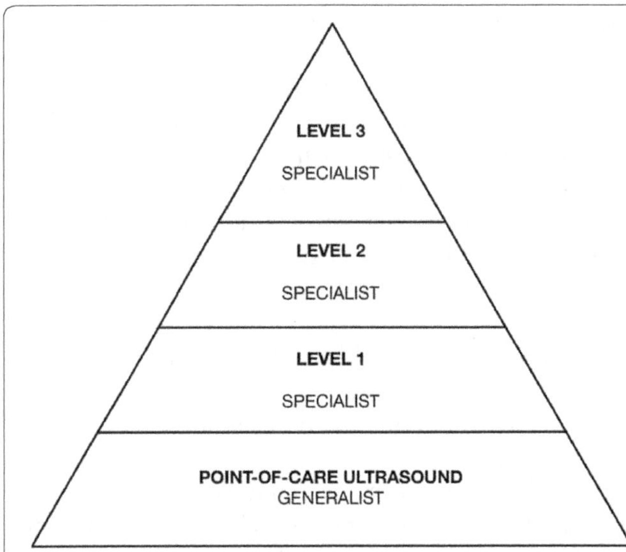


**Fig. 2** The expertise pyramid. The conventional perception of ultrasound competency expressed in the expertise pyramid. The point-of-care examination is placed as the lowest level of expertise, and the pyramid visualizes how the physician can extend their expertise to advance to more sophisticated levels. The underlying assumption is that PoCUS is an inferior examination. The pyramid does not permit point-of-care ultrasound to possess strengths, such as speed, cost, and availability, which are superior to the layers above it (Adapted from Oxorn and Pearlman [1])

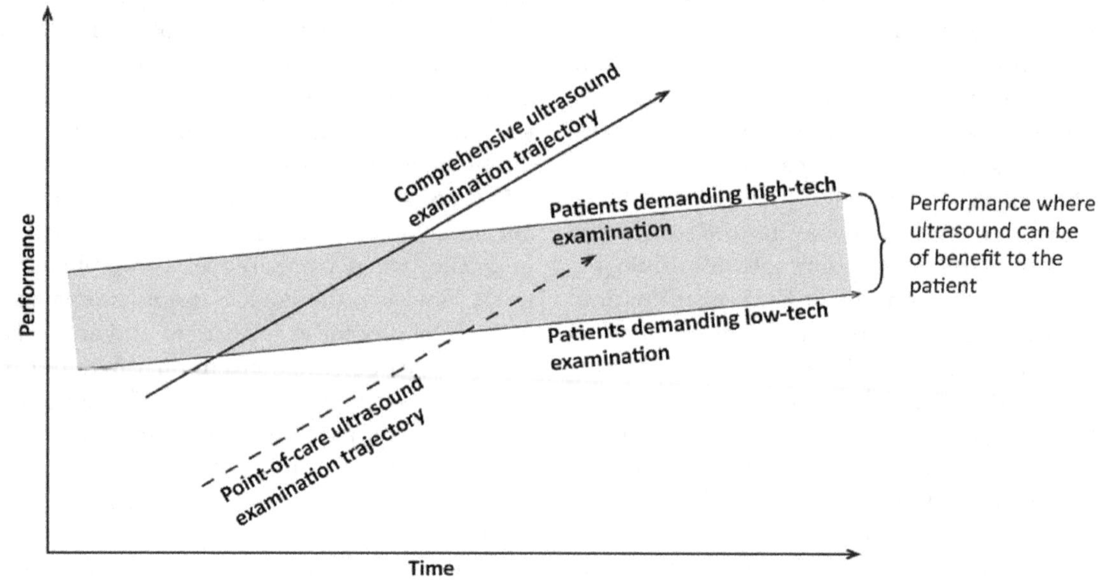


**Fig. 3** Point-of-care Ultrasound Expressed as a Disruptive Innovation. In this context, the conventional comprehensive ultrasound examination and the point-of-care examination are two parallel trajectories. PoCUS examination is a disruptive innovation, as its speed, cost, and availability differ from that of the conventional comprehensive examination. The speed and availability enable the examination to become an extension to any physical examination at any time. The point-of-care examination is inferior to comprehensive examinations, but meets the low end of customer demand (Adapted from Christensen [7])

will reflect the level of expertise: higher expertise is considered higher performance. This places the level-3 expert sonographer from the pyramid in Fig. 2 at the top of (or maybe above) the market region's ability to absorb technology. In this presentation, levels 2 and 1 will follow further down on the same trajectory. PoCUS is placed on its own trajectory, as the examination is fast and available but inferior in range. Depending on the examiner's skill, the examination performed will be placed somewhere along the trajectory. Due to high availability, the indication for the examination becomes wider, resembling a much larger customer base; however, the high-end customer will still exist and demand highly specialized examinations.

## How stakeholders should act and react

For all medical specialties performing ultrasound or PoCUS, it is paramount to understand the differences between the services.

For the disrupter, this means understanding the advantages but also the limitations of PoCUS. Hence, the disrupter should be cautious in evolving PoCUS toward the standards of comprehensive examinations, as the examination will lose speed and availability. The time-consuming comprehensive examinations will obstruct patient flow.

The disrupted (e.g., cardiology or radiology) must focus on the core values of the high-quality product and cultivate these. The disrupted parties should also promote knowledge of the potential gains from a conventional examination over a PoCUS examination. This will enable providers of PoCUS to identify the highly demanding customer and recognize when referrals can create value for the patient. At the same time, the disrupted parties should find delight in the fact that even more patients will now have the privilege of ultrasound examinations performed.

Aspiring to increase quality should also inspire to increase standards of education for providers. The PoCUS examinations are faster and simpler; however, this does not necessarily mean they are easier to master. The providers must receive appropriate training to avoid overconfidence and potential wrongful interpretation. The commodity must stay above the low end of customer demands (Fig. 3) or it loses its definition as a disruptive innovation.

## Conclusion

PoCUS examination is in a process of disruptive innovation. This knowledge provides a theoretical basis to segregate PoCUS from comprehensive ultrasound examinations.

Perceiving PoCUS as a disruptive innovation challenges the conventional view of the PoCUS examination being inferior on the expertise pyramid. This perspective leads to viewing PoCUS and conventional ultrasound as two parallel trajectories with different strengths, opportunities, and patients.

The innovation is vulnerable to up-market movements due to the physician performing over the means of existence, with the disruptive innovation losing the strengths of speed and availability. The innovation is also vulnerable to down-market movement if the performing physician does not possess sufficient competency.

The disrupter and the disrupted should both embrace the similarities and differences in the comprehensive specialized examinations and PoCUS. The core values of each examination should be recognized and cultivated [5, 6].

**Authors' contributions**

All authors contributed to the paper's conception and design. JW drafted the manuscript. All authors critically revised drafts and contributed with important intellectual content. All authors read and approved the final manuscript.

**Author details**

[1] Emergency Department, Regional Hospital Herning, Herning, Denmark. [2] Research Center for Emergency Medicine, Aarhus University Hospital, Aarhus, Denmark. [3] Department of Learning& Philosophy, Research Group for Evaluation & Capacity Building, Aalborg University, Aalborg, Denmark.

**References**

1. Oxorn D, Pearlman A (2012) CON: physician-performed ultrasound: the time has come for routine use in acute care medicine. Anesth Analg 115(5):1004–1006
2. Abu-Zidan FM (2012) Point-of-care ultrasound in critically ill patients: where do we stand? J Emerg Trauma Shock 5(1):70–71
3. Lewiss R (2014) How an old technology became disruptive innovation, TEDMED. http://www.tedmed.com/talks/show?id=293054. Accessed 28 Nov 2017
4. Christensen CM, Bohmer R, Kenagy J (2000) Will disruptive innovations cure health care? Harv Bus Rev 78(5):102–112
5. Wessel M, Christensen CM (2012) Surviving disruption. Harv Bus Rev 90(12):56–64
6. Charitou CD, Markides CC (2002) Responses to disruptive strategic innovation. MIT Sloan Manag Rev 44(2):55–64
7. Christensen CM (1997) The innovator's dilemma: when new technologies cause great firms to fail. Harvard Business School Press, Boston
8. South J, Blass B (2001) The future of modern genomics. Blackwell, London. http://money.cnn.com/2013/04/25/technology/itunes-music-decline/index.html
9. Breitkreutz R et al (2010) Focused echocardiographic evaluation in life support and peri-resuscitation of emergency patients: a prospective trial. Resuscitation 81(11):1527–1533
10. Breitkreutz R et al (2007) Focused echocardiographic evaluation in resuscitation management: concept of an advanced life support-conformed algorith. Crit Care Med 35(5 Suppl):S150–S161
11. Jensen MB et al (2004) Transthoracic echocardiography for cardiopulmonary monitoring in intensive care. Eur J Anaestesiol 21:700–707
12. Picard MH et al (2011) American Society of Echocardiography recommendations for quality echocardiography laboratory operations. J Am Soc Echocardiogr 24(1):1–10
13. Wharton G et al (2015) A minimum dataset for a standard adult transthoracic echocardiogram: a guideline protocol from the British Society of Echocadiography. Echo Res Pract 2(1):G9–G24

# 19

# Which ultrasound transducer type is best for diagnosing pneumothorax?

R. Ketelaars[1,2*], E. Gülpinar[1], T. Roes[1], M. Kuut[1] and G. J. van Geffen[1,2]

**Abstract**

**Background:** An accurate physical examination is essential in the care of critically ill and injured patients. However, to diagnose or exclude a pneumothorax, chest auscultation is unreliable compared to lung ultrasonography. In the dynamic prehospital environment, it is desirable to have the best possible ultrasound transducer readily available. The objective is to assess the difference between a linear-array, curved-array, and phased-array ultrasound transducer in the assessment for pneumothorax and to determine which is best.

**Methods:** In this double-blinded, cross-sectional, observational study, 15 observers, experienced in lung ultrasonography, each assessed 66 blinded ultrasound video clips of either normal ventilation or pneumothorax that were recorded with three types of ultrasound transducers. The clips were recorded in 11 adult patients that underwent thoracoscopic lung surgery immediately before and after the surgeon opened the thorax. The diagnostic accuracy of the three transducers, elapsed time until a diagnosis was made, and the perceived image quality was recorded.

**Results:** In total, 15 observers assessed 990 ultrasound video clips. The overall sensitivity and specificity were 98.2% and 97.2%, relatively. No significant difference was found in the diagnostic performance between transducers. A diagnosis was made slightly faster in the linear-array transducer clips, compared to the phased-array transducer ($p = .031$). For the linear-, curved-, and phased-array transducer, the image quality was rated at a median (interquartile range [IQR]) of 4 (IQR 3–4), 3 (IQR 2–4), and 2 (IQR 1–2), relatively. Between the transducers, the difference in image quality was significant ($p < .0001$).

**Conclusions:** There was no difference in diagnostic performance of the three transducers. Based on image quality, the linear-array transducer might be preferred for (prehospital) lung ultrasonography for the diagnosis of pneumothorax.

**Keywords:** Ultrasonography, Transducer, Pneumothorax, Emergency medical services

## Background

In the critically ill and injured patient, an accurate physical examination is essential in the care of the patient. However, auscultating for breath sounds in a respiratory distressed patient is often difficult or even impossible, especially in a noisy accident scene, or patient compartment of a (moving) ambulance or helicopter.

The sensitivity of auscultation for the diagnosis of hemothorax, hemopneumothorax, and pneumothorax is only 58–66% [1–3]. Unilateral decreased or absent breath sounds are often interpreted as a pneumothorax. However, conditions such as splinting from rib pain, lung contusion, atelectasis, pneumonia, pleural effusion, and tumor growth may account for the same abnormal auscultation.

Lung ultrasonography (US) for the diagnosis of pneumothorax was first described in 1986 [4]. It may rule-in pneumothorax with a sensitivity ranging from 81 to 98% and rule it out with a specificity approaching 99–100% [5–7]. Additionally, pleural effusion, lung contusion, and atelectasis may be detected [7]. It has even been suggested that US might 1 day replace the stethoscope [8, 9].

*Correspondence: Rein.Ketelaars@radboudumc.nl
[1] Department of Anesthesiology, Pain and Palliative Medicine, Radboud University Medical Center, Radboud Institute for Health Sciences, Geert Grooteplein-Zuid 10, 6525 GA Nijmegen, The Netherlands
Full list of author information is available at the end of the article

US is feasible in the prehospital setting including inside ground ambulances and a helicopter emergency medical service (HEMS) [10–12]. Similar to most diagnostic and therapeutic procedures, US requires training and regular practice. Time pressure and limited working space are additional challenges [12]. To facilitate the best possible images, it is important that optimally set-up US equipment is readily available. In an optimal configuration, the most suitable transducer is connected to the US machine.

Lung US can be performed with high-frequency linear-array, curved-array, or phased-array transducers. However, it is not known which one is preferable and provides the best images.

We hypothesized that a linear-array transducer is the optimal transducer for the appreciation of the pleural line for diagnosing pneumothorax. The aim of the study is to compare three transducer types on diagnostic accuracy, speed of the diagnosis, and image quality in the assessment for pneumothorax.

## Methods

We performed a double-blinded, cross-sectional, observational study to compare three types of ultrasound transducers for the diagnosis of two conditions: normal ventilation, and pneumothorax. Ethical approval was obtained from the institutional ethics review board of the Radboud university medical center, Nijmegen. Written informed consent was asked and obtained from every patient and from every observer.

At the preoperative outpatient evaluation clinic of the Radboud university medical center, Nijmegen, the Netherlands, from September to October 2017, we recruited a consecutive series of eleven eligible patients that were scheduled for video-assisted thoracoscopic surgery (VATS) for pulmonary, mainly neoplastic, pathology. The inclusion criteria were a body mass index < 30 kg m$^{-2}$ and the absence of pathology of the chest wall, visceral or parietal pleura.

Lung US is a valuable test for the detection or exclusion of a pneumothorax [13, 14]. A US transducer is positioned on the chest wall perpendicular to two adjacent ribs. Between the acoustic shadows of two ribs, a hyperechoic line is visible representing the interface of the parietal and visceral pleura. With normal ventilation, lung sliding is observed as a to-and-fro movement at the pleural line as a result of the sliding of the visceral pleura against the inner chest wall. B-lines may be observed as hyperechoic lines radiating down from the pleural line. Their presence excludes pneumothorax (at the transducer position). Horizontal repetitions of the pleural line appearing below at multiples of the skin-pleural line distance are called A-lines. Their appearance is more prominent in the presence of a pneumothorax when B-lines are absent and no longer obscuring the A-lines.

We used a portable X-Porte ultrasound system (Fujifilm SonoSite Inc., Bothell, WA, USA) equipped with three transducers: a high-frequency linear-array 15–6 MHz (HFL50xp), a curved-array abdominal 5–2 MHz (C60xp) and a phased-array cardiac 5–1 MHz (P21xp) transducer. The footprints of the transducers are 5 cm, 6 cm, and 2.1 cm, respectively.

For the VATS procedure, isolated ventilation of the dependent lung via a double-lumen endotracheal tube was necessary. First, all patients underwent general anesthesia, were intubated and ventilated, and placed in a lateral decubitus position. The ventilator was set to deliver a tidal volume of 5 ml kg$^{-1}$ at a rate of 20 min$^{-1}$. The anesthesiologist verified the position and depth of the double-lumen endotracheal tube with fiberoptic bronchoscopy.

Second, the linear array, curved-array, and phased-array transducer were positioned over the fourth or fifth intercostal space at the axillary line in a craniocaudal orientation. 15-second ultrasound video clips were recorded of normal ventilation at a respiratory rate of 20 min$^{-1}$. The zone of interest was the pleural line with its two adjacent ribs. A typical clip was framed as shown in Fig. 1.

Third, after the chest was prepped and draped, ventilation of the non-dependent lung was interrupted while the surgeon opened the chest, introduced the videoscope and visually confirmed the collapse of the lung. Thereafter, the surgeon recorded three similar 15-s video clips of the established pneumothorax with the three transducers wrapped in sterile transducer covers (Fig. 2). Hence, six clips were recorded in every patient. The time interval between the induction of the pneumothorax (reference test) and the performance of the three ultrasound

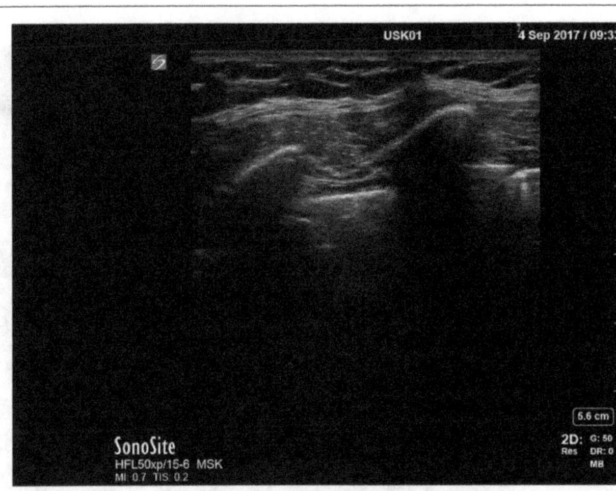


**Fig. 1** A typical uncropped image of the pleural interface, acquired with the phased-array transducer. On the right, the cropped version is displayed as is was played back to the observers

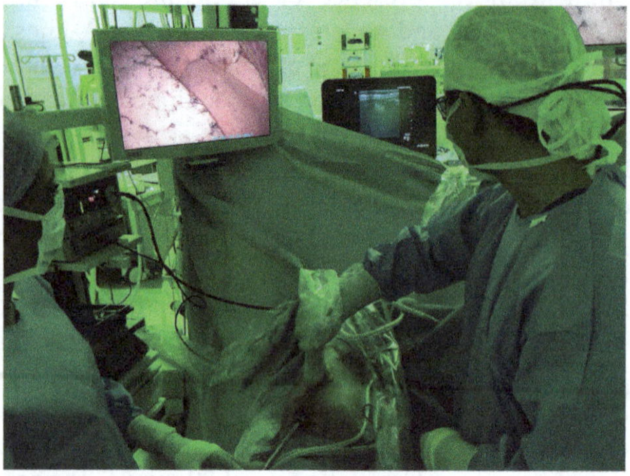

**Fig. 2** The surgeon performs lung ultrasonography in a patient with a confirmed pneumothorax and the videoscope in situ. The video screen displays an image of the inside of the right hemi-thorax and the collapsed right lung. The surgeon is handling the wrapped-up ultrasound transducer. The ultrasound device is shown in the back of the image

video clips was no longer than 2 min. No adverse events occurred.

We cropped the video clips using iMovie for OS X, version 10.1.8 (Apple Inc., Cupertino, CA, USA). After we cropped and removed the text from the captured video clips, it was now no longer possible for the observers and the researchers to reliably recognize the transducer type by the image shape (rectangular or sector-shaped). An uncropped still image of the video clip and its cropped version are displayed in Fig. 3.

The Nijmegen physician-staffed HEMS carries a portable US machine since 2006. All HEMS physicians were trained in lung US either at the introduction of the US machine or at the start of their employment. They use lung US regularly in their prehospital practice.

We recruited all 13 HEMS physicians (except the author, RK) and two anesthesiology residents with extensive experience in lung ultrasonography as observers to assess a randomized set of 66 15-s ultrasound clips. We used PotPlayer for Windows, version 1.7 (Kakao Corp., Jeju, South Korea) to separately randomize and playback the cropped set of clips for each observer (Fig. 4). Before the observers assessed the set of video clips, they were informed about how we acquired the clips and about the two possible conditions (normal ventilation and pneumothorax). Due to the cropping and randomization, the observers were blinded for the diagnosis and for the transducer type.

The observers were requested to pause the playback themselves when they were certain about the diagnosis based on the presence or lack of lung sliding, A-line sign, or B-lines. The equally blinded researcher recorded the elapsed time (s), the observer's diagnosis and perceived image quality rated on a 1–5 Likert scale (1, very poor; 5, very good). For every observer, their experience (years) with lung US and preferred transducer type for lung US was recorded.

### Statistical analysis

Normally distributed data are reported as mean and standard deviation (SD). Data with an asymmetrical distribution are reported as median and interquartile range (IQR). We calculated the difference in elapsed time and image quality between transducers in every patient and observer: linear-array vs curved-array; linear-array vs phased-array; curved-array vs phased-array. Then, we

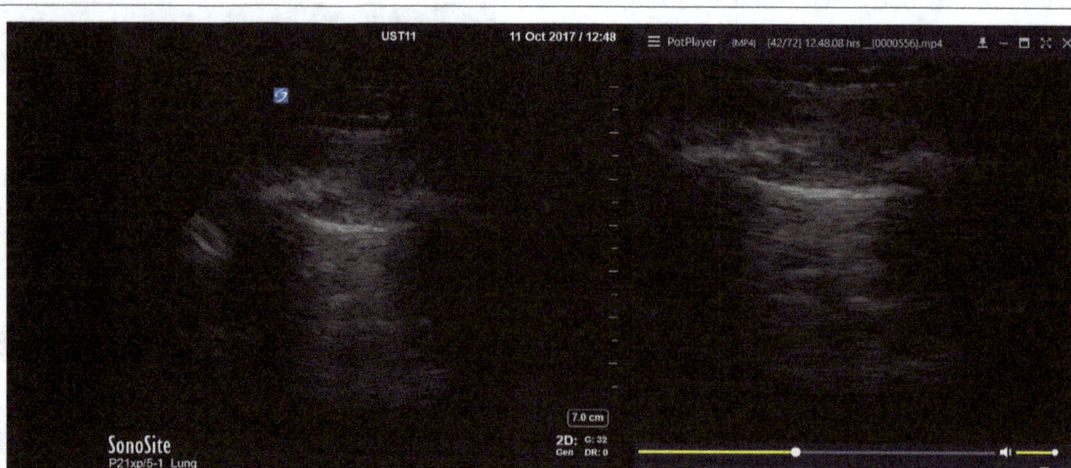


**Fig. 3** A typical uncropped and cropped image of the pleural interface, acquired with the phased-array transducer. On the right, the cropped version is displayed as it was played back to the observers

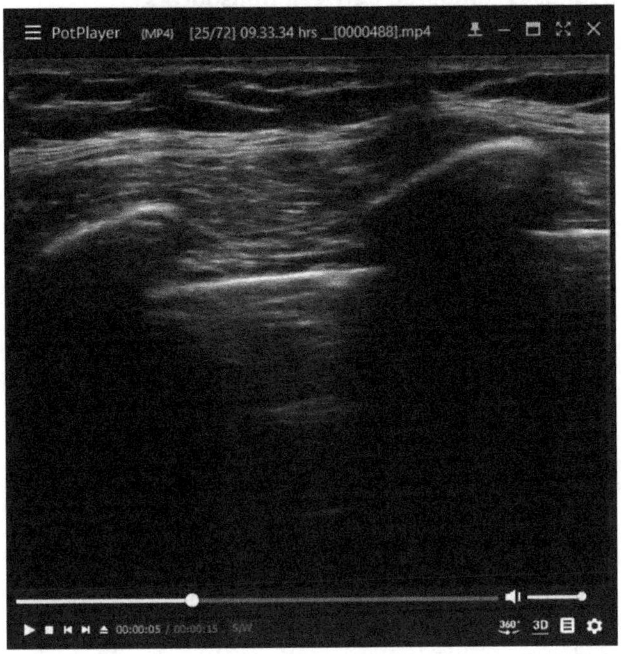


**Fig. 4** A cropped 15-s clip played in a random order to the observers

fitted a linear mixed model with a random intercept to these differences to account for clustering within each observer. A two-tailed McNemar's test for clustered data (Durkalski's Chi-square test) was used to test for differences between the transducers in diagnostic performance. The Wilcoxon signed-rank test was used to test for differences in time until final diagnosis between diagnoses (normal ventilation and pneumothorax). For all statistical tests, significance level was set to .05. For statistical analysis, IBM SPSS Statistics for Windows, version 25.0 (IBM Corp., Armonk, NY, USA) and R, version 3.4.1, lme4 package installed (R Foundation for Statistical Computing, Vienna, Austria) were used.

## Results

### Patients

Sixty-six lung US video clips were acquired in 11 patients, of whom eight women, with a mean age of 64.0 years (±9.03). Their mean weight was 66.1 kg (±9.30) and the mean body mass index (BMI) was 24.3 kg $m^{-2}$ (±2.98). Surgery was performed on the left and right chest in four and seven cases, respectively. All participants had a pneumothorax after the surgeon opened the thorax.

### Observers

The video clips were observed by 15 physicians of whom 13 HEMS physicians (nine anesthesiologists, and four trauma surgeons) and two anesthesiology residents. These observers all had extensive experience (a mean of 7.1 years [±3.58]) in lung ultrasonography.

Prior to the observations, six observers indicated to prefer a linear-array transducer for lung ultrasonography. Seven preferred a phased-array transducer and two had no preference. The curved-array transducer was preferred by none.

Each observer assessed the 66 cropped clips in a random order. There was no significant difference between their different backgrounds for success rate (correct or incorrect diagnosis) or time they needed to assess the video clips.

In 10 of the 990 judged clips, an observer could not decide on the diagnosis because the image quality was perceived to be too bad. Therefore, for data analysis where the diagnosis is a factor we used the data on 980 clips. The time was recorded from the start of video playback to the moment the observer declared to be unable to state a diagnose.

### Diagnostic performance

The overall sensitivity and specificity was 98.2% and 97.2%, positive predictive value (PPV) and negative predictive value (NPV) was 97.2% and 98.2%, respectively. A cross tabulation of the correct and incorrect diagnosis compared between transducers are displayed in Table 1.

The diagnostic performance measures for the different transducers for pneumothorax were calculated for 980 assessed clips and are displayed in Table 2.

McNemar's test for clustered data showed no significant difference in diagnostic performance between the different transducers. (Linear- vs curved-array: $p=.706$, linear- vs phased-array: $p=.537$, curved- vs phased-array: $p=.515$).

### Time

The time the observers needed to reach a diagnosis is displayed in Table 3 and Fig. 5.

After we fitted the linear mixed model, we found a significant difference between the times that elapsed until a final diagnosis was made. Whit the linear-array transducer the diagnosis was made .51 s ($p=.031$) faster compared with the phased-array transducer. The curved-array transducer was .15 s ($p=.049$) faster than the phased-array transducer. We found no significant difference between the linear- and curved-array transducers. These comparisons between transducers are displayed in Table 4.

Normal ventilation was diagnosed significantly faster than the diagnosis of a pneumothorax, regardless of transducer type. The Wilcoxon signed-rank test showed a significant difference overall ($p<.0001$) and within the three transducer groups as shown in Fig. 5 ($p<.0001$ in all three groups).

**Table 1 Cross tabulation of the number of correct and incorrect diagnoses compared between transducers**

| | Diagnosis | Correct | Incorrect | Total |
|---|---|---|---|---|
| | | Curved-array transducer | | |
| Linear-array transducer | Correct | 313 | 7 | 320 |
| | Incorrect | 8 | 2 | 10 |
| Total | | 321 | 9 | 330 |
| | | Phased-array transducer | | |
| Linear-array transducer | Correct | 308 | 12 | 320 |
| | Incorrect | 8 | 2 | 10 |
| Total | | 316 | 14 | 330 |
| | | Phased-array transducer | | |
| Curved-array transducer | Correct | 309 | 12 | 321 |
| | Incorrect | 7 | 2 | 9 |
| Total | | 316 | 14 | 330 |

**Table 2 Diagnostic performance of the three ultrasound transducers for pneumothorax**

| | Linear-array transducer (%) | Curved-array transducer (%) | Phased-array transducer (%) | All transducers combined (%) |
|---|---|---|---|---|
| Sensitivity | 97.5 | 98.2 | 98.8 | 98.2 |
| Specificity | 97.6 | 96.4 | 97.5 | 97.2 |

**Table 3 Time elapsed until a final diagnosis was made**

| Diagnosis | Linear-array transducer | Curved-array transducer | Phased-array transducer | All transducers combined |
|---|---|---|---|---|
| Normal ventilation | 2 (1–5) | 3 (1–5.5) | 3 (2–5.5) | 3 (1–5) |
| Pneumothorax | 5 (3–7) | 5 (3–7) | 6 (3.5–8.5) | 5 (3–7) |
| All diagnoses[a] | 4 (2–6) | 4 (2–6) | 4 (2–7) | 4 (2–6.25) |

The data are presented as median seconds (interquartile range)

[a] This includes the ten clips without diagnosis

### Image quality

Image quality was scored on a 5-point Likert scale. The image quality of the linear-, curved-, and phased-array transducers was appreciated at a median of 4 (IQR 3–4), 3 (IQR 2–4); 2 (IQR 1–2), respectively. Overall image quality was rated a median of 3 (IQR 2–4). The distribution of the image quality scores per transducer type is displayed in Fig. 6.

The Wilcoxon signed-rank test showed a significant difference in image quality between all three transducers ($p<.0001$).

After we fitted the linear mixed model, we found significant differences in image quality between all three transducers. The image quality with the linear-array transducer was 1.78 higher than the image quality with the phased-array transducer on a 5-point Likert scale. These comparisons in image quality between transducers are displayed in Table 5.

The image quality was deemed too bad to make a diagnosis in ten cases: 8 of 330 phased-array transducer clips and 2 of 330 linear-array transducer clips. Of those, seven clips showed a pneumothorax and three showed normal lung sliding.

## Discussion

In this study, we found no difference in the diagnostic performance of the linear-array, curved-array, and phased-array transducer. The diagnostic performance was very good: sensitivity, specificity, PPV, and NPV were all between 96.4 and 98.8%. The observers needed an additional .51 s to reach a final diagnosis with the phased-array transducer compared to the linear-array transducer. A final diagnosis was reached much faster when lung sliding was present regardless of the transducer type.

The image quality scored by the observers on a 1–5 scale was significantly different between all three transducers; the linear-array transducer achieved the best scores, the phased-array transducer the worst. Moreover, the image quality was too bad to reach a diagnosis in eight phased-array transducer clips and two linear-array transducer clips.

These findings suggest that the actual diagnostic performance of the three transducers for pneumothorax is comparable. However, these experienced observers perceived the best image quality and needed the

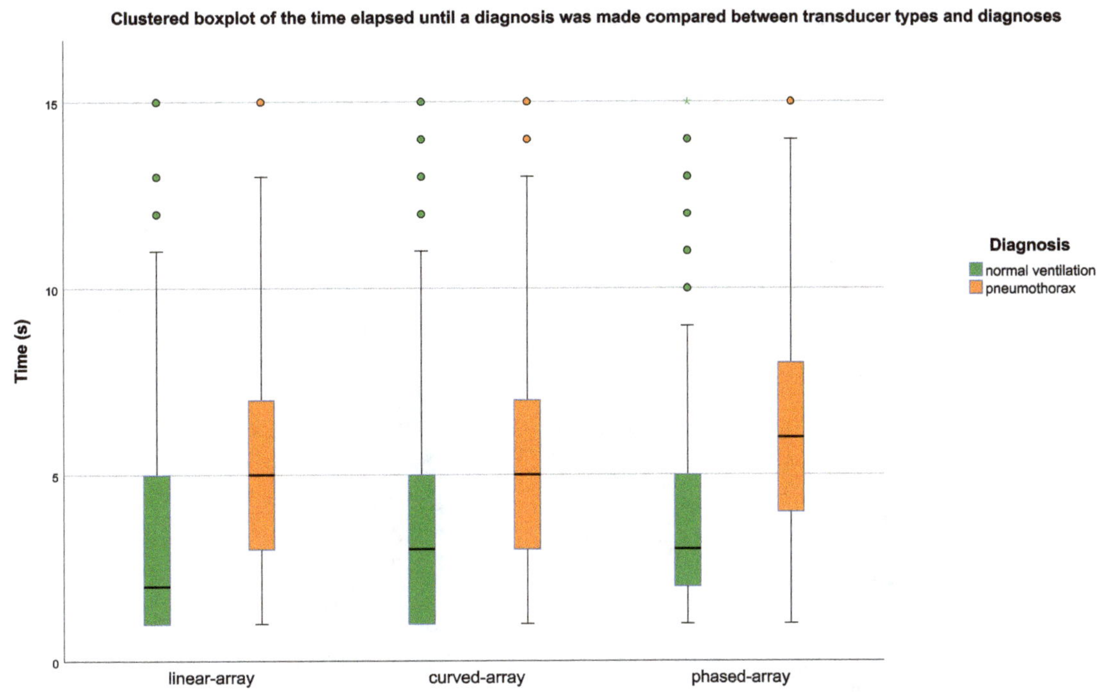


**Fig. 5** Boxplot of the elapsed time until a diagnosis was made compared between transducer types and diagnoses. The elapsed time until a diagnosis was stated by the observers. The time is represented in median seconds. The box represents the 25–75% interquartile range. The whiskers indicate the 95% confidence interval. There is a significant difference in the elapsed time until a diagnosis was made between normal ventilation and pneumothorax within all three transducers ($p < .0001$)

**Table 4 Difference in time elapsed until a diagnosis was made between transducer types**

| Compared transducers | Estimate [95% CI] | *p* value |
|---|---|---|
| Linear-array vs curved-array | − .35 [− .78, .07] | .105 |
| Linear-array vs phased-array | − .51 [− .97, − .05] | .031 |
| Curved-array vs phased-array | − .15 [− .59, .28] | .049 |

This table presents the differences in elapsed time until a diagnosis was made between a combination of two transducers, using a linear mixed model with a random intercept

The differences are presented in seconds

A negative value indicates that less time elapsed using the left of the two compared transducers

least amount of time when they judged the linear-array transducer clips. Based on these findings, the linear-array transducer might qualify as the preferred transducer for lung ultrasonography. However, the transducer choice may depend on more important factors such as the intended gamut of indications US is used for and whether the machine will be equipped with one or more transducers. In a single transducer setup, the best choice is probably a curved-array or a phased-array transducer to be able to evaluate both the abdomen and pericardium, in addition to the chest.

To our knowledge, there are no studies that have compared US transducers for diagnosing pneumothorax in a similar study design.

In a study with a comparable design, but not focused on pneumothorax, the authors compared a 10–5 MHz and a 14–5 MHz linear-array transducer for a wide array of emergency department point-of-care ultrasound indications [15]. However, lung ultrasonography was discussed only briefly. Overall, their observers most frequently preferred the 10–5 MHz transducer over the 14–5 MHz transducer.

In another study, the investigators compared a 5–10 MHz linear-array and a 1–5 MHz phased-array sector transducer in 55 patients scheduled for a thoracic-computed tomography (CT) scan [16]. The authors evaluated the diagnostic performance for pneumothorax, pleural effusion, consolidation, and interstitial syndrome. In six patients with a pneumothorax, confirmed with CT, they found that the linear-array transducer performed best with a sensitivity and specificity of 83% and 100%, respectively. The phased-array transducer showed a sensitivity and specificity of 67% and 100%. Sensitivity of both auscultation and chest radiography was only 50%. In our study, the gold standard was a thoracoscopically induced and confirmed pneumothorax. Because we assessed 495 ultrasound

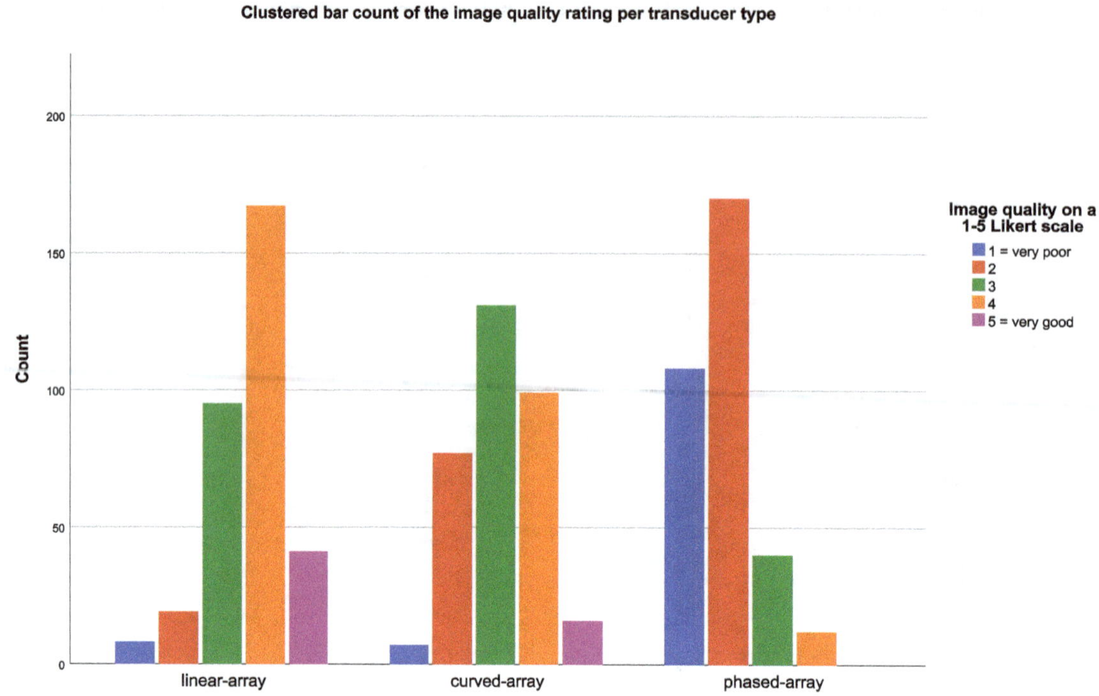


**Fig. 6** Clustered bar count of the image quality rating per transducer type. The Wilcoxon signed-rank test showed a significant difference in image quality between all three transducers ($p<.0001$)

**Table 5 Difference in image quality between transducer types**

| Compared transducers | Estimate [95% CI] | *p* value |
|---|---|---|
| Linear-array vs curved-array | .53 [.29, .76] | <.0001 |
| Linear-array vs phased-array | 1.78 [1.56, 2.01] | <.0001 |
| Curved-array vs phased-array | 1.25 [1.09, 1.42] | <.0001 |

This table presents the differences in reported image quality between a combination of two transducers, using a linear mixed model with a random intercept

The image quality was reported on a 5-point Likert scale: 1, very poor; 5, very good

A positive value indicates that the image quality was better with the left of the two compared transducers

clips showing pneumothorax, the diagnostic performance we found is more reliable.

We hypothesized that the linear-array transducer would have the best diagnostic performance. This study, however, showed no difference in diagnostic accuracy between the transducers.

The Nijmegen HEMS introduced prehospital ultrasonography to the Netherlands in 2006 and used a phased-array transducer ever since. Only years later, a linear-array transducer was added. A curved-array transducer has never been used. This history might explain the transducer preferences of the observers and the high and equal diagnostic performance between transducers.

Although diagnostic performance is equal, we recommend the linear-array transducer for (prehospital) lung ultrasonography. The diagnosis is made faster and with a better image quality. These are important advantages in the dynamic prehospital environment, HEMS physicians encounter challenges such as time pressure, limited working space, residual clothing, defibrillator pads, and Velcro® straps. Most importantly, the interpretation of US images may be hampered by sunlight or precipitation. When the HEMS physicians have the best possible image quality, they can better deal with these factors and do the best possible for our patients.

Furthermore, when the linear-array transducer is installed as the default transducer, it may have additional advantages. It is the preferred transducer for vascular access and assessment of the airway and endotracheal tube position [15]. These matters often take precedence over detailed assessment of breathing, although it may be of vital importance to be informed about a significant pneumothorax before airway management is commenced.

In addition, the linear-array transducer is superior for ultrasound-guided regional anesthesia (UGRA) in severely injured or trapped extremities and for optic nerve sheath diameter (ONSD) measurements in traumatic brain injury (TBI) patients [17]. For abdominal ultrasound and echocardiography, however, the phased-array or curved-array transducer is still invaluable.

The observers were able to successfully assess the video clips of normal ventilation and pneumothorax without having access to the US machine or the patient. This situation is comparable to a telemedicine setup in which the US operator could be at a different physical location than the observer of the images. Therefore, we agree that lung ultrasound can be successfully used in telemedicine setups [18].

### Strengths and limitations

We chose a unique approach to select VATS patients with a freshly induced and visually confirmed pneumothorax as the gold standard. In addition, we included the video clips of the same patients with normal anatomy before surgery. Another unique aspect was the cropping of the video clips thus transducers could not be identified by any text or image or sector shape.

A limitation of this study is that it might be underpowered because we could not demonstrate a difference in diagnostic performance between transducers. It could also mean the difference is close to none.

Another limitation is that we informed the observers that all patients were ventilated similarly and that besides a pneumothorax in half of the video clips, no other pathology was present. This could be an advantage for them judging the clips and might have resulted in an overestimation of the diagnostic performance and time needed. The performance could have been even better when we acquired M-mode clips looking for lung pulse or clips that included the lung point [14].

Conversely, most observers were uncomfortable with the fact that they had to assess video clips and that they were therefore unable to reposition or adjust the transducer, adjust the gain or depth, or compare with the contralateral chest. In addition, it was regarded a disadvantage that no additional clinical parameters were provided. The setting of pulmonary surgery introduced some minor challenges. In some clips, lung sliding was minimal, probably due to the lung-protective ventilator settings. B-lines were still present, obviously. In contrast to the normal clips, the pneumothorax clips were recorded with the transducer wrapped in a sterile cover. In theory, this might result in a slightly degraded US image.

Image quality might be overstated in video clips in which the diagnosis was made fast and perceived to be easy. Those clips might be scored good quality because they were 'easy' to assess.

A suggestion for future studies comparing ultrasound transducers might be to include subjects of all BMIs to better represent the general population of critically ill and injured patients.

## Conclusion

In conclusion, we found no difference in the effectiveness of detecting or excluding a pneumothorax between a high-frequency linear-array ultrasound transducer, a curved-array, and a phased-array transducer. Besides many indications for which it is essential, the linear-array transducer produces the best image quality in lung ultrasonography. Based only on image quality, the linear-array transducer might qualify as the preferred transducer for lung ultrasonography and the preferred default in our prehospital setting.

#### Abbreviations

CT: computed-tomography; IQR: interquartile range; HEMS: helicopter emergency medical service; NPV: negative predictive value; ONSD: optic nerve sheath diameter; PPV: positive predictive value; SD: standard deviation; TBI: traumatic brain injury; UGRA: ultrasound-guided regional anesthesia; US: ultrasonography; VATS: video-assisted thoracoscopic surgery.

#### Authors' contributions

RK, EG, and GvG designed the study. RK, EG, and MK included the patients and assisted in data acquisition. RK, EG, and TR recorded the ultrasound video clips. RK analyzed the data. All authors contributed to writing and revising the manuscript. All authors read and approved the final manuscript.


#### Author details

[1] Department of Anesthesiology, Pain and Palliative Medicine, Radboud University Medical Center, Radboud Institute for Health Sciences, Geert Grooteplein-Zuid 10, 6525 GA Nijmegen, The Netherlands. [2] Helicopter Emergency Medical Service-Lifeliner 3, Radboud University Medical Center, Radboud Institute for Health Sciences, Geert Grooteplein-Zuid 10, 6525 GA Nijmegen, The Netherlands.



#### Acknowledgements

We would like to thank the thoracic surgeons, scrub nurses, cardiothoracic anesthesiologists, nurse anesthetists, respiratory physicians, and respiratory nurse specialists of the Radboud university medical center for their invaluable assistance in the acquisition of the ultrasound clips.

We would like to thank Eva Cillessen for meticulously editing and cropping the ultrasound clips and Ewald Bronkhorst for his assistance with the statistical calculations. A sincere thank to all the HEMS physicians and expert anesthesiology residents (Loes Didden and Michiel van Lieshout) for their assessment of the video clips.

Many thanks to Roel van Vugt and Jouke Landman for their diligent proofreading of the manuscript.


#### References


1. Chen SC, Markmann JF, Kauder DR, Schwab CW (1997) Hemopneumothorax missed by auscultation in penetrating chest injury. J Trauma 42(1):86–89
2. Kong VY, Sartorius B, Clarke DL (2015) The accuracy of physical examination in identifying significant pathologies in penetrating thoracic trauma. Eur J Trauma Emerg Surg 41(6):647–650
3. Hirshberg A, Thomson SR, Huizinga WK (1988) Reliability of physical examination in penetrating chest injuries. Injury 19(6):407–409
4. Rantanen NW (1986) Diseases of the thorax. Vet Clin North Am Equine Pract 2(1):49–66
5. Blaivas M, Lyon M, Duggal S (2005) A prospective comparison of supine chest radiography and bedside ultrasound for the diagnosis of traumatic pneumothorax. Acad Emerg Med 12(9):844–849

6. Nagarsheth K, Kurek S (2011) Ultrasound detection of pneumothorax compared with chest X-ray and computed tomography scan. Am Surg 77(4):480–484
7. Lichtenstein DA, Meziere GA (2008) Relevance of lung ultrasound in the diagnosis of acute respiratory failure: the BLUE protocol. Chest 134(1):117–125
8. Gillman LM, Kirkpatrick AW (2012) Portable bedside ultrasound: the visual stethoscope of the 21st century. Scand J Trauma Resusc Emerg Med 20:18
9. Wittenberg M (2014) Will ultrasound scanners replace the stethoscope? BMJ 348:g3463
10. Price DD, Wilson SR, Murphy TG (2000) Trauma ultrasound feasibility during helicopter transport. Air Med J 19(4):144–146
11. Nelson BP, Melnick ER, Li J (2011) Portable ultrasound for remote environments, part I: feasibility of field deployment. J Emerg Med 40(2):190–197
12. Roline CE, Heegaard WG, Moore JC et al (2013) Feasibility of bedside thoracic ultrasound in the helicopter emergency medical services setting. Air Med J 32(3):153–157
13. Lichtenstein DA, Menu Y (1995) A bedside ultrasound sign ruling out pneumothorax in the critically ill: lung sliding. Chest 108(5):1345–1348
14. Lichtenstein DA (2014) Lung ultrasound in the critically ill. Ann Intensive Care 4(1):1
15. Adhikari S (2014) High-frequency transducers for point-of-care ultrasound applications: what is the optimal frequency range? Intern Emerg Med 9(4):463–466
16. Tasci O, Hatipoglu ON, Cagli B, Ermis V (2016) Sonography of the chest using linear-array versus sector transducers: correlation with auscultation, chest radiography, and computed tomography. J Clin Ultrasound 44(6):383–389
17. Rajajee V, Vanaman M, Fletcher JJ, Jacobs TL (2011) Optic nerve ultrasound for the detection of raised intracranial pressure. Neurocrit Care 15(3):506–515
18. Biegler N, McBeth PB, Tiruta C et al (2013) The feasibility of nurse practitioner-performed, telementored lung telesonography with remote physician guidance—'a remote virtual mentor'. Crit Ultrasound J 5(1):5

# 20

# An easier and safe affair, pleural drainage with ultrasound in critical patient: a technical note

Luigi Vetrugno[1], Giovanni Maria Guadagnin[1*], Daniele Orso[1], Enrico Boero[2], Elena Bignami[3] and Tiziana Bove[1]

**Abstract**

Thoracic ultrasound is a powerful diagnostic imaging technique for pleural space disorders. In addition to visualising pleural effusion, thoracic ultrasound also helps clinicians to identify the best puncture site and to guide the drainage insertion procedure. Thoracic ultrasound is essential during these invasive manoeuvres to increase safety and decrease potential life-threatening complications. This paper provides a technical description of pigtail-type drainage insertion using thoracic ultrasound, paying particular attention to indications, contraindications, ultrasound guidance, preparation/equipment, procedure and complications.

**Keywords:** Pleural effusion, Thoracic ultrasound, Ultrasound guidance, Pleural drainage

## Background

Percutaneous pleural drainage is the third most commonly performed procedure in the intensive care unit (ICU) after vascular catheterisation and tracheal intubation [1–3]. Forty-one percent of patients admitted to the ICU have pleural effusion at the time of admission, while 21% will develop it during hospitalisation [4]. The gold standard technique for pleural effusion (PLEFF) diagnosis is computed tomography (CT), which requires transporting critical patients outside the ICU [5]. Thoracic ultrasound (TUS) allows a bedside approach for PLEFF diagnosis with a sensitivity of 92%, a specificity of 93% and a diagnostic accuracy of 93% [6], thus showing better reliability and accuracy than chest X-ray, without using ionising radiation. The use of bedside ultrasound (US) not only leads to an improvement in the diagnosis [7], but also allows the detection of the best puncture site and the fluid quantification of PLEFF [8, 9]. The positioning of percutaneous pleural drainage with TUS guidance increases the procedure's success rate and safety [10]. International guidelines recommend ultrasound guidance for pleural drainage procedures and the usage of small-bore catheters [11]. Our technical note describes the pigtail insertion using ultrasound, paying particular attention to indications, contraindications, preparation/equipment, ultrasound guidance, procedure and complications.

## Indications

Pleural effusions drainage theoretically improves oxygenation by enhancing the ventilation–perfusion ratio and by reducing arteriovenous shunt, re-expanding areas of a collapsed, poorly ventilated lung [4]. Consequently, drainage of PLEFF seems to accelerate the weaning process from mechanical ventilation [4]. Respiratory mechanics could significantly improve after effusion drainage because it leads to an increase in end-expiratory transpulmonary pressure, respiratory system compliance, end-expiratory lung volume and a decrease in plateau pressure [12]. Pleural drainage also provides a chance to obtain chemical-physical-cytological samples to guide the differential diagnosis of PLEFF and any follow-up therapy. Indications [11, 13] and relative contraindications [14] are shown in Table 1.

*Correspondence: giovannimaria.guadagnin@gmail.com
[1] Anesthesiology and Intensive Care Clinic, Department of Medicine, University of Udine, P.le S. Maria della Misericordia n.15, 33100 Udine, Italy
Full list of author information is available at the end of the article

**Table 1 Indications and contraindications to pleural drainage positioning**

| Indications | Contraindications (relative) |
|---|---|
| Recurrent malignant pleural effusion | Coagulopathy, thrombocytopenia |
| Symptomatic patients caused by the effusions | Small to medium size pleural effusions in cardiac patients with more than moderate left ventricular dysfunction |
| Massive transudative or exsudative pleural effusion | Pulmonary bullae |
| Parapneumonic effusions | Pulmonary, pleural or thoracic adhesions |
| Weaning from mechanical ventilation | Loculated pleural effusion or empyema |
| | Recurrent pleural infections |
| | Skin infection over the chest tube insertion site |

## Preparation and equipment

The position of the patients is dependent on the operator preference [11]. To increase safety margin (depth of pleural effusion) [15, 16], whenever possible, place the patient in supine position with trunk elevation of 40–45° (in this position effusion gravitates down to the lower part of the chest pushing up the lung) and with arm elevated behind the head. However, as critically ill patients may often have limited mobility and also upright sitting position can generate haemodynamic side-effects (i.e., requirements of vasopressors) in a short time, the procedure will be described in a supine rather than a seated position. Considering that, some patients are limited ability to elevate the arm above the shoulder; it can be fixed in a soft bandage to the other side of the bed in a direction to the opposite shoulder.

Never rotate patient to the opposite site to create room for the procedure, as the fluid moves towards the paravertebral zone. The puncture might be more dangerous and patient could then lie on the insertion site which relates to infection complications. In patients with mechanical ventilation, do not take down PEEP or disconnect patient during drainage insertion because those manoeuvers can be associated with severe alveolar de-recruitment, especially in a patient that required high mean airway pressure and high PEEP to expand a poor compliance lung. On the other hand, the possibility of sudden reduction of intrapleural pressure due to puncture with risk of puncture of the visceral pleura is unlikely, especially in the case of ultrasound-guided puncture. Pigtail insertion is a sterile procedure; consequently, the operator should wear sterile gloves and use sterile drapes, sterilised materials on a sterilised puncture site. The necessary materials are listed in Table 2 and shown in Fig. 1. About pain management, pleura could be the most painful portion of the procedure, as it is highly innervated. For patients who are intubated you have the benefits of general anesthesia. For awake patient, pleural drainage insertion can be performed in a pain free manner if local anesthesia is performed properly, especially just above the upper rib edge.

## Ultrasound guidance

### Identification of puncture site

Pigtail insertion should be carried out in the *safety triangle,* almost always at the posterior axillary line if aiming for effusion [11], and performed under image guidance [11, 17]. The safety triangle is bordered by the lateral edge of the *pectoralis major*, the lateral edge of the *latissimus dorsi* and a line along the fifth intercostal space at the level of the nipple. However, ultrasound guidance allows the operator to better decide where to

**Table 2 Percutaneous pigtail drainage insertion equipment**

| For the operator | Over the tray | Patient |
|---|---|---|
| Medical hat | Sterile drapes | Disinfection of puncture site |
| Medical mask | Sterile towels | Sterile drapes |
| Hand disinfection | Syringes (5–10 mL) | Informed consent (when possible) |
| Sterile gown | Local anaesthetics | |
| Sterile gloves | Sterile water | |
| | Phased array probe or convex and linear probe<br>Sterile US probe cover | |
| | Introducer needle | |
| | Guidewire | |
| | Scalpel and dilator | |
| | Catheters (8–14F) | |
| | Trocar | |
| | Suture and medical dressing | |

*US* ultrasound, *F* French (1 F = 0.33 mm)

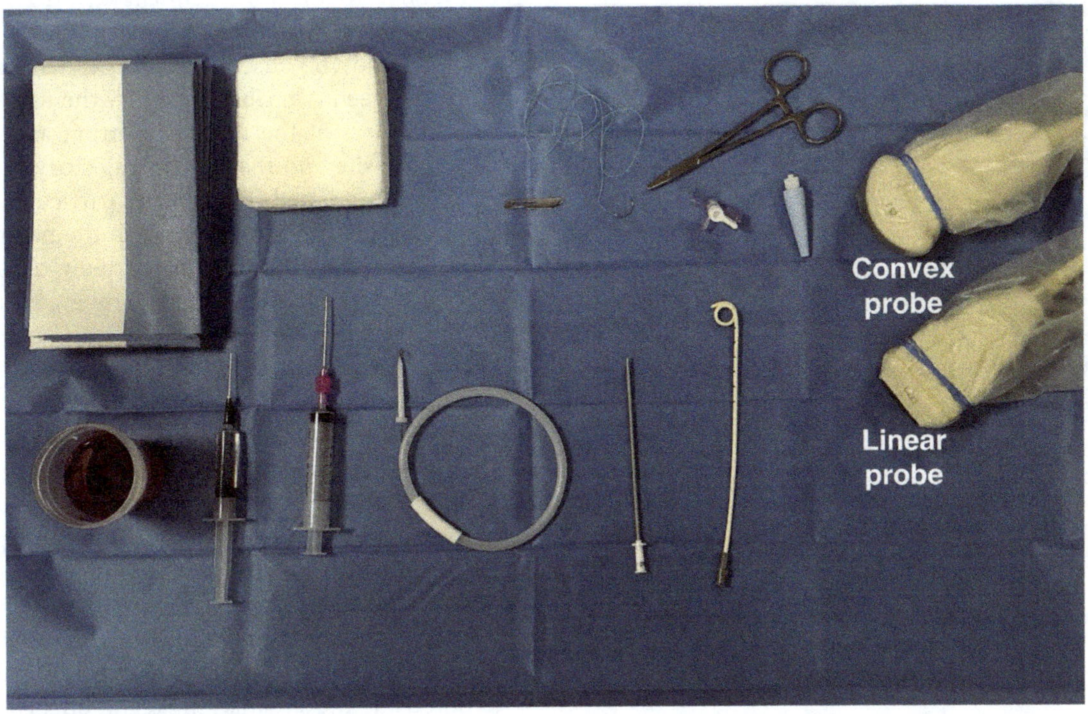


**Fig. 1** A set of pleural drainage tools on the tray

insert the pigtail. The best puncture site is, in fact, the place where the operator can visualise each anatomical structure (i.e., diaphragm, pleural, and organs) and where the operator can measure the maximum distance between visceral and parietal pleural (increasing the safety margin). One of the most commonly used US method for estimation of pleural effusion volume (*V*) is represented by the Balik equation: $V\,(\text{mL}) = 20 \times \text{Sep}\,(\text{mm})$ [8]. To obtain separation (Sep), the operator has to measure the maximal vertical distance between the parietal and visceral pleura in end-expiration at the lung base, in supine patient with trunk elevation of 10–15°. The patient's position greatly influences the extent of PLEFF [18]. In addition, for pleural effusion when measuring the maximal end-expiratory distance between the parietal and visceral pleura at the thoracic base the area under the curve, as reported by Vignon et al. [19], was greater for right-sided pleural effusions, on the left side the heart increases the fluid level, like a stone in a water recipient. The operator should also examine the ultrasound features of the effusion; the presence of hyperechoic material within the effusion indicates an exsudative effusion.

#### Intercostal artery visualisation

It was once thought that ultrasound was incapable of identifying intercostal vessels [10]. However, some studies have shown that Doppler ultrasound can be used to visualise intercostal vessels [20–23] helping prevent vessel injury and ensure a procedure with a low risk of bleeding, even in patients with abnormal pre-procedural coagulation parameters [24]. The colour Doppler box should be placed on the bottom edge of the rib and the depth reduced so the rib does not occupy the entire screen. Reduce the pulse repetition frequency (PRF) until pulsation is detected (Fig. 2, Additional file 1: Video S1). Take care the more posteriorly puncture site is performed, the greater the risk of puncture of the intercostal artery which is not covered by the lower rib edge approaching to the paravertebral line [25–28].

#### Site marking or direct needle guidance

Ultrasound guidance during pigtail insertion is performed using either *site marking* or *direct needle guidance* [29]. In the first case, the physician defines the optimal location point and marks it on the skin, then carries out the procedure without using real-time visualisation through US. Remember that patient repositioning can lead to fluid reallocation, so drain insertion has to be performed instantly after "*site marking*". In "*direct needle guidance*" ultrasound is used in real-time to guide the pleural puncture; some operators prefer to perform needle insertion under real-time ultrasound guidance even though this approach is more technically challenging [29]. Advantages and limitations of ultrasound guidance are enlisted in Table 3.

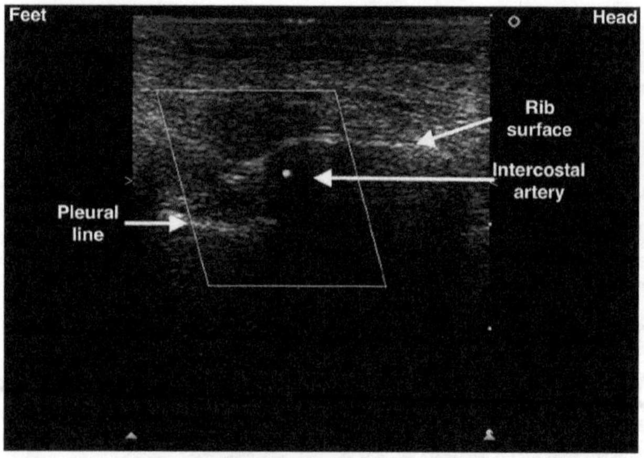


**Fig. 2** Visualisation of intercostal vessels using Doppler ultrasound. The probe marker is facing the patient's head (on the right of the screen). The colour Doppler box should be placed on the bottom edge of the rib and the depth reduced until the rib does not occupy the entire screen. Pulse repetition frequency (PRF) should be reduced until pulsation is detected

**Table 3 Advantages and limitations of ultrasound guidance**

| Advantage | Limitations |
|---|---|
| Can be performed in any position | Thickness of ribcage and soft tissues (i.e., obese patients) |
| Identification of the best site of puncture and best safety margin | Subcutaneous emphysema or large thoracic dressings |

## The procedure

The following steps may also be performed with a single phased array probe, according to the local transducers availability. In the case of a single transducer the point IV will be performed without changing the probe.

A. Identify the best site for the puncture. Use a low-frequency (3.5–5 MHz) ultrasound transducer *(convex or phased array probe)* to identify the best puncture site evaluating these following steps. The probe should be used in the transverse position between two ribs (Fig. 3, Additional file 2: Video S2):

   I. *Diaphragm.* The position of the diaphragm should always be marked at end-expiration when it is the most cranial in position;
   II. *Organs.* Subdiaphragmatic (liver, spleen, kidneys) and over-diaphragmatic (visceral and parietal pleura, heart, lungs);
   III. *Maximum distance between visceral and parietal pleura.* This increases the safety margin;
   IV. *Shift to the high-frequency* (7–15 MHz) *ultrasound transducer* (linear probe). The probe should be used in the transverse position between two ribs to identify the upper and lower borders of the needle insertion area. The puncture site and the needle trajectory must be carefully designed (Fig. 3), with particular attention to the depth required to reach the pleural fluid and avoid lung injuries. In morbidly obese with limited rib palpation, linear probe can also be used to help to be perpendicular and over the upper rib edge with great safety.
   V. *Intercostal artery.*

B. Ultrasound-guided puncture. To minimize the risk of neurovascular bundle injury the needle must aim to the upper rib margin perpendicular to pleura, with the transducer to follow the needle trajectory under direct needle guidance (Fig. 4). The needle must be advanced slowly under direct visualisation. Aspiration of fluid with a syringe confirms the correct position using the site marking technique. For direct needle guidance, the correct position of the needle tip is visualised in real-time and constantly monitored (Fig. 4).
C. Guidewire insertion and guidewire position check. Remove the syringe from the needle and pass the guidewire through the needle. Then remove the needle, leaving the guidewire in place (Fig. 5). It is mandatory to define the final position of the guidewire using US prior to proceeding with dilation (Fig. 5, Additional file 3: Video S3). It can be visualised as a hyperechoic linear structure from the insertion point at the skin surface to the hypoechoic effusion. Vertical rotation of the probe over the intercostal space allows for visualisation of the guidewire (leading towards the costophrenic space). Check that the guidewire is moving freely in and out of the dilator throughout this process to avoid kinking the guidewire.
D. Dilation. Make a small incision adjacent to the guidewire with the scalpel, then pass the dilator through the guidewire into the pleural space (Fig. 6). The dilator should not be introduced further than 1 cm beyond the depth from skin to parietal pleura; excessive dilator insertion increases the risk of visceral injury [24]; this depth can be safely taken with ultrasound.
E. Pigtail insertion. The pigtail is passed over the guidewire, making sure that the last side hole is within the pleural space. Remove the guidewire, leaving the pigtail catheter in place (Fig. 7). After the guidewire has been removed, the drain is connected to the drainage

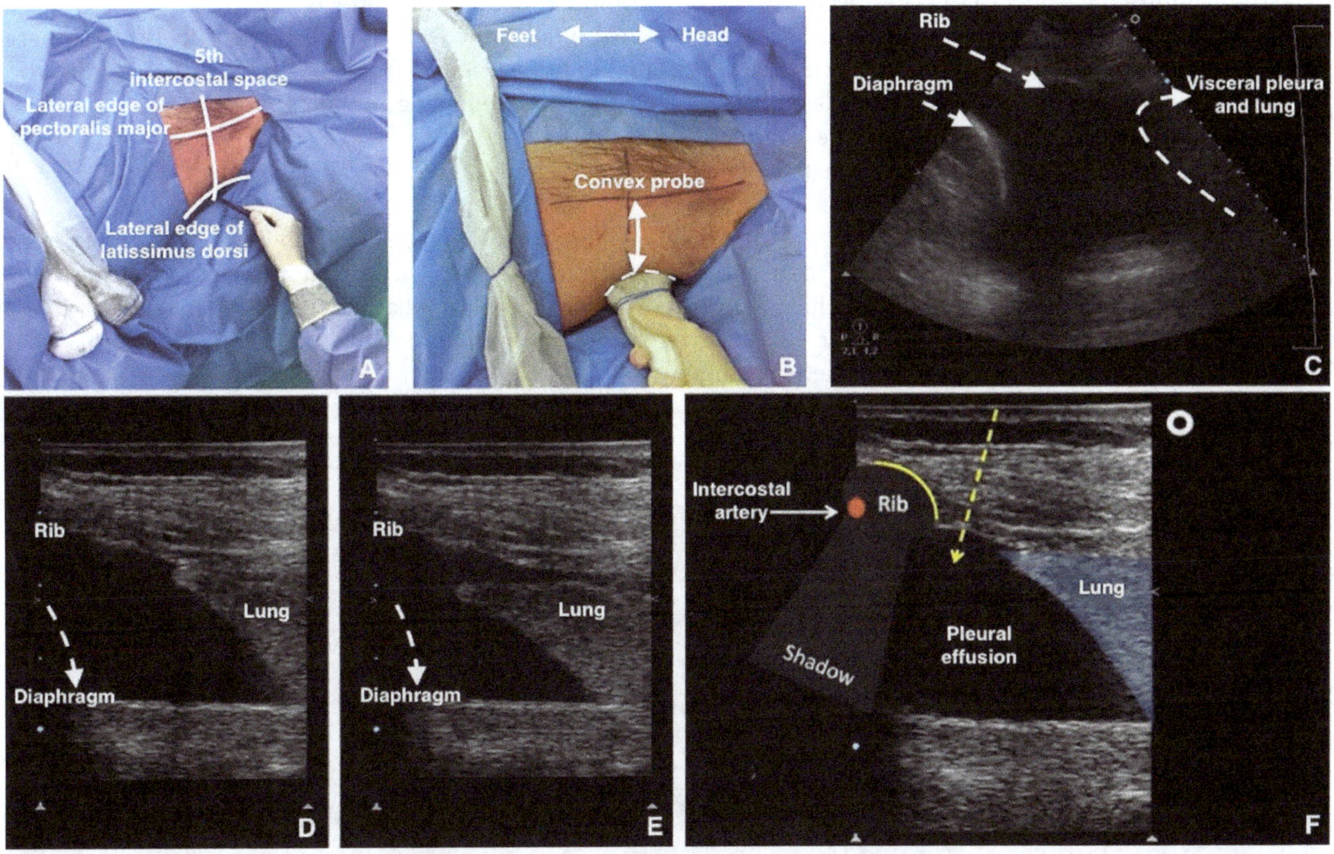


**Fig. 3** **A** Identify and draw the safety triangle. Note both convex and linear probes are present. **B, C** Use a low-frequency US transducer (convex or phased array probe) to identify the best puncture site. The best puncture site is where the operator can visualise each anatomical structures (i.e., diaphragm, pleural, organs) and can measure the maximum distance between visceral and parietal pleural (increasing the safety margin). The probe should be used in the transverse position between two ribs. The probe marker is facing the patient's head (on the right of the screen). **D** At the end-expiration (high-frequency US transducer) diaphragm reaches the most cranial position. **E** At the end inspiration (high-frequency US transducer) lung reaches the most caudal position. **F** A high-frequency US transducer (linear probe) should be used in the transverse position, between two ribs to understand the upper and lower border of the needle insertion area. The probe marker is facing the patient's head (on the right of the screen). The operator designs the course of the needle within the expected insertion area

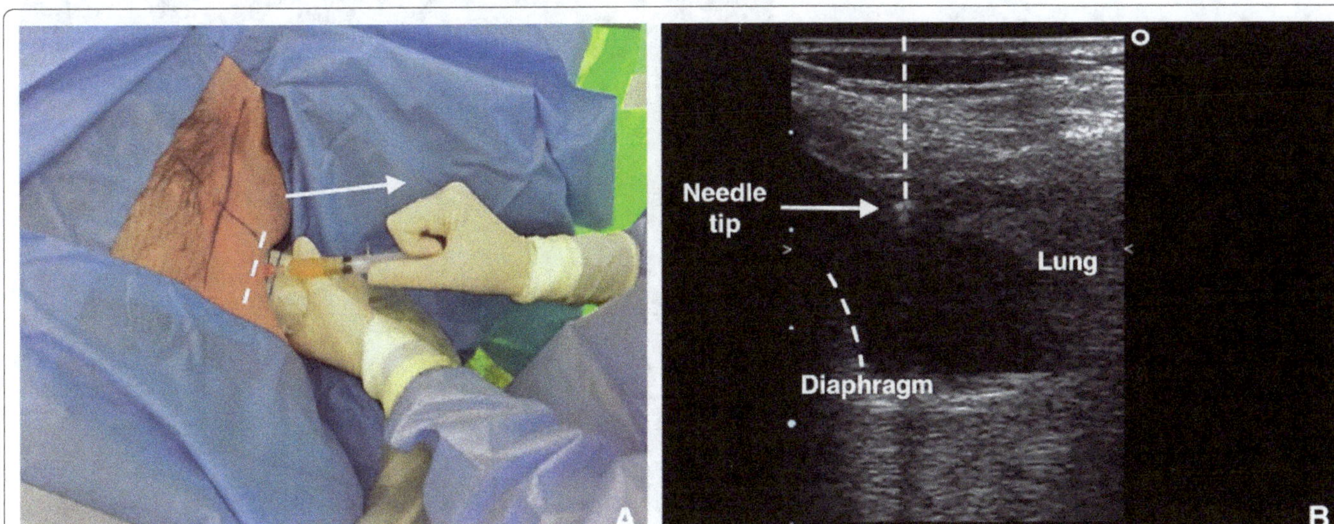


**Fig. 4** **A** Using the high-frequency US transducer (linear probe) in the transverse position, the puncture is performed employing short axis ultrasound-guidance (out of plane technique) at the point previously identified. Aspiration of fluid with a syringe confirms correct position of the needle tip. **B** With direct needle guidance, the correct position of the needle tip is visualised in real-time and is monitored constantly

system. Suture the pigtail to the chest wall in a manner similar to conventional chest tubes.

F. Ultrasound confirmation. At the end of the procedure, it is mandatory to perform a complete bilateral lung ultrasound scan to exclude possible complications (e.g., pneumothorax) and confirm the pigtail position.

A step-by-step guide for pigtail insertion effusion is provided in Additional file 4: Video S4. It includes ultrasound guidance, insertion of the introducer needle to ultrasound confirmation of the pigtail catheter within PLEFF.

**Complications and side-effects**

The pigtail catheter is a smaller drain (8–14F) compared to traditional chest tubes. Pigtail catheters insertion includes the following complications:

- Pneumothorax;
- Dry tap;
- Subdiaphragmatic insertion (injury to the diaphragm, liver or spleen with significant haemorrhage);
- Laceration of adjacent structures (pleural or cardiac laceration);
- Intercostal artery laceration;
- Catheter malposition;

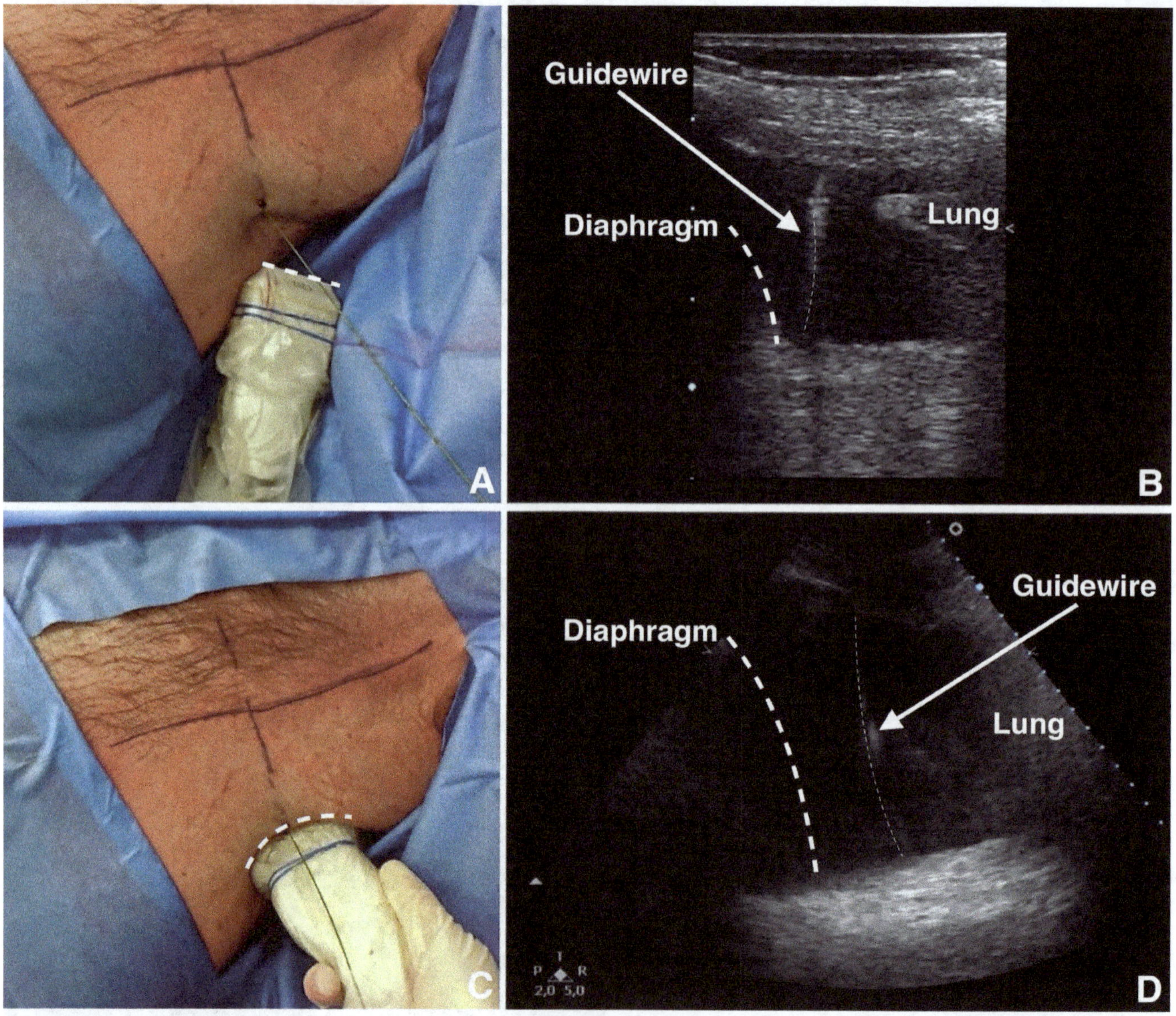


**Fig. 5** **A** Remove the syringe from the needle and pass the guidewire through the needle. After inserting the guidewire, remove the needle, leaving the guidewire in place. **B** Employing a high-frequency US transducer (linear probe) it is possible to visualise the insertion of the guidewire in real-time. **C** Shift to low-frequency US transducer (convex probe) to define the final position of the guidewire using US. It is mandatory to check the correct insertion of the guidewire at the end of the procedure. **D** As shown, the guidewire is correctly positioned within pleural effusion

- Catheter dislodgement or kinking;
- Catheter blockage;
- Wound infection and empyema;
- Re-expansion pulmonary edema.

Insertional complications, dry taps and procedure failure are less common with ultrasound guidance [11].

The main complications linked to small-bore catheters are blockade, dislodgement, malposition, and kinking [30]. The disconnection of the tubing system represents another possible complication. For infected pleural-fluid effusions, the efficacy and safety of intrapleural fibrinolytic agents are still debatable [11, 31].

Wound infection and empyema may occur if the chest tube (a foreign object) introduces bacteria into the pleural space.

The etiopathogenesis of the re-expansion oedema (RPO) is relatively unknown. Over the years different hypotheses have arisen about increased permeability of pulmonary blood vessels damaged by fast re-expansion of lung tissue [32], blood vessels damaging by free oxygen radicals generated by reperfusion of ischemic lung [33], pulmonary hydrostatic pressure caused by increased venous return, pressure-induced disruption of the alveolar capillaries and altered lymphatic clearance [34]. Mokotedi postulated that RPO could be due to decreased pleural and intrathoracic pressure and left ventricular afterload increased after pleural drainage with a detrimental effect on LV performance in patient with more than moderate compromised LV systolic function [35]. Rapid lung re-expansion in the following settings [36] has been described as a risk factor:

- Young patients 20–39 aa [37]
- Large pneumothorax
- Large volume pleural drainage (> 3 L) or high negative pressure suction (more than − 20 cm $H_2O$) [38]
- Lung collapsed for over 7 days.

Due to the fact that the etiology of re-expansion pulmonary oedema is unclear, there is concern that re-expansion pulmonary oedema may occur if larger volumes of fluid are withdrawn. Despite BTS guidelines, consensus statement of American College of Chest Physicians and most authors advise to drain no more than 1–1.5 L of fluid at one time, the amount of fluid safely removed continues to be debated as in several studies volumes greater than 1.5 L up to 6 L were safely aspirated.

Cause the RPO mortality rate has been quoted as high as 20%, preventive strategies include limiting drainage of pleural fluid, if the patient reports chest pressure or discomfort during thoracentesis, and using low negative pressure (less than − 20 cm $H_2O$) for

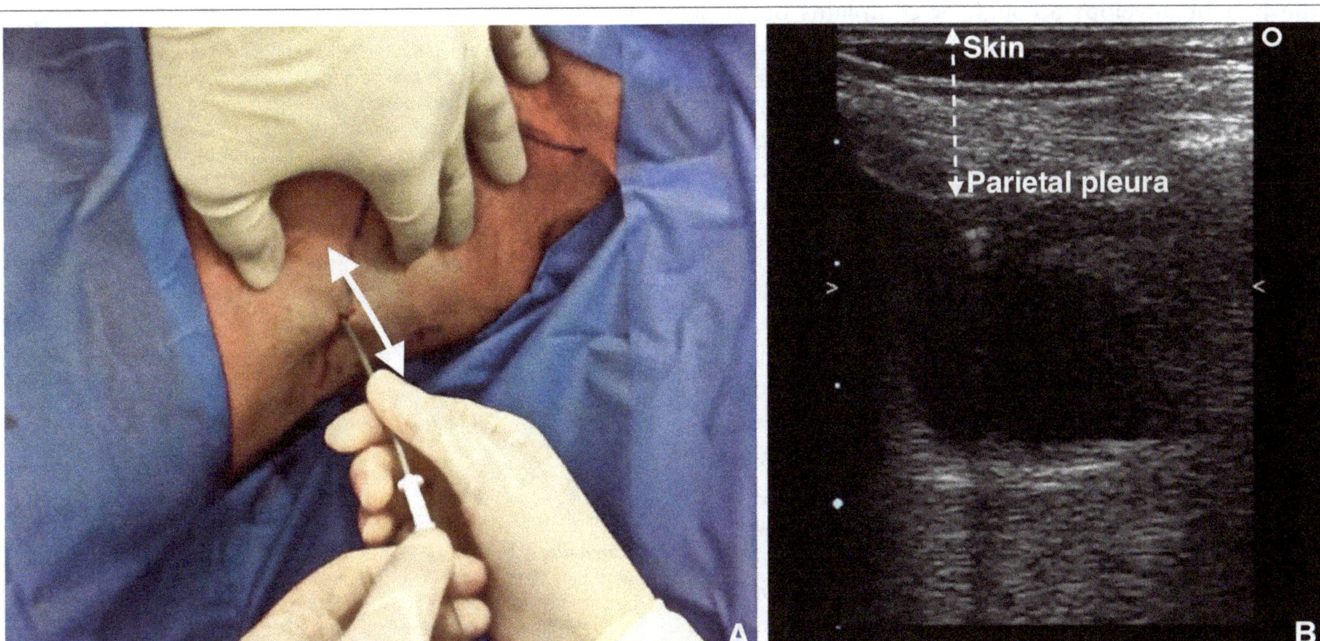


**Fig. 6** **A** Using the high-frequency probe, it is possible to calculate the distance between the skin and parietal pleura. **B** The dilator should not be inserted further than 1 cm beyond the depth from skin to pleural space

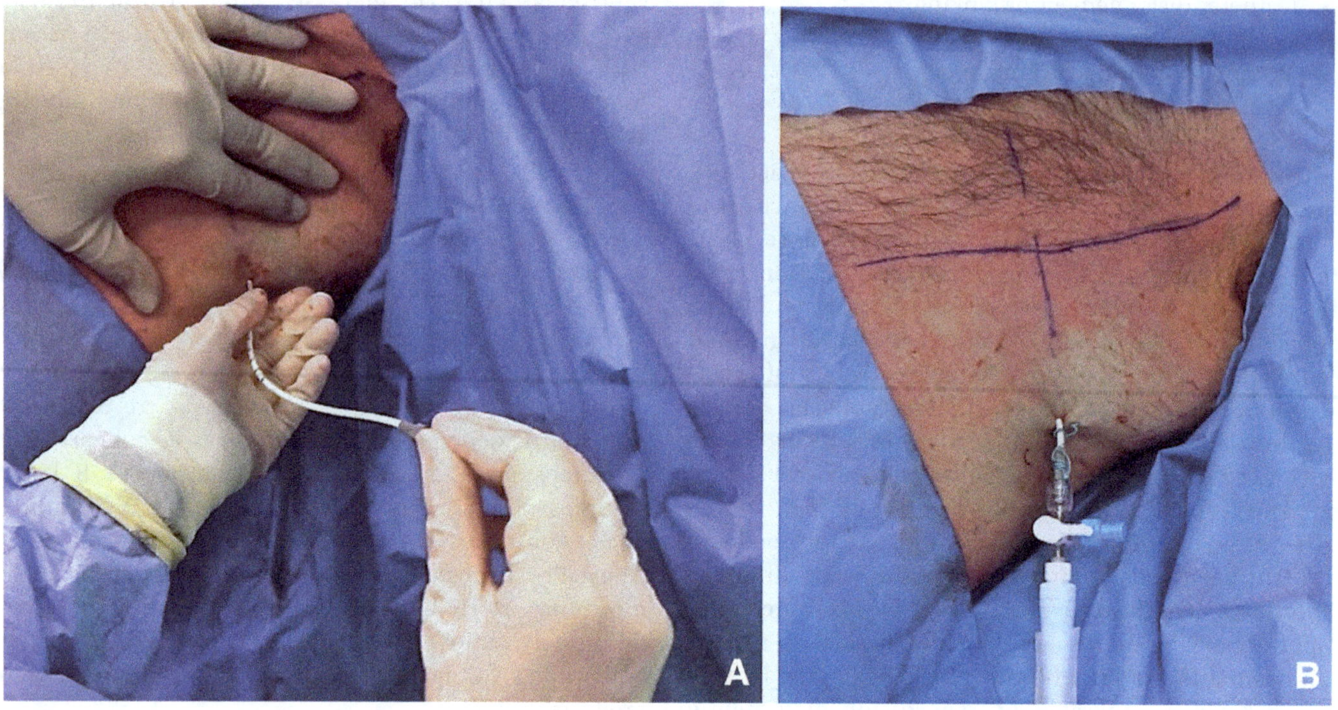


**Fig. 7** **A** The pigtail is passed over the guidewire, making sure that the last side hole is within the pleural space. Remove the guidewire, leaving the pigtail catheter in place. After the guidewire has been removed, the drain is connected to the drainage system. **B** Suture the pigtail to the chest wall in a manner similar to conventional chest tubes

suction with serial measures of pleural pressure can lead to prevention and early recognition of complication. Pleural manometry is not currently in clinical practice and there are no randomised controlled trials. Two important warning signs to end the aspiration are if the patient develops a cough or complains of chest discomfort [11].

Remember that pigtails can easily be drawn back, but cannot be inserted farther in after the procedure is completed.

## Conclusions

Placement of a pigtail catheter is a therapeutic manoeuvre in the presence of a pleural effusion that may noticeably improve gas exchange and respiratory mechanisms (i.e., respiratory system compliance, increase of functional residual capacity). Ultrasound guidance allows the operator to increase the rate of success of the procedure and reduce its associated risks. Consequently, usage of the ultrasound guidance during pleural drainage has become mandatory. Training programs, using appropriate manikins [39], must be encouraged to teach residents and clinicians how to use US during a pleural procedure.

## Additional files

**Additional file 1: Video S1.** Ultrasound allows for the visualisation of the vascular bundles, thus minimising the risk of damage to nerves and vessels. As shown, the intercostal neurovascular bundle is easily visible below the lower margin of the rib.

**Additional file 2: Video S2.** Ultrasound guidance allows the operator to decide where to insert the pigtail. The best puncture site is the place where the operator best visualises each anatomical structures (i.e., diaphragm, pleural, organs) and where the operator can measure the maximum distance between visceral and parietal pleural (increasing the safety margin). The probe should be used in the transverse position between two ribs. The probe marker is facing the patient's head (on the right of the screen).

**Additional file 3: Video S3.** Check the position of the guidewire using thoracic ultrasound (TUS) before introducing the dilator. As shown, the guidewire is positioned correctly within the pleural effusion. The operator can insert the dilator.

**Additional file 4: Video S4.** The use of ultrasound allows identification of the best puncture site and for recheck, at all times, the correct position of the devices used. In this video, we can see all the procedure previously descripted.

**Abbreviations**

TUS: thoracic ultrasound; PLEFF: pleural effusion; ICU: intensive care unit; CT: computed tomography; US: ultrasound; PEEP: positive end-expiratory pressure; PRF: pulse repetition frequency; MHz: megahertz; RPE: re-expansion pulmonary edema.

**Authors' contributions**
LV and GMG planned the study and drafted the manuscript. LV, GMG, DO and EB collected images and video clips, helped develop the bibliography, and drafted the manuscript. EB and TB helped to draft the manuscript. All authors read and approved the final manuscript.

**Author details**
[1] Anesthesiology and Intensive Care Clinic, Department of Medicine, University of Udine, P.le S. Maria della Misericordia n.15, 33100 Udine, Italy. [2] Anesthesiology and Intensive Care, Department of Surgical Sciences, University of Turin, Turin, Italy. [3] Anesthesiology, Critical Care and Pain Medicine Division, Department of Medicine and Surgery, University of Parma, Parma, Italy.

**Acknowledgements**
We would like to thank our colleague Lolita Fasoli who provided valuable insight and language expertise that greatly assisted the drafting of our manuscript.

**References**
1. Azoulay E (2003) Pleural effusions in the intensive care unit. Curr Opin Pulm Med 9(4):291–297
2. Fartoukh M, Azoulay E, Galliot R et al (2002) Clinically documented pleural effusions in medical ICU patients: how useful is routine thoracentesis? Chest 121(1):178–184
3. Mattison LE, Coppage L, Alderman DF et al (1997) Pleural effusions in the medical ICU: prevalence, causes, and clinical implications. Chest 111(4):1018–1023
4. Goligher EC, Leis JA, Fowler RA et al (2011) Utility and safety of draining pleural effusions in mechanically ventilated patients: a systematic review and meta-analysis. Crit Care 15:R46
5. Gargani L, Picano E (2015) The risk of cumulative radiation exposure in chest imaging and the advantage of bedside ultrasound. Crit Ultrasound J 7:4. https://doi.org/10.1186/s13089-015-0020-x
6. Lichtenstein D, Goldstein I, Mourgeon E et al (2004) Comparative diagnostic performances of auscultation, chest radiography, and lung ultrasonography in acute respiratory distress syndrome. Anesthesiology 100(1):9–15
7. Brogi E, Barbariol F, Marra A et al (2017) Thoracic ultrasound for pleural effusion in the intensive care unit: a narrative review from diagnosis to treatment. Crit Care 21:325. https://doi.org/10.1186/s13054-017-1897-5
8. Balik M, Plasil P, Waldauf P et al (2006) Ultrasound estimation of volume of pleural fluid in mechanically ventilated patients. Intensive Care Med 32(2):318. https://doi.org/10.1007/s00134-005-0024-2
9. Diacon AH, Brutsche MH, Solèr M (2003) Accuracy of pleural puncture sites: a prospective comparison of clinical examination with ultrasound. Chest 123(2):436
10. Liang SJ, Tu CY, Chen HJ et al (2009) Application of ultrasound-guided pigtail catheter for drainage of pleural effusions in the ICU. Intensive Care Med 35(2):350–354. https://doi.org/10.1007/s00134-008-1314-2
11. Havelock T, Teoh R, Laws D et al (2010) Pleural procedures and thoracic ultrasound: British Thoracic Society pleural disease guideline 2010. Thorax 65(Suppl 2):ii61–ii76. https://doi.org/10.1136/thx.2010.137026
12. Talmor M, Hydo L, Gershenwald JG et al (1998) Beneficial effects of chest tube drainage of pleural effusion in acute respiratory failure refractory to positive end-expiratory pressure ventilation. Surgery 123(2):137–143
13. Colice GL, Curtis A, Deslauriers J et al (2000) Medical and surgical treatment of parapneumonic effusions: an evidence-based guideline. Chest 118(4):1158–1171
14. Yu H (2011) Management of pleural effusion, empyema, and lung abscess. Semin Intervent Radiol 28(1):75–86. https://doi.org/10.1055/s-0031-1273942
15. Ko JM, Kim J, Park SA et al (2016) Depth of pleural effusion in thoracentesis: comparison of lateral, posterolateral and posterior approaches in the supine position. Iran J Radiol 13(2):e20919. https://doi.org/10.5812/iranjradiol.20919
16. Mayo PH, Doelken P (2006) Pleural ultrasonography. Clin Chest Med 27:215–217
17. Keeling AN, Leong S, Logan PM et al (2008) Empyema and effusion: outcome of image-guided small-bore catheter drainage. Cardiovasc Intervent Radiol 31(1):135–141
18. Vetrugno L, Brogi E, Barbariol F et al (2018) A message in the bottle. Anesthesiology 128:677. https://doi.org/10.1097/ALN.0000000000002039
19. Vignon P, Chastagner C, Berkane V et al (2005) Quantitative assessment of pleural effusion in critically ill patients by means of ultrasonography. Crit Care Med 33(8):1757–1763
20. Salamonsen M, Dobeli K, McGrath D et al (2013) Physician-performed ultrasound can accurately screen for a vulnerable intercostal artery prior to chest drainage procedures. Respirology 18(6):942–947. https://doi.org/10.1111/resp.12088
21. Salamonsen M, Ellis S, Paul E et al (2012) Thoracic ultrasound demonstrates variable location of the intercostal artery. Respiration 83(4):323–329. https://doi.org/10.1159/000330920
22. Hew M, Rahman N (2013) Preventing intercostal vessel trauma: ultrasound to the rescue once more? Respirology 18:891–892. https://doi.org/10.1111/resp.12136
23. Koyanagi T, Kawaharada N, Kurimoto Y et al (2010) Examination of intercostal arteries with transthoracic Doppler sonography. Echocardiography 27(1):17–20
24. Hibbert RM, Atwell TD, Lekah A et al (2013) Safety of ultrasound-guided thoracentesis in patients with abnormal preprocedural coagulation parameters. Chest 144(2):456–463. https://doi.org/10.1378/chest.12-2374
25. Olinger A, Shurtleff E (2012) Posterior intercostal artery tortuosity and collateral branch points: a cadaveric study. Folia Morphol 71(4):245–251
26. Carney M, Ravin CE (1979) Intercostal artery laceration during thoracocentesis: increase risk in elderly patients. Chest 75(4):520–522
27. DeBiasi EM, Puchalski J (2016) Thoracentesis: state-of-the-art in procedural safety, patient outcomes, and physiologic impact. Pleura 3:1–10. https://doi.org/10.1177/2373997516646554
28. Dancel R, Schnobrich D, Puri N (2017) Recommendations on the use of ultrasound guidance for adult thoracentesis: a position statement of the Society of Hospital Medicine. J Hosp Med 13(2):126–135. https://doi.org/10.12788/jhm.2940
29. Wrightson JM, Fysh E, Maskell NA et al (2010) Risk reduction in pleural procedures: sonography, simulation and supervision. Curr Opin Pulm Med 16(4):340–350. https://doi.org/10.1097/MCP.0b013e32833a233b
30. Davies HE, Merchant S, McGown A (2008) A study of the complications of small bore 'Seldinger' intercostal chest drains. Respirology 13(4):603–607
31. Davies HE, Davies RJ, Davies CW (2010) Management of pleural infection in adults: British Thoracic Society pleural disease guideline 2010. Thorax 65(Suppl 2):ii41–ii53
32. Sohara Y (2008) Reexpansion pulmonary edema. Ann Thorac Cardiovasc Surg 14(4):205–209
33. Gumus S, Yucel O, Gamsizkan M et al (2010) The role of oxidative stress and effect of alpha-lipoic acid in reexpansion pulmonary edema: an experimental study. Arch Med Sci 6(6):848–853
34. Mahfood S, Hix WR, Aaron BL et al (1988) Reexpansion pulmonary edema. Ann Thorac Surg 45:340–345
35. Mokotedi CM, Balik M (2017) Is the mechanism of re-expansion pulmonary oedema in a heart–lung interaction? BMJ Case Rep. https://doi.org/10.1136/bcr-2017-219340
36. Echevarria C, Twomey D, Dunning J et al (2008) Does re-expansion pulmonary oedema exist? Interact Cardiovasc Thorac Surg 7(3):485–489. https://doi.org/10.1510/icvts.2008.178087
37. Matsuura Y, Nomimura T, Murakami H et al (1991) Clinical analysis of reexpansion pulmonary edema. Chest 100(6):1562–1566
38. Kasmani R, Irani F, Okoli K et al (2010) Re-expansion pulmonary edema following thoracentesis. Can Med Assoc J 182(18):2000–2002. https://doi.org/10.1503/cmaj.090672
39. Vetrugno L, Volpicelli G, Barbariol F et al (2016) Phantom model and scoring system to assess ability in ultrasound-guided chest drain positioning. Crit Ultrasound J 8:1. https://doi.org/10.1186/s13089-016-0038-8

# 21

# A simplified lung ultrasound approach to detect increased extravascular lung water in critically ill patients

Antonio Anile[1], Jole Russo[2], Giacomo Castiglione[1*] and Giovanni Volpicelli[3]

**Abstract**

**Background:** The quantification of B-lines at lung ultrasonography is a valid tool to estimate the extravascular lung water (EVLW) in patients after major cardiac surgery. However, there is still uncertainty about the correlation between B-lines and EVLW in a general population of critically ill.

**Aim:** To evaluate a simplified lung ultrasonographic assessment as a tool to estimate the EVLW in critically ill patients admitted to a polyvalent intensive care unit (ICU).

**Methods:** Nineteen consecutive critically ill patients requiring mechanical ventilation and hemodynamic monitoring were enrolled. Lung ultrasonography and the thermodilution methodology (PiCCO system) were performed by two independent operators. The positive scan at lung ultrasound was defined by visualization of at least 3 B-lines. We then compared the number of chest areas positive for B-lines with the EVLW index obtained by the invasive procedure.

**Results:** A significant correlation was found between the number of lung quadrants positive for B-lines and EVLW indexed using both actual body weight ($rho = 0.612$ $p = 0.0053$) and predicted body weight ($rho = 0.493$ $p = 0.032$). Presence of more than 3 positive lung quadrants showed a good performance in identifying an EVLW index value >10 ml/kg of actual body weight(area under the ROC 0.894; 95% CI 0.668–0.987 $p < 0.0001$). Presence of of more than 4 positive lung quadrants indentified an EVLW index value >10 ml/kg of predicted body weight (area under the ROC 0.8; 95% CI 0.556–0.945 $p = 0.0048$).

**Conclusion:** A simplified lung ultrasound approach can by used as a reliable noninvasive bedside tool to predict EVLW in emergency and critically ill patients.

## Background

The early evaluation of haemodynamic status and need for fluid treatment are essential in the management of patients presenting with severe cardio-pulmonary failure, both those who are spontaneously breathing and those who are mechanically ventilated [1].

Accurate assessment and monitoring of haemodynamic status often require the placement of a pulmonary artery catheter or other invasive vascular lines. Transpulmonary thermodilution is often used for measuring volumetric haemodynamic parameters, of which the most commonly used are the global end diastolic volume and extra vascular lung water (EVLW) [2, 3]. This procedure is based on a central venous access and femoral arterial line, without the need for pulmonary artery catheterization.

The change in EVLW is a useful parameter for monitoring the evolution of cardiogenic pulmonary oedema, acute lung injury and acute respiratory distress syndrome (ARDS). In previous studies, the EVLW index showed a statistically significant correlation with $PaO_2/FiO_2$ ratio in ARDS patients [4].

In recent years, ultrasonography has shown to be useful as a "new eye" to look inside the lung [5, 6]. A change in the balance between air and fluids in the lung parenchyma determines a significant and corresponding

*Correspondence: giacomo.castiglione@tin.it
[1] Intensive Care Unit, Ospedale Vittorio Emanuele, AOU Policlinico–Vittorio Emanuele, Catania, Italy
Full list of author information is available at the end of the article

change in the acoustic patterns that can be easily detected and measured.

After studying the artefacts that the air/fluid imbalance creates, it is possible to diagnose some pulmonary conditions, ranging from lung consolidations to an increased interstitial water content [7]. The B-lines are vertical echoic comet-tail artefacts detected by lung ultrasonography, and they are typically correlated with the loss of pulmonary aeration and an increase in lung water [8].

Lichtenstein was the first who published about B-lines as a sign of interstitial lung water in 1997 [9].

In 2004, Jambrik et al. published the first paper showing the use of lung ultrasonography to assess interstitial lung water in the lung [10].

In 2005, Agricola et al. found a good correlation between the number of B-lines at lung ultrasonography and EVLW in a selected group of 20 post-operative cardiac surgery patients [11]. Their data demonstrated, for the very first time, a correlation between lung ultrasonography and invasive measurements of EVLW. However, the limitation of their study was that the data were obtained from only a specific subgroup of post-surgical patients that represents a minority of the population usually submitted to invasive haemodynamic monitoring in the intensive care unit (ICU). Moreover, the ultrasound technique proposed in their study is quite time consuming, which has also been suggested by recent evidence-based recommendations [7].

In the years following these studies, more studies have showed the ability of lung ultrasonography to reliably assess lung water or, in general, the aeration of the lungs [12, 13].

In 2015, Zhao et al. showed a very good correlation between lung ultrasound score (LUS) and EVLW, as measured using trans-pulmonary thermodilution, in a population of 21 ARDS patients [14].

The aim of our study is to evaluate the correlation between B-lines and EVLW in a general population of mechanically ventilated ICU patients. Moreover, a further aim is to assess the possibility of using a very simplified ultrasound approach based on a technique that is easily reproducible at the bedside.

## Methods

### Patients

The study was performed between June and August in 2010 in an 8 bed adult general ICU of the university-affiliated Vittorio Emanuele Hospital in Catania, Italy. All consecutive adult ICU patients requiring mechanical ventilation and haemodynamic monitoring with trans-pulmonary thermodilution in the opinion of the attending physician were enrolled. Our critically ill patients are admitted to the ICU from the emergency department, from post-surgery and post-procedure settings, and from the trauma centre. These patients are referred from all of the ordinary wards in the hospital when their haemodynamic status worsens to a level with the critical need for invasive ventilation. A lung ultrasound study was performed in all patients immediately after they obtained a trans-pulmonary thermodilution haemodynamic profile (PiCCO System). The two methodologies were performed separately by two independent operators. Particularly, the operator performing the lung ultrasound study was totally unaware of the results of the haemodynamic invasive analysis. Lung ultrasonography was performed by an anaesthesiology resident trained in lung ultrasonography under the direct supervision of a senior physician who had more than 5 years of experience in critical care ultrasonography.

Both lung ultrasonography and haemodynamic monitoring are part of routine management protocols in our ICU, and their application was totally independent from the study protocol. All data were treated anonymously, as represented by the standardized protocol applied in our institution for any patient admitted for treatment. The informed consent of patients was waived because the patients were all unconscious and the study did not involve additional procedures to the standardized clinical protocols, apart from the anonymous treatment of data.

### Lung ultrasound

The sonographic examinations were performed with the patients in the supine position. Four quadrants were examined in each hemithorax: anterior–superior, anterior-basal (between the parasternal line and the anterior axillary line), lateral-superior and lateral-basal (between the anterior axillary line and the posterior axillary line). A longitudinally oriented probe was used. In total, 8 quadrants were studied in each patient. As previously defined, the B-lines are an "echoic, coherent bundle with a narrow basis, spreading from the pleural line to the edge of the screen without fading". When 3 or more B-lines were visualized in a single chest area, the quadrant was defined as "positive," as defined in recently published guidelines.

The ultrasound examinations were performed using a single ultrasound system (Acuson Cypress, Siemens Medical Solutions USA Inc., Mountain View, CA, USA) equipped with a 5–7 MHz phased-array probe (Acuson 3V2c).

### PiCCO system

The trans-pulmonary thermodilution technique (Pulsion PiCCO Plus, Pulsion Medical Systems, München, Germany) was used for haemodynamic monitoring.

In all patients, a 5 Fr arterial catheter was placed in the femoral artery (PV2015LZQ-A Pulsion Medical Systems, München, Germany), and an 8.5 Fr multi-lumen central venous catheter was placed in the internal jugular vein or subclavian vein (Arrow International, Reading, CA, USA). The position of the central venous catheter was verified using a standard chest radiogram.

For the calibration of the system, 3 injections of 15 ml cold saline were performed. Cardiac output was measured, whereas EVLW was computed by the machine. For the calculation of the EVLW index, the actual and predicted body weights were used. For the predicted body weight (PBW) calculation, the following formulas were used: PBW (kg) = 0.91 (height cm—152.4) +50 (for males) and PBW (kg) = 0.91 (height cm—152.4) +45.5 (for females) [14].

**Table 2 Admission clinical diagnosis**

| | |
|---|---|
| Acute myocardial infarction | 1 |
| Septic shock | 4 |
| Acute respiratory failure | 6 |
| Acute pancreatitis | 1 |
| Cardiogenic shock | 1 |
| Inhalation pneumonitis | 1 |
| Acute on chronic hearth failure | 1 |
| Acute pulmonary edema following hepatectomy | 1 |
| Hemorrhagic shock | 1 |
| Pulmonary edema following tricuspid valve plasty | 1 |
| Bowel perforation | 1 |

### Statistical analysis

Data are expressed as the median and the range.

The Spearman (rho) rank correlation test was used to analyse the correlation between the number of chest quadrants positive for B-lines at lung ultrasound and the EVLW index values.

Sensitivity and specificity of the number of positive quadrants predictive of the EVLW index >10 ml/kg were adjudicated by using the receiver operative characteristic (ROC) curve. A $p$ value of $<0.05$ was considered statistically significant. The statistical analysis was performed using the software MedCalc version 11.6.1.0 (MedCalc Software, Mariakerke, Belgium).

## Results

Nineteen consecutive adult patients requiring mechanical ventilation and haemodynamic monitoring with transpulmonary thermodilution were enrolled in the study.

The patient characteristics are shown in Table 1, and the diagnoses of their admission in the ICU are listed in Table 2.

In all patients, lung ultrasound examination was feasible. The median number of chest quadrants positive for B-lines was 4 (range 0–8). The median EVLW index was 10 ml/kg actual body weight (ABW) (range 4–20) and 11 ml/kg PBW (range 6–22). A significant correlation was found between the number of positive quadrants at lung ultrasound examination and EVLW index ($rho = 0.612$ and $p = 0.0053$ for ABW; $rho = 0.493$ and $p = 0.032$ for PBW) (Figs. 1, 2).

The detection of more than 3 positive chest quadrants upon lung ultrasound examination showed the best specificity (70%) and sensitivity (100%) for predicting an EVLW index >10 ml/kg ABW (area under ROC curve: 0.894; 95% CI 0.668–0.987, $p < 0.0001$, see Fig. 3).

Detection of more than 4 positive chest quadrants at lung ultrasound examination showed the best specificity (100%) and sensitivity (50%) for predicting an EVLW index >10 ml/kg PBW (area under ROC curve: 0.8; 95% CI 0.556–0.945, $p = 0.0048$, see Fig. 4).

**Table 1 Patient characteristics**

| | Median | Range |
|---|---|---|
| Age (years) | 61 | 23–77 |
| Height (cm) | 165 | 155–180 |
| Actual body weight (kg) | 74 | 50–100 |
| Predicted body weight (kg) | 60 | 47–75 |
| APACHE II | 15 | 10–41 |
| CVP (mmHg) | 13.5 | 7–22 |
| PEEP ($cmH_2O$) | 10 | 0–14 |
| Tidal volume (ml/kg) | 8 | 5.7–10 |
| $PaO_2/FiO_2$ | 164 | 100–335 |

## Discussion

Our study confirms the correlation between B-lines and EVLW in critically ill patients with various haemodynamic conditions and diseases. Moreover, we found that the presence of more than 3 B-line positive chest quadrants correlates well with EVLW superior to the threshold of normality when EVLW is indexed for the actual body weight. When using the predicted body weight, as is what is reported in some papers in the literature, the number of B-line positive quadrants that best predicts EVLW >10 ml/kg was 4.

In recent years, ultrasonography has been increasingly used in daily practices in the ICU and has showed its usefulness in monitoring the pulmonary aeration and haemodynamic condition of critically ill patients [14, 15]. Haemodynamic evaluation using a bedside ultrasound offers a large number of advantages to invasive monitoring, including the absence of risks, not needing costly disposable devices, and rapid and easy repeatable assessments.

Some studies demonstrated the reliability of ultrasound evaluation in detecting lung oedema.

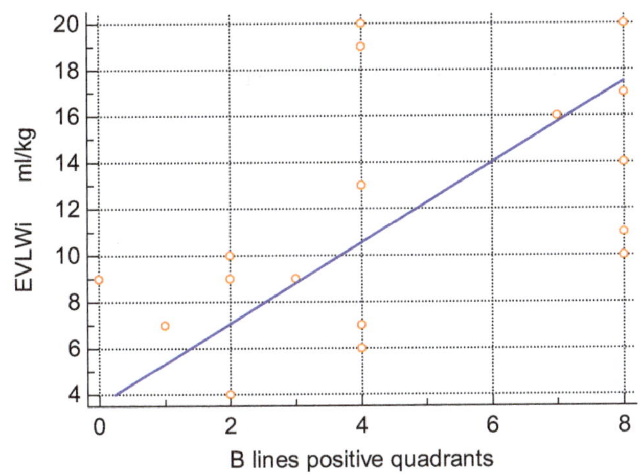


**Fig. 1** Correlation between the number of chest quadrants positive for B-lines at lung ultrasound and the values of EVLW/kg ABW. Spearman (rho) rank correlation test: sample size—19; Spearman's coefficient of rank correlation (rho)—0.162; significance level—$p = 0.0053$; 95% confidence interval for rho—0.219 to 0.834

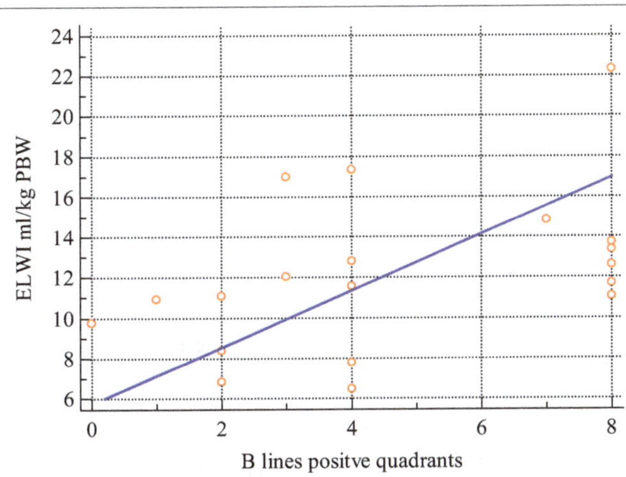


**Fig. 2** Correlation between the number of chest quadrants positive for B-lines at lung ultrasound and the values of EVLW/kg PBW. Spearman (rho) rank correlation test: sample size—19; Spearman's coefficient of rank correlation (rho)—0.493; significance level—$p = 0.032$; 95% confidence interval for rho—0.499 to 0.774

A seminal study by Agricola et al. showed a good correlation between lung ultrasound B-lines and EVLW measured by trans-pulmonary thermodilution. This method is widely used in haemodynamic monitoring and is minimally invasive in comparison to pulmonary artery catheterization because of its capability to measure not only "pressures" but also "volumes." Extravascular lung water is one of the many important parameters that become available when this technique is applied at the bedside, and it is universally considered as one of the most important parameters to predict the real haemodynamic status and response to treatment of the critically ill. The potential of lung ultrasound examination to predict EVLW allows for the hypothesis that it can be used as an alternative to invasive procedures when the PiCCO methodology is not yet available at the bedside, as it usually occurs in the emergency setting before admission to the ICU. The study of Agricola et al. already demonstrated the correlation between the invasive EVLW and B-lines, but it evaluated only a selected population of post-operative cardiac surgery patients and excluded patients with lung diseases. In our opinion, this selection prevents the generalization of the results of the study to other patient populations. In a similar study, our group assessed the correlation between a positive lung ultrasound examination for B-lines and high EVLW or wedge pressure in a wide and multifaceted population of critically ill patients using a multi-centre enrolment scheme [16]. While Agricola et al. used a time consuming chest count of B-lines to find the linear correlation with EVLW, Volpicelli et al. applied only a dichotomous evaluation based on the positivity of lung ultrasound evaluation for B-lines, without investigating a numeric correlation between the artefacts and EVLW values.

Our study was designed to evaluate a general ICU population requiring mechanical ventilation and haemodynamic monitoring, without exclusion criteria. For this specific reason, but compatible with our sample size, our results may be better generalized to the real practice of a polyvalent ICU and in general to emergency and critical care medicine. Moreover, the ultrasound technique that we applied in our study, the simple counting of positive chest quadrants, is less labourious than Agricola's technique but still allows for the analysis of a linear numeric correlation between the artefacts and EVLW values.

We chose 10 ml/kg as a cut-off value for an elevated EVLW index, which is in agreement with previous literature [17]. Only one of our patients with an EVLW index >10 ml/kg showed a $PaO_2/FiO_2$ >200. This observation is a further demonstration that EVLW has a very close association with clinically relevant gas exchange impairment.

One practical application of our limited fast lung ultrasound examination at the bedside may be in the extreme emergency setting, when the critically ill patients are still in the very early initial phase of diagnostic evaluation. In this situation, lung ultrasound examination may be very helpful in confidently ruling out the condition of elevated EVLW, possibly allowing the treating physician to be more confident in applying an intensive fluid treatment, when indicated, and in monitoring the effect on pulmonary function [18]. The new appearance of B-lines during this early phase may be considered a sign of rapidly increasing EVLW, which is a condition that demands for a stop in fluid administration [19]. On the other hand, a

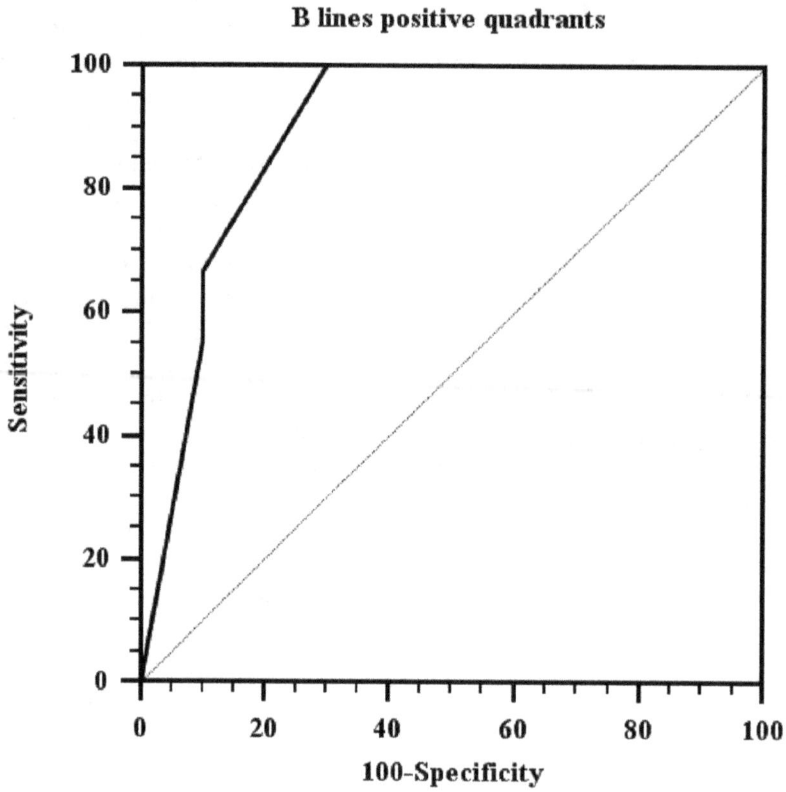


| Sample size | | 19 |
|---|---|---|
| Positive group : | ELWI>10 = 1 | 9 |
| Negative group : | ELWI>10 = 0 | 10 |

| Area under the ROC curve (AUC) | 0.894 |
|---|---|
| Standard Error [a] | 0.0759 |
| 95% Confidence Interval [b] | 0.668 to 0.987 |
| z statistic | 5.197 |
| Significance level P (Area=0.5) | <0.0001 |

[a] DeLong et al., 1988
[b] Binomial exact

**Criterion values and coordinates of the ROC curve**

| Criterion | Sensitivity | 95% CI | Specificity | 95% CI |
|---|---|---|---|---|
| >=0 | 100.00 | 66.4 - 100.0 | 0.00 | 0.0 - 30.8 |
| >0 | 100.00 | 66.4 - 100.0 | 10.00 | 0.3 - 44.5 |
| >1 | 100.00 | 66.4 - 100.0 | 20.00 | 2.5 - 55.6 |
| >2 | 100.00 | 66.4 - 100.0 | 50.00 | 18.7 - 81.3 |
| >3 * | 100.00 | 66.4 - 100.0 | 70.00 | 34.8 - 93.3 |
| >4 | 66.67 | 29.9 - 92.5 | 90.00 | 55.5 - 99.7 |
| >7 | 55.56 | 21.2 - 86.3 | 90.00 | 55.5 - 99.7 |
| >8 | 0.00 | 0.0 - 33.6 | 100.00 | 69.2 - 100.0 |

**Fig. 3** Receiver operative characteristic (ROC) *curve* for EVLW/kg ABW

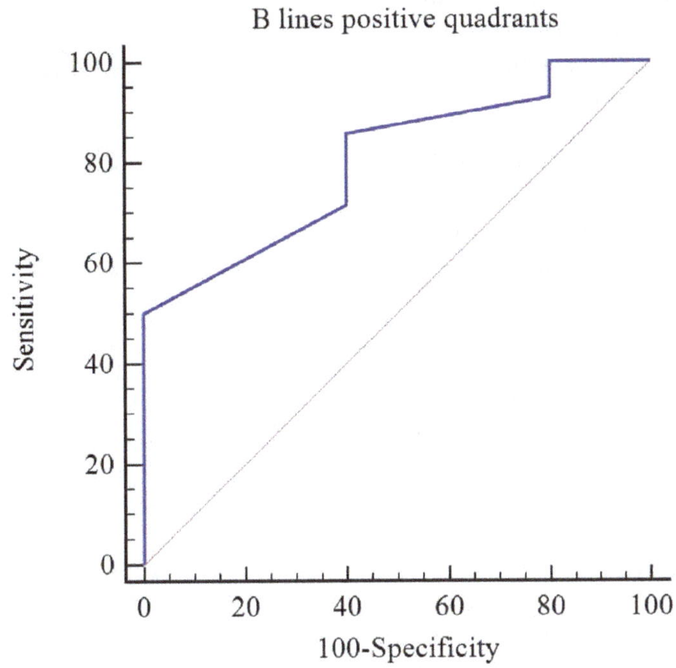


| | |
|---|---|
| Variable | tot_linee_B<br>tot linee B |
| Classification variable | ELWI_10<br>ELWI>10 |

| | |
|---|---:|
| Sample size | 19 |
| Positive group [a] | 14 (73,68%) |
| Negative group [b] | 5 (26,32%) |

[a] ELWI_10 = 1
[b] ELWI_10 = 0

**Area under the ROC curve (AUC)**

| | |
|---|---:|
| Area under the ROC curve (AUC) | 0,800 |
| Standard Error [a] | 0,106 |
| 95% Confidence interval [b] | 0,556 to 0,945 |
| z statistic | 2,822 |
| Significance level P (Area=0.5) | 0,0048 |

[a] Hanley & McNeil, 1982
[b] Binomial exactCriterion values and coordinates of the ROC curve

**Criterion values and coordinates of the ROC curve** [Hide]

| Criterion | Sensitivity | 95% CI | Specificity | 95% CI | +LR | 95% CI | -LR | 95% CI |
|---|---:|---|---:|---|---:|---|---:|---|
| ≥0 | 100,00 | 76,8 - 100,0 | 0,00 | 0,0 - 52,2 | 1,00 | 1,0 - 1,0 | | |
| >0 | 100,00 | 76,8 - 100,0 | 20,00 | 0,5 - 71,6 | 1,25 | 0,8 - 1,9 | 0,00 | |
| >1 | 92,86 | 66,1 - 99,8 | 20,00 | 0,5 - 71,6 | 1,16 | 0,7 - 1,8 | 0,36 | 0,03 - 4,7 |
| >2 | 85,71 | 57,2 - 98,2 | 60,00 | 14,7 - 94,7 | 2,14 | 0,7 - 6,4 | 0,24 | 0,05 - 1,0 |
| >3 | 71,43 | 41,9 - 91,6 | 60,00 | 14,7 - 94,7 | 1,79 | 0,6 - 5,5 | 0,48 | 0,2 - 1,4 |
| >4 | 50,00 | 23,0 - 77,0 | 100,00 | 47,8 - 100,0 | | | 0,50 | 0,3 - 0,8 |
| >7 | 42,86 | 17,7 - 71,1 | 100,00 | 47,8 - 100,0 | | | 0,57 | 0,4 - 0,9 |
| >8 | 0,00 | 0,0 - 23,2 | 100,00 | 47,8 - 100,0 | | | 1,00 | 1,0 - 1,0 |

**Fig. 4** Receiver operative characteristic (ROC) *curve* for EVLW/kg PBW

positive lung ultrasound examination with more than 3 or 4 positive quadrants at the very early stage should lead to a more careful consideration of the haemodynamic state before any definitive conclusion is made on the fluid treatment.

A great limitation of our study is the relatively low number of patients enrolled. The significance of our results should be read under this limited perspective. However, while we cannot exclude that increasing the number of enrolled patients may have a significant influence on the best numeric correlation between the lung ultrasound cut-off and elevated EVLW, our data represent a further confirmation of the tight relationship that exists between B-lines and EVLW detected by the PiCCO technique.

## Conclusion

In conclusion, we showed a correlation between the number of lung quadrants positive for the presence of B-lines at lung ultrasound examination and extravascular lung water. We also showed that the detection of more than 3 B-line positive chest quadrants, when using ABW for indexing EVLW, or more than 4 B-line positive chest quadrants, when using PBW, allows for the prediction of abnormal EVLW value, with strong sensitivity and specificity. Results from our study support the use of lung ultrasonography as a screening tool in the emergency and critical care settings with an acceptable performance at the bedside in identifying patients without a significant condition of increased EVLW, with encouraging rapidity and reliability.

### Authors' contributions

AA: study design, data collection, and manuscript preparation. JR: study design, data collection, and manuscript preparation. GC: study design, manuscript preparation, and data analysis. GV: manuscript review. All authors read and approved the final manuscript.

### Author details

[1] Intensive Care Unit, Ospedale Vittorio Emanuele, AOU Policlinico–Vittorio Emanuele, Catania, Italy. [2] Department of Anesthesia and Intensive Care, Ospedale Vittorio Emanuele, ASP Caltanissetta, Gela, Italy. [3] Department of Emergency Medicine, San Luigi Gonzaga University Hospital, Orbassano, Turin, Italy.

### References

1. Pinsky MR (2003) Hemodynamic monitoring in intensive care unit. Clin Chest Med 24:549–560
2. Combes A et al (2004) Estimation of left ventricular systolic function by single transpulmonary thermodilution. Intensive Care Med 30:1377–1383
3. Bindels AJ, van der Hoeven JG, Meinders AE (1999) Pulmonary artery wedge pressure and extravascular lung water in patients with acute cardiogenic pulmonary edema requiring mechanical ventilation. Am J Cardiol 84:1158–1163
4. Berkowitz DM, Danai PA, Eaton S, Moss M, Martin GS (2008) Accurate characterization of extravascular lung water in acute respiratory distress syndrome. Crit Care Med 36:1803–1809
5. Volpicelli G (2013) Lung sonography. J Ultrasound Med 32:165–171
6. Lichtenstein D (2004) Comparative diagnostic performance of auscultation, chest radiography and lung ultrasonography in acute respiratory distress syndrome. Anesthesiology 100:9–15
7. Volpicelli G et al (2012) International evidence-based recommendations for point-of-care lung ultrasound. Intensive Care Med 38:577–591
8. Lichtenstein DA (2007) Ultrasound in the management of thoracic disease. Crit Care Med 35(Suppl):S250–S261
9. Lichtenstein D, Mézière G, Biderman P, Gepner A, Barré O (1997) The comet-tail artifact. An ultrasound sign of alveolar-interstitial syndrome. Am J Respir Crit Care Med 156(5):1640–1646
10. Jambrik Z, Monti S, Coppola V, Agricola E, Mottola G, Miniati M, Picano E (2004) Usefulness of ultrasound lung comets as a non radiologic sing of extravascular lung water. Am J Cardiol 93:1265–1270
11. Agricola E, Bove T, Oppizzi M, Marino G, Zangrillo A, Margonato A, Picano E (2005) "Ultrasound comet—tail images": a marker of pulmonary edema. A comparative study with wedge pressure and Extravascular lung water. Chest 127:1690–1695
12. Bouhemad B et al (2011) Bedside ultrasound assessment of positive end-expiratory pressure induced lung recruitment. Am J Respir Crit Care Med 183:341–347
13. Bouhemad B et al (2010) Ultrasound assessment of antibiotic-induced reaeration in ventilator induced pneumonia. Crit Care Med 38:84–92
14. Zhao Z, Jiang L, Xi X, Jiang Q, Zhu B, Wang M, Xing J, Zhang D (2015) Prognostic value of extravascular lung water assessed with lung ultrasound score by chest sonography in patients with acute respiratory distress syndroma. BMC Pulm Med 15:98
15. Via G, Storti E, Gulati G, Neri L, Mojoli F, Braschi A (2012) Lung ultrasound in the ICU: from diagnostic instrument to respiratory monitoring tool. Minerva Anestesiol 78:1282–1296
16. Volpicelli G, Skurzak S, Boero E, Carpinteri G, Tengattini M, Stefanone V, Luberto L, Anile A, Cerutti E, Radeschi G, Frascisco MF (2014) Lung ultrasound predicts well extravascular lung water but is of limited usefulness in the prediction of wedge pressure. Anesthesiology 121:320–327
17. Tagami T, Sawabe M, Kushimoto S, Marik PE, Mieno MN, Kawaguchi T, Kusakabe T, Tosa R, Yokota H, Fukuda Y (2013) Quantitative diagnosis of diffuse alveolar damage using extravascular lung water. Crit Care Med 41:2144–2150
18. Lichtenstein DA (2015) BLUE-protocol and FALLS-protocol: two applications of lung ultrasound in the critically ill. Chest 147:1659–1670
19. Caltabeloti FC, Monsel A, Arbelot C, Brisson H, Lu Q, Gu WJ, Zohu GJ, Auler JOC Jr, Rouby JJ (2014) Early fluid loading in acute respiratory distress syndrome with septic shock deteriorates lung aeration without impairing arterial oxygenation: a lung ultrasound observational study. Crit Care 18(3):R91

# 22

# Bedside transcranial sonography monitoring in a patient with hydrocephalus post subarachnoid hemorrhage

Ahmed Najjar[1], André Y. Denault[2,3*] and Michel W. Bojanowski[1]

**Abstract**

**Background:** Development of hydrocephalus can occur after subarachnoid hemorrhage (SAH). Typically, it is diagnosed with computed tomography, CT, scan. However, transcranial sonography (TCS) can be used particularly in patients with craniotomy which removes the acoustic interference of the skull and allows a closer up visualization of brain structures through the skin.

**Case presentation:** We report a 73-year-old woman who was hospitalized for SAH and developed acute hydrocephalus requiring an external ventricular drain (EVD). In this patient, detection and monitoring of hydrocephalus was done and monitored with a small pocket-sized TCS device. Nine days after surgery, weaning of the EVD was attempted. Prior to EVD closure and removal, TCS showed a measurement of the 3rd ventricle at around 1.16 cm. On the third day, the patient deteriorated clinically and the TCS showed a dilated 3rd ventricle measuring 1.37 cm which correlated well with computed tomography and with clinical signs of active hydrocephalus as both her sensorium and communication were affected. Subsequently following EVD re-installation, on the next day, TCS showed that the 3rd ventricle dimension was reduced to 0.99 cm and the following day it went down to 0.69 cm.

**Conclusions:** Patients with SAH and in particular those with a craniotomy can be monitored easily at the bedside with hand-held TCS for the development and monitoring of hydrocephalus.

**Keywords:** Transcranial ultrasound, Subarachnoid hemorrhage, Intracranial hypertension, Bedside ultrasound, Transcranial sonography

## Background

Hydrocephalus in patients with subarachnoid hemorrhage (SAH) is a frequent cause of clinical deterioration. In addition to clinical evaluation, computed tomography (CT) scans are used regularly to monitor for the appearance of hydrocephalus. The use of bedside ultrasound for imaging has expanded to multiple clinical applications especially in the acute critical patient care. We describe a case for which we used a hand-held two-dimensional (2D) transcranial sonography (TCS) probe to follow-up a patient with hydrocephalus after subarachnoid hemorrhage demonstrating high accuracy and clinical correlation. Permission to use the following figures was granted by the patient's family.

*Correspondence: andre.denault@umontreal.ca
[3] Department of Anesthesiology, Montreal Heart Institute, Université de Montréal, 5000 Belanger Street, Montreal, QC H1T 1C8, Canada
Full list of author information is available at the end of the article

## Case report

A 73-year-old woman was admitted to our hospital in coma after having an acute thunder clap headache. Her vitals were stable apart from high blood pressure and other signs of increased intracranial pressure (ICP). Her CT showed extensive SAH with acute hydrocephalus and signs of elevated ICP. An anterior communicating artery aneurysm was identified on CT angiogram. Patient underwent urgent surgery including insertion of external ventricular drain (EVD), right-sided craniectomy and clipping of the aneurysm at the same time. She had a fair good outcome after the surgery immediately with improvement in consciousness and good control of her

ICP. An intensivist with bedside ultrasound experience followed the patient with daily TCS using a hand-held pocket ultrasound device (GE Vingmed Ultrasound AS, Horten, Norway) (Fig. 1a). Image acquisition was facilitated by the absence of bone on the site of the craniectomy which allows close contact with the brain structure through the skin. The technique is usually straight forward. In contrast to CT scan no preparation is required except for good head position. The head is cleaned with saline where the probe is applied if necessary. The TCS probe is applied directly on the skin where the craniotomy defect (in the temporal region) is and images in coronal plane are obtained. To visualize the brain images, as described by Seidel et al. [1] and by Couture et al. [2]: we positioned the ultrasound probe over the temporal area in an axial orientation with the marker pointing toward the occiput. Then using 2D imaging, we adjusted the display depth to see the opposite skull border. Following these initial steps, we scanned in a cranial to caudal direction to identify the intracranial bone artifacts: contralateral skull, foramen lacerum, petrous ridge, and sphenoid bone. Then we tilted at about 10° cranially to identify the 3rd ventricle. Color Doppler using a low-velocity scale is then used to visualize the main cerebral arteries along the Circle of Willis. Nine days after surgery, weaning of the EVD was attempted. Prior to EVD closure, TCS showed a measurement of the 3rd ventricle at around 1.16 cm (Fig. 1b). On the 3rd day of weaning, she deteriorated clinically and the TCS showed a dilated 3rd ventricle measuring 1.37 cm (Fig. 1c). This correlated well with the CT scan (Fig. 1d) and with clinical signs of active hydrocephalus as both her sensorium and communication were affected. Subsequently following EVD re-opening, on the next day using TCS the 3rd ventricle dimension was reduced to 0.99 cm (Fig. 1e) and the following day it went down to 0.69 cm (Fig. 1f). After 20 days from the hemorrhage, the EVD was clamped and removed because her sensorium and ICP were well preserved during the EVD weaning process. Patient had a favorable outcome and was transferred to a rehabilitation center.

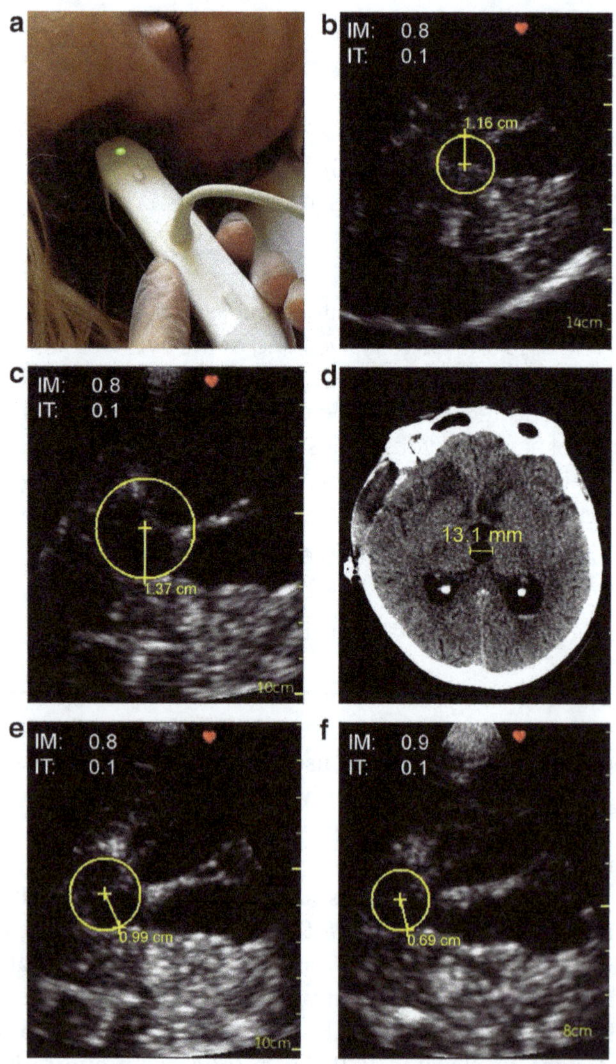


**Fig. 1** **a** TCS using hand-held pocket ultrasound device (GE Vingmed Ultrasound AS, Horten, Norway). **b** Prior to EVD closure, TCS showed a measurement of the 3rd ventricle at around 1.16 cm. **c** On the third day, TCS showed a dilated 3rd ventricle measuring 1.37 cm. **d** CT scan showed a dilated 3rd ventricle measuring 13.1 mm. **e** Subsequently following EVD re-opening, on the next day using TCS the 3rd ventricle dimension was reduced to 0.99 cm. **f** The following day it went down to 0.69 cm

## Discussion

Hydrocephalus is a common problem after subarachnoid hemorrhage SAH [3]. It is a devastating complication and can occur in up to 30% of patients. Its onset can be acute, within 48 h of SAH or, less frequently chronic, developing weeks or even months after SAH. The pathophysiology is most likely due to acute or chronic obstruction of cerebrospinal fluid (CSF) flow either by clot burden or induced inflammation and arachnoiditis. There are no current guidelines on how to manage or follow these patients in the acute stage and how to prevent the development of chronic symptomatic hydrocephalus. CT scan is used frequently in the management and monitoring of acute hydrocephalus of SAH as these patients often comatosed or sedated and clinical examination is not the safest method to monitor for hydrocephalus. According to the Food and Drug Administration, there is no amount of radiation that is completely without risk of radiation related cancer [4]. Moreover, transfer from and to intensive care units pose a real problem to medical care staff. Therefore, alternative monitoring strategies should be developed. The role of TCS has evolved as an imaging modality for the brain parenchyma in the setting of multiple pathologies, including movement disorders, parkinsonism and follow up of vasospasm post

SAH using transcranial Doppler [5]. The diagnosis and monitoring for hydrocephalus has been used in young children because of the possibility of using the fontanelle as an acoustic window to the brain. The advantages of TCS in the management of hydrocephalus in adult have not been fully studied to date. But according to sporadic papers, the advantages of using TCS even in adults to follow hydrocephalus could encompass ease of use, low cost, wide acceptance by patients, no radiation risk, high mobility and relative independence from movement artifacts. Specifically, bedside availability and reliability has made critical care intensivists interested to use it with increasing frequency [6].

The accuracy of ultrasound compared to CT scan is not well established in adults and no known large studies confirming or infirming the utility of ultrasound in adults with hydrocephalus. Most of the literature comparing ultrasonography and computed tomography has been done in infants and children because of the natural acoustic windows of the brain through the fontanelles [7–12]. A report in 1984 by Rubenstein describes 19 adult patients the correlation between ultrasound images of the brain obtained post-operatively through a burr-hole and computed tomography [13]. The quality of the image was, however, much inferior to what we are able to see now. Recently, a comparison of the two techniques was performed in 15 brain-injured patients [14]. In 15 patients with brain injury, the 3rd ventricle was 35.5 ± 12 mm using TCS versus 33.1 ± 14 mm with computed tomography with an intraclass correlation of 0.88 and 95% confidence interval of 0.63–0.96, $p < 0.01$. There were no systematic biais using the Bland–Altman plot. In our case, the craniectomy site allowed direct skin dura matter contact which helps clarify more the brain structures and decreases the distance and eliminates artifacts caused by bone. To our knowledge, so far not many case reports and or case series evoked the possibility to use ultrasound instead of CT scan to monitor these patients' hydrocephalus. Recently, a case series was published and showed that TCS using B-sonography mode was effective in decision making regarding removal of external ventricular drainage in patients with post-hemorrhagic malabsorption hydrocephalus with good specificity and sensitivity [15, 16].

This case illustrates the usefulness of hand-held bedside ultrasound for follow-up of patients with subarachnoid hemorrhage as a non-invasive, simple and safe method to monitor for the development of hydrocephalus and may be to guide management.

## Conclusion

Patients with SAH and particular those with a craniotomy can be monitored easily at the bedside with hand-held TCS for the development of hydrocephalus. Further studies with larger number of patients should be performed to evaluate the feasibility, sensitivity and specificity of TCS in the detection of hydrocephalus in adult patients after SAH.

#### Abbreviations

CSF: cerebrospinal fluid; CT: computed tomography; EVD: external ventricular drain; ICP: intracranial pressure; SAH: subarachnoid hemorrhage; TCS: transcranial sonography.

#### Authors' contributions

AN: made substantial contributions to (a)conception and design, (b)acquisition of data, (c)analysis and interpretation of data; involved in drafting the manuscript and revising it critically for important intellectual content. AYD: made substantial contributions to (a)conception and design, (b)acquisition of data, and (c)analysis and interpretation of data; involved in drafting the manuscript and revising it critically for important intellectual content. MWB: made substantial contributions to (a)conception and design, (b)acquisition of data, and (iii)analysis and interpretation of data. All authors read and approved the final manuscript.

#### Author details

[1] Department of Neurosurgery, Centre Hospitalier de l'Université de Montréal, Montreal, QC, Canada. [2] Division of Critical Care, Centre Hospitalier de l'Université de Montréal, Montreal, QC, Canada. [3] Department of Anesthesiology, Montreal Heart Institute, Université de Montréal, 5000 Belanger Street, Montreal, QC H1T 1C8, Canada.

#### References

1. Seidel G, Kaps M, Gerriets T, Hutzelmann A (1995) Evaluation of the ventricular system in adults by transcranial duplex sonography. J Neuroimag 5(2):105–108
2. Couture EJ, Desjardins G, Denault AY (2017) Transcranial doppler monitoring guided by cranial two-dimensional ultrasonography. Can J Anesth 64(8):885–887. doi:10.1007/s12630-017-0898-9
3. Germanwala AV, Huang J, Tamargo RJ (2010) Hydrocephalus after aneurysmal subarachnoid hemorrhage. Neurosurg Clin N Am 21(2):263–270. doi:10.1016/j.nec.2009.10.013
4. Food and Drug Administration (2002) FDA public health notification: reducing radiation risk from computed tomography for pediatric and small adult patients. Pediatr Radiol 32(4):314–316. doi:10.1007/s00247-002-0687-6
5. Caricato A, Pitoni S, Montini L, Bocci MG, Annetta P, Antonelli M (2014) Echography in brain imaging in intensive care unit: state of the art. World J Radiol 6(9):636–642. doi:10.4329/wjr.v6.i9.636
6. Harrer JU, Eyding J, Ritter M, Schminke U, Schulte-Altedorneburg G, Kohrmann M, Nedelmann M, Schlachetzki F (2012) The potential of neurosonography in neurological emergency and intensive care medicine: monitoring of increased intracranial pressure, brain death diagnostics, and cerebral autoregulation- part 2. Ultraschall Med 33(4):320–331. doi:10.1055/s-0031-1299498
7. Rumack CM, Johnson ML (1983) Role of computed tomography and ultrasound in neonatal brain imaging. J Comput Tomogr 7(1):17–29
8. Taylor GA (2001) Sonographic assessment of posthemorrhagic ventricular dilatation. Radiol Clin N Am 39(3):541–551
9. Brouwer MJ, de Vries LS, Pistorius L, Rademaker KJ, Groenendaal F, Benders MJ (2010) Ultrasound measurements of the lateral ventricles in neonates: why, how and when? A systematic review. Acta Paediatr 99(9):1298–1306. doi:10.1111/j.1651-2227.2010.01830.x
10. Jary S, Kmita G, Wroblewska J, Whitelaw A (2012) Quantitative cranial ultrasound prediction of severity of disability in premature infants with post-haemorrhagic ventricular dilatation. Arch Dis Child 97(11):955–959. doi:10.1136/archdischild-2012-301778
11. Deeg KH (2015) Sonographic and doppler sonographic diagnosis of posthemorrhagic hydrocephalus. Ultraschall Med 36(4):318–333. doi:10.1055/s-0034-1398855
12. Benavente-Fernandez I, Lubian-Gutierrez M, Jimenez-Gomez G, Lechuga-Sancho AM, Lubian-Lopez SP, Neonatal Neurology Foundation

(2017) Ultrasound lineal measurements predict ventricular volume in posthaemorrhagic ventricular dilatation in preterm infants. Acta Paediatr 106(2):211–217. doi:10.1111/apa.13645

13. Rubenstein JB, Pasto ME, Rifkin MD, Goldberg BB (1984) Real-time neurosonography of the brain through calvarial defects with computed tomographic correlation. J Ultrasound Med 3(10):443–448
14. Oliveira RA, de Oliveira Lima M, Paiva WS, de Sa Malbouisson LM, Teixeira MJ, Bor-Seng-Shu E (2017) Comparison between brain computed tomography scan and transcranial sonography to evaluate third ventricle width, peri-mesencephalic cistern, and sylvian fissure in traumatic brain-injured patients. Front Neurol 8:44. doi:10.3389/fneur.2017.00044
15. Harrer JU, Tsivgoulis G (2011) Transcranial sonography for monitoring hydrocephalus: an underestimated imaging modality. Neurology 76(10):852–853. doi:10.1212/WNL.0b013e31820f2e8a
16. Kiphuth IC, Huttner HB, Struffert T, Schwab S, Kohrmann M (2011) Sonographic monitoring of ventricle enlargement in posthemorrhagic hydrocephalus. Neurology 76(10):858–862. doi:10.1212/WNL.0b013e31820f2e0f

23

# The Area method: a new method for ultrasound assessment of diaphragmatic movement

Søren Helbo Skaarup[1*], Anders Løkke[1] and Christian B. Laursen[2,3]

**Abstract**

**Background:** Ultrasound can be used to assess diaphragm movement. Existing methods focus on movement at a single point at the hemidiaphragm and may not consider the anatomic and functional complexity. We aimed to develop an ultrasound method, the Area method, to assess movement of the entire hemidiaphragm dome and to compare it with existing methods to evaluate accuracy, inter-rater agreement, and feasibility.

**Methods:** Movement of the diaphragm was evaluated by ultrasonography in 19 healthy subjects and correlated with simultaneously performed spirometry. Two existing methods, the M-mode excursion at the posterior part of diaphragm and the B-mode at the top of the diaphragm, were compared with the Area method. Two independent raters reviewed film clips to analyze inter-rater agreement. Feasibility was tested by novice ultrasound operators.

**Results:** Correlation with expired lung volume was higher with the Area method, 0.88 (95% CI 0.81–0.95), $p < 0.001$, and with the M-mode measurement, 0.84 (95% CI 0.75–0.92), $p < 0.001$, than with the B-mode measurement, 0.71 (95% CI 0.59–0.83), $p < 0.001$. Inter-rater agreement was highest with the Area method, 0.9, $p < 0.001$, and M-mode measurement 0.9, $p < 0.001$, and lower with the B-mode measurement, 0.8, $p < 0.001$. The M-mode measurement could be done in only 20% at the left side. The Area method could be performed in all participants at both hemidiaphragms, and novice operators found it easy to perform.

**Conclusion:** A new method to evaluate diaphragm movement is introduced. Accuracy and inter-rater agreement are high. The Area method is equally feasible at both hemidiaphragms in contrast to existing methods. However, additional studies should include more participants, different types of pulmonary diseases, and investigate the role of patient position to validate the Area method fully.

## Background

The diaphragm is the primary respiratory muscle. It has a complex structure and function. Contraction of the peripheral diaphragm musculature results in a cranio-caudal movement of the central fibrous parts [1]. Decreased diaphragm movement is seen in central neurological diseases, motor neuron diseases, and in traumatic injuries to the phrenic nerve [2, 3]. Pulmonary conditions such as pleural effusion [4], chronic obstructive pulmonary disease (COPD) [5, 6], and interstitial lung diseases [7] also affect diaphragm function. Symptoms of diaphragm dysfunction are often non-specific. Patients may suffer from acute hypercapnic respiratory failure, unexplained dyspnea, prolonged weaning from mechanic ventilation, recurrent pneumonia, or they may be asymptomatic with elevation of the diaphragm as an incidental finding on conventional chest X-ray images [8]. The non-specific nature of symptoms and wide spectrum of causal diseases emphasize the need for a feasible and accurate diagnostic method in diaphragm dysfunction. Ultrasonography can be used to evaluate diaphragm movement, diaphragm thickness, and thickening [9, 10].

Different methods to measure diaphragm movement exist but there is no consensus on choice of method. The

*Correspondence: soeska@gmail.com; soeska@rm.dk
[1] Department of Respiratory Diseases and Allergy, Aarhus University Hospital, Nørrebrogade 44, 8000 Aarhus C, Denmark
Full list of author information is available at the end of the article

most widely used method is the M-mode measurement of diaphragm movement [11–14]. It is easily performed at the right hemidiaphragm but is very often difficult at the left hemidiaphragm [12]. Another method, the B-mode, measures the cranial–caudal movement of the top point of the diaphragm and can be used on both sides [5, 15]. However, problems with methods exist; M-mode has low feasibility at the left hemidiaphragm; for B-mode is accuracy insufficiently studied. Thus, a new method without these limitations is needed.

The aim of this study was to develop a new ultrasound method with high accuracy, inter-rater agreement, and feasibility to measure diaphragm movement at both left and right hemidiaphragms. The new method, the Area method, was compared with existing methods, M-mode and B-mode methods.

## Methods

The study was designed as a prospective, observational study. The first part of the study compared the new method with the two previously described ultrasound methods to assess diaphragm movement, using exhaled air volume as reference test. The second part evaluated agreement between two expert ultrasound operators. The third part examined feasibility of the different methods performed by novice ultrasound operators.

### First part

#### *Participants*

Healthy volunteers were eligible for inclusion after giving oral informed consent. Exclusion criteria were diaphragm dysfunction, any neuromuscular, neurological, or pulmonary disease. Nineteen individuals were enrolled.

#### *Breathing pattern and participant positioning*

Participants were placed in erect position, allowing simultaneous spirometry measurement and ultrasound recording of film clips and images. Participants performed several breathing maneuvers that all were recorded and analyzed. Participants were instructed to inhale and exhale slowly to allow simultaneous ultrasound examination during the entire breathing cycle. Forced exhalation was avoided not to displace the ultrasound transducer. Measurements were performed with different breathing patterns decided by the participants, ranging from maximal inspiration to shallow breathing.

#### *Spirometry measurement*

All participants exhaled through a Vitalograph, Spirotrac (Hamburg, DE) spirometer. The spirometer was calibrated before analysis following manufacturer's instruction. Volume of exhaled air was measured with the spirometer in a "slow vital capacity" modus. In this way, total volume was quantified.

#### *Ultrasound measurement*

A single experienced ultrasound operator performed all ultrasound examinations. All ultrasound examinations were done simultaneously with spirometry recordings of exhaled volume. The ultrasound operator was blinded to spirometry measurement results. Film clips were saved for later analysis. A curvilinear 3–5 MHz probe and a General Electric Vivid S8 (Little Chantfort, UK) ultrasound machine with a standard abdominal preset were used for ultrasound measurements. Analysis of diaphragm movement performed on ultrasound films and images was done blinded to volume of exhaled air measured by spirometry. The following three different methods were performed in all participants.

#### *M-mode measurement*

The M-mode measurement has been described in several studies [11–14]. Right hemidiaphragm was visualized using a subcostal view in the mid-clavicular line with the probe tilted cranially. The liver served as an acoustic window to identify the posterior part of the diaphragm. A M-mode line was placed over the posterior part of the diaphragm with maximal movement, and the excursion was measured in millimeters during breathing (Fig. 1).

#### *B-mode measurement*

The B-mode was performed in accordance with Gethin-Jones et al. [15]. In a mid-axillary view, the cranial top of right hemidiaphragm was visualized. A film clip was saved during respiration, and maximal cranial–caudal movement of the diaphragm top was measured in millimeters (Fig. 2).

#### *Area method*

Changes in the intra-thoracic area during respiration were calculated using the Area method, which is described in detail here. A further instruction on how the Area method is performed is available in the Additional file 1: Video 1 and Additional file 2: Video 2. The same film clip of the respiration as used to in the B-mode measurement, a recording of the diaphragm movement from a mid-axillary lateral view, was used. At the right side, the liver was used as a sonographic landmark to identify the right hemidiaphragm. At the left side, the spleen was the landmark. Scrolling through the film an image frame with maximal diaphragm contraction, corresponding to end-inspiration, was identified. With the ultrasound machine's build-in area-calculation function, the entire visible portion of the diaphragm was traced (Fig. 3). In case of limited view to a part of the

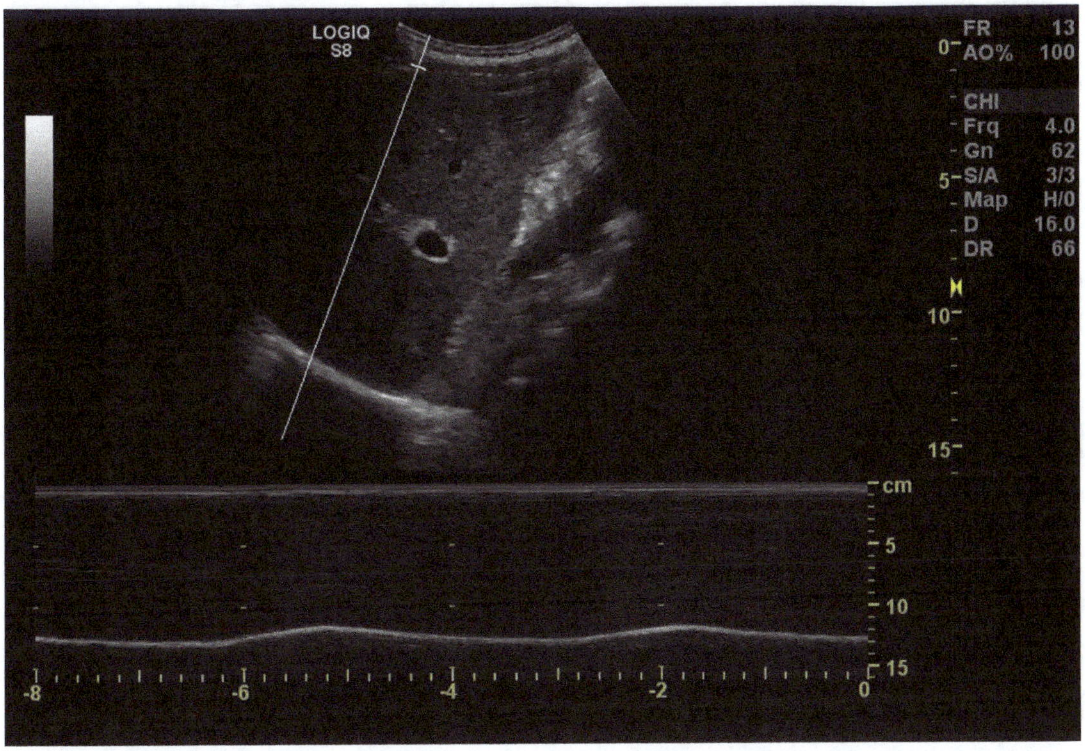


**Fig. 1** Subcostal ultrasound image in mid-clavicular line with M-mode measuring diaphragm excursion

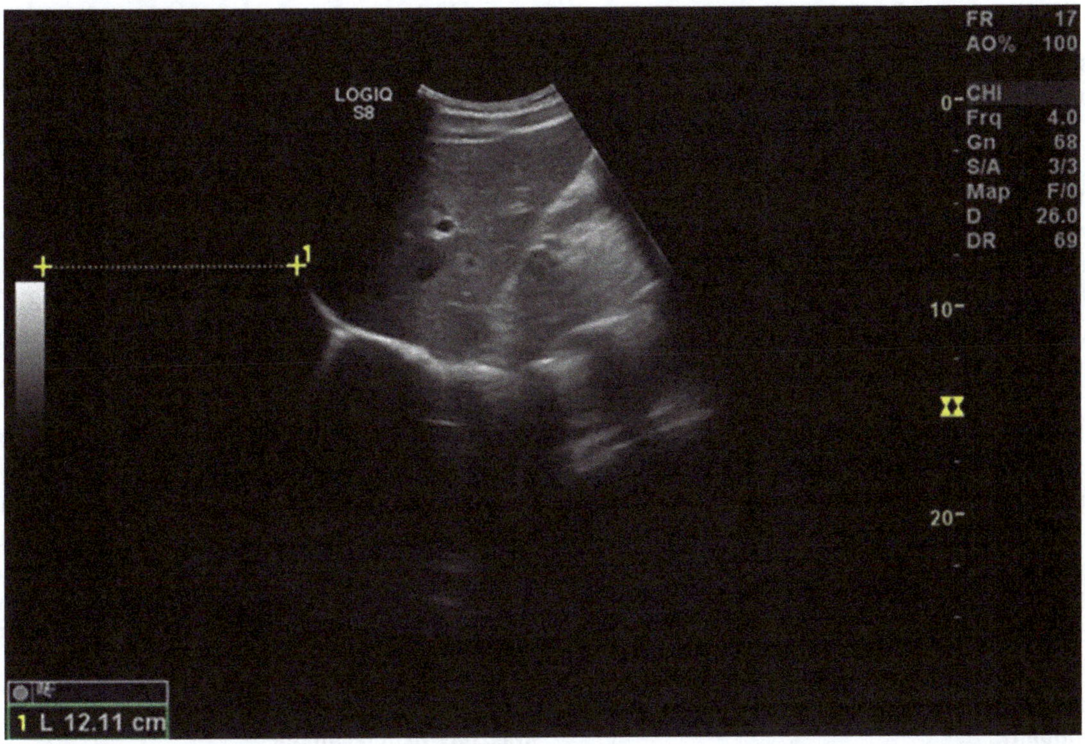


**Fig. 2** Lateral ultrasound view in the mid-axillary line assessing the cranio-caudal diaphragm movement with B-mode using ultrasound machine's inbuilt distance measure function

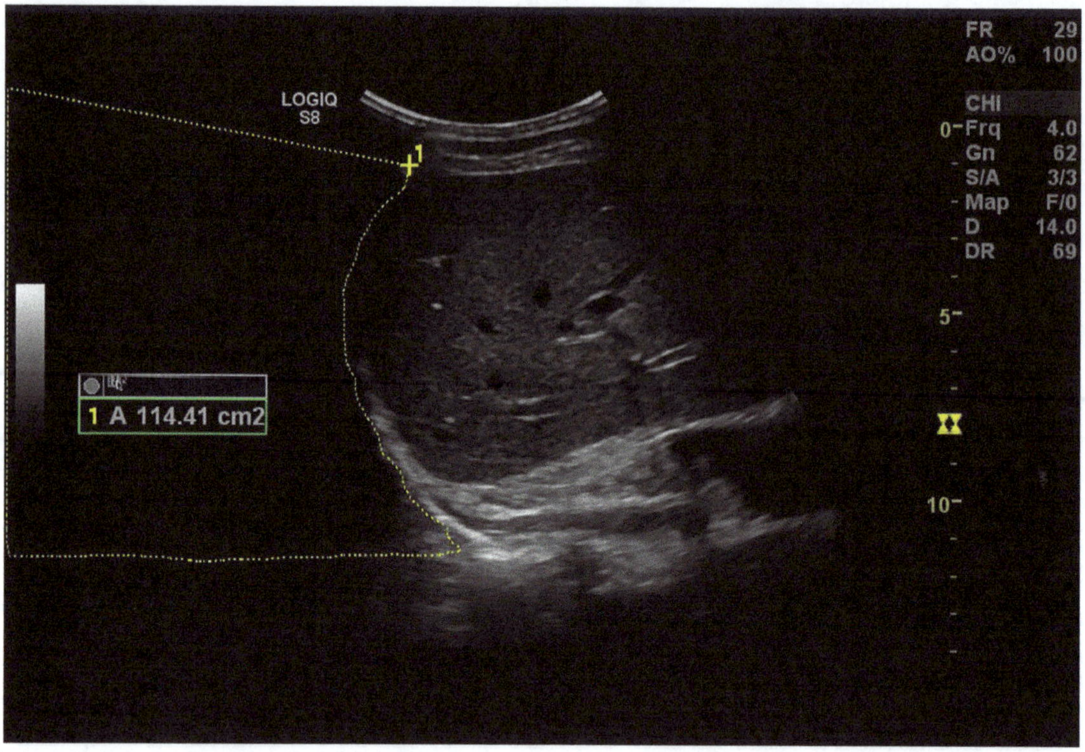


**Fig. 3** Lateral ultrasound view in the mid-axillary line. Diaphragm is identified behind the liver. With the ultrasound machine's inbuilt area function the area over the diaphragm is measured in maximal inspiration

diaphragm, tracing continued the curve obtained from visible parts. The ultrasound transducer was kept in a fixed position during the respiratory maneuver, allowing the borders of the ultrasound image to be used as limits of the area. These limits did not change during the respiratory maneuver. The only change in area was due to the change in position of the diaphragm with respiration. In this manner, the intra-thoracic area was calculated in maximal diaphragm contraction. Then, scrolling through the film, the frame with minimal diaphragm contraction, corresponding to pre-inspiration, was identified. The intra-thoracic area was calculated by tracking the diaphragm in the same way (Fig. 4). Subtraction of the area with maximal diaphragm contraction from the area with minimal diaphragm contraction gave the change in intra-thoracic area during the breathing maneuver: *Δ intra-thoracic area during respiration = intra-thoracic area in maximal diaphragm contraction − intra-thoracic area in minimal diaphragm contraction.*

**Second part**

***Inter-rater variability***

To evaluate the inter-rater variability, two independent observers (SHS, CBL) viewed 40 ultrasound film clips. Observers analyzed film clips and measured diaphragm movement using all three methods. The analysis was blinded to the other observer and blinded to volume of exhaled air.

**Third part**

***Feasibility***

The feasibility to obtain ultrasound images of the diaphragm in the different scanning positions was studied in healthy volunteers. Novice ultrasound operators completed a 1-day course in point-of-care ultrasonography and were introduced to ultrasound examination of the diaphragm in a 1-h practical training session.

***Scanning positions and imaging technique***

The novice operators were asked to produce ultrasound images of both hemidiaphragms needed to make the different measurements. Ultrasound examination of the right and left mid-clavicular lines was performed to do the M-mode measurements. Ultrasound examination of the right and left mid-axillary lines was performed to do the B-mode and Area measurements.

***Measurement technique***

The novice ultrasound operators were asked to do M-mode and Area measurements on stored images or film clips, following instructions of an expert operator. They were asked to rate difficulty of each method on a

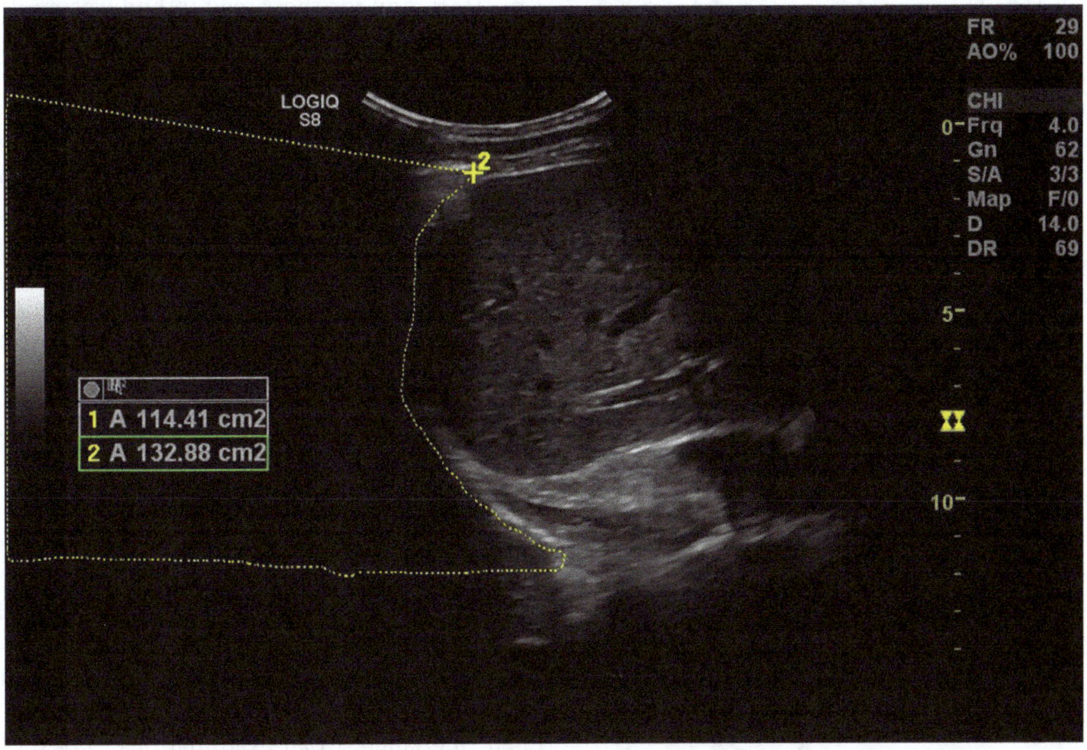


**Fig. 4** Lateral ultrasound view in the mid-axillary line. Diaphragm is identified behind the liver. With the ultrasound machine's inbuilt area function the area over the diaphragm is measured in minimal inspiration

5-point Likert scale, where 1 was given if the measurement was very easy to perform, 2 if it was easy, 3 if it was moderately difficult, 4 if it was difficult, and 5 if it was very difficult to perform.

### Statistics

Statistics were performed using Stata vs.14.2 (StataCorp, TX, USA). For continuous data, quantile–quantile plots were done to assess parametric distribution. Spearman's ranked-order correlation coefficient ($r_s$) was used to analyze associations between non-parametric variables. Agreement between raters was calculated with one-way intra-class correlation. Binominal data were analyzed using exact methods. Estimates are presented with 95% confidence intervals. Significance level was set to equal $p \leq 0.05$. Graphs were made using GraphPad Prism (GraphPad Software, CA, USA). No prior studies could be used to provide data for sample size calculations.

## Results

Nineteen healthy young men and women were included. Mean age was 23 years (SD 1.6). Mean BMI was 23.2 (SD 1.23). All participants completed the planed spirometry and ultrasound measurements; 36.6% were women (see Table 1).

**Table 1 Mean values for volumes of expired air and mean for all three ultrasound methods to measure diaphragm movement**

| | Mean | SD | Minimum | Maximum | *n*, observation |
|---|---|---|---|---|---|
| M-mode, cm | 6.6 | 2.4 | 1.9 | 10.8 | 79 |
| Volume of expired air, l | 4.5 | 2.3 | 0.8 | 8.4 | 79 |
| B-mode, cm | 3.0 | 1.8 | 0.4 | 7.4 | 79 |
| Volume of expired air, l | 3.8 | 2.3 | 0.4 | 7.3 | 79 |
| Area Method, cm$^2$ | 89.8 | 51.0 | 17.0 | 197.0 | 72 |
| Volume of expired air, l | 3.8 | 2.2 | 0.4 | 7.3 | 72 |

### First part: correlation between diaphragm movement and exhalation volumes

All methods showed a significant linear correlation between the movement of the diaphragm and the expired volume. The correlation between expired air volumes and movement of the diaphragm is shown in Figs. 5, 6, and 7. The correlation coefficient for the M-mode measurement was $r_s = 0.84$ (95% CI 0.75–0.92), $p < 0.001$, for the B-mode measurement was $r_s = 0.71$ (95% CI 0.59–0.83),

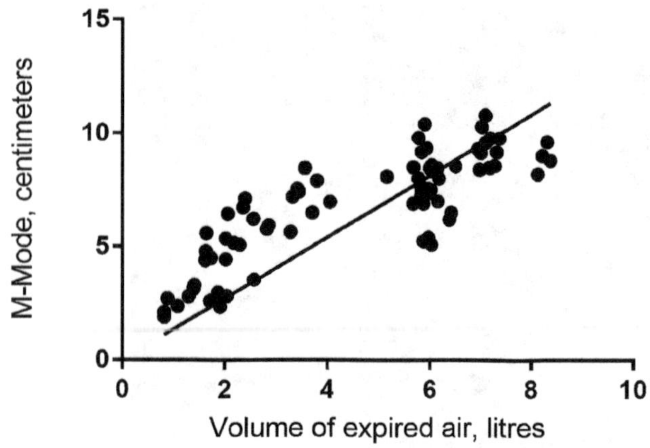


**Fig. 5** Correlation between diaphragm movement with M-mode and volume of expired air

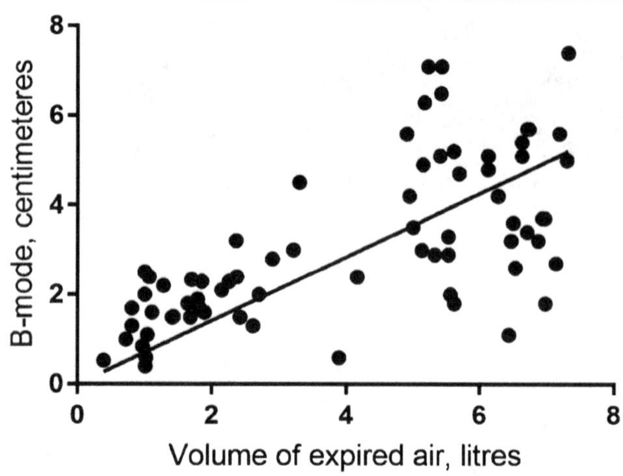


**Fig. 6** Correlation between diaphragm movement with B-mode and volume of expired air

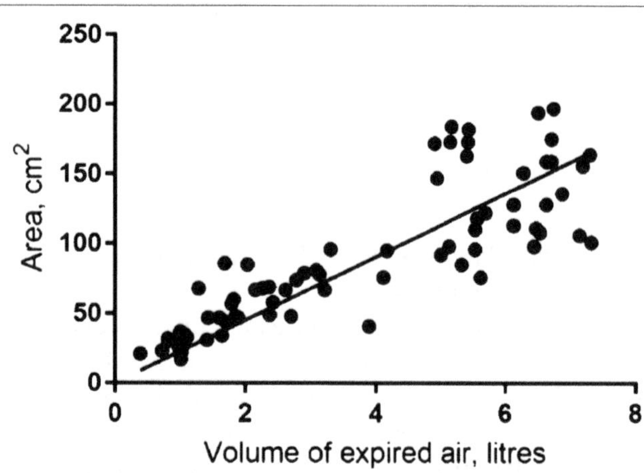


**Fig. 7** Correlation between diaphragm movement with Area measurement and volume of expired air

$p < 0.001$, and for the Area method was $r_s = 0.88$ (95% CI 0.81–0.95), $p < 0.001$.

For each ultrasound method, it is seems as correlation coefficient is different at low and high volumes of expired air (Figs. 5, 6, 7). Air volumes were separated into low and high by the mean value and correlation coefficient calculated. Results are present in Table 2.

**Second part: inter-rater variability**

There was a high inter-rater agreement for the Area method, intra-class correlation $= 0.9$, $p < 0.001$, and for the M-mode measurement, intra-class correlation $= 0.9$, $p < 0.001$. Agreement was lower for the B-mode measurement, intra-class correlation $= 0.8$, $p < 0.001$.

**Third part: feasibility**

Five novice operators performed ultrasound examinations of the diaphragm in three healthy volunteers. They failed to produce an ultrasound image of the left hemidiaphragm in 80% (95% CI 0.44–0.97) of the examinations at the left mid-clavicular line. Conversely, only 10% (95% CI 0–0.45) of the examinations at the right mid-clavicular line failed. In all examinations (95% CI 0.69–1), the diaphragm could be visualized in both the right and left sides from a mid-axillary view. Results for operator's ability to identify the left and right hemidiaphragms are shown in Table 3.

On a 5-point Likert scale, all novice operators rated the difficulty in performing the Area measurement to 2 (easy) and the M-mode to 1 (very easy), $p = 0.003$, mostly due to operator uncertainty to identify the maximal and minimal inspiration at the film clip of the respiratory maneuver.

## Discussion

In the present study, a new method to evaluate diaphragm movement is introduced. Results show that the Area method has high accuracy, inter-rater agreement, and feasibility.

The Area method assesses diaphragm movement in two dimensions: cranio-caudal and posterior–anterior movement. This gives a precise measurement of the complex diaphragmatic movement. M- and B-modes simply analyze movement in one dimension. The B-mode only measures the cranio-caudal movement, and movement of the anterior and posterior parts is not assessed. Likewise, the M-mode exclusively measures movement of the posterior hemidiaphragm toward the transducer. Furthermore, the sample area is small, as the B-mode just measures movement at the top point of the diaphragm and the M-mode measures only a single point at the posterior part.

**Table 2 Correlation coefficients for low and high volumes of expired air and the three ultrasound methods to measure diaphragm movement**

| | Mean | Low volume | | | High volume | | |
|---|---|---|---|---|---|---|---|
| | | Correlation coefficient | 95% CI | *p* value | Correlation coefficient | 95% CI | *p* value |
| M-mode | 4.49 | 0.85 | (0.74–0.96) | <0.01 | 0.43 | (0.17–0.68) | <0.01 |
| Area method | 3.78 | 0.84 | (0.71–0.96) | <0.01 | 0.29 | (0.07–0.64) | 0.11 |
| B-mode | 3.82 | 0.61 | (0.35–0.86) | <0.01 | 0.14 | (−0.19–0.48) | 0.4 |

**Table 3 Feasibility**

| | Mid-clavicular | Mid-axillary | *p* value |
|---|---|---|---|
| Right hemidiaphragm | 90% (0.55–0.99) | 100% (0.69–1) | 0.61 |
| Left hemidiaphragm | 20% (0.03–0.56) | 100% (0.69–1) | >0.001 |

The table shows distribution of useable ultrasound images from the different views. Visualization of the right/left mid-clavicular line is required to do M-mode measurement of the right/left hemidiaphragm. Likewise, visualization of the right/left mid-axillary line was required to do B-mode and Area measurements of the right/left hemidiaphragm. Numbers are given in percentages and 95% CI

We found highly accurate linear correlation with volume of expired air volume for Area and M-mode methods. Correlation was slightly lower for B-mode. Previous studies on M-mode are in line with this result [12, 13, 16, 17]. All three methods are found to be less precise at very high lung volumes probably due to the involvement of secondary respiratory muscles when maximal diaphragm contraction is reached. Correlation between diaphragm movement and volume of exhaled air may be less accurate in patients who have extensive use of secondary respiratory musculature.

Regarding inter-observer agreement, high levels are reported for the M-mode method [12]. Data from the current study confirm this and show similarly high inter-observer agreement for the Area method. B-mode seems to hold a lower inter-observer agreement possible due to obscureness of the diaphragm top caused by the air-filled lung during respiration. This may lower accuracy of B-mode measurement.

Ultrasound images of diaphragm can be made in various ways. M-mode method requires a subcostal mid-clavicular view to the hemidiaphragm, which is easily accomplished through the liver at the right side. A subcostal mid-clavicular view to the left hemidiaphragm, however, is very often obstructed by air–fluid content of the ventricle and hindered by the more posterior location of the spleen making it much more difficult to acquire an ultrasound view of the left hemidiaphragm [12]. This fact raises a question about the level of feasibility for the three different methods. In our study, novice operators could only identify the left hemidiaphragm in an unacceptably low percentage of the mid-clavicular examinations, making M-mode evaluation impossible. In contrast, B-mode and Area method measurements are acquired from a lateral mid-axillary view. Both right and left mid-axillary ultrasound views to the respective hemidiaphragm were highly feasible to novice ultrasound operators in our study. This result may be explained by that, in the lateral mid-axillary view, the spleen and liver function as ultrasound acoustic windows straightforward to the respective hemidiaphragm.

Calculations are easily performed with M-mode and B-mode measurements, as excursion is read with the standard M-mode and caliber function. The Area method requires tracking of the diaphragm dome, and may be more complicated to perform for the operator. Nevertheless, novice ultrasound operators found it easy to perform the calculations in our study.

The Area method presented and tested in this paper is the first step for developing a better ultrasound tool to evaluate diaphragm movement. The Area method quantifies the difference in intra-thoracic area during respiration. While an absolute number of the area in, e.g., maximal inspiration, is not related to any anatomic area, we show that change between inspiration and expiration is physiologically correlated with volume of expired air. The Area method has potential relevant clinical implications as it is just as accurate as the widely used M-mode method and has the advantage of being able to evaluate both hemidiaphragms in contrast to M-mode that is only feasible at the right hemidiaphragm in most cases. Thus, the Area method offers the clinician a highly accurate diagnostic tool to evaluate the complete diaphragm movement, which is not available with the M-mode method.

Some important limitations have to be addressed in additional studies prior to clinical implementation of the Area method. First, larger studies including participants with a range of different pulmonary diseases are warranted since only a limited number of healthy subjects were included in this pilot study. The present results may not be valid in diseases such as emphysema, where hyperinflation causes flattening of the diaphragm and substantial use of secondary respiratory muscles. Second, future studies should also focus on patients on mechanical ventilation since positive pressure ventilation may affect the normal diaphragm movement, and evaluation in such patients is often performed in supine position. In our study, all examinations were done with participants with spontaneous ventilation in the erect position to ease simultaneous spirometry.

## Conclusion

In conclusion, a new method to evaluate diaphragm movement is introduced, tested, and compared to existing methods. Results show that the Area method is accurate, has a high inter-rater agreement, is equally highly feasible at both hemidiaphragms, and is easy to perform, even for novice ultrasound operators. However, future studies should include more participants, different types of pulmonary diseases, and investigate the role of patient position to validate the Area method fully.

## Additional files

**Additional file 1: Video 1.** Video explaining how calculations of the area method is performed.

**Additional file 2: Video 2.** Video showing how ultrasound film clips for area method calculations are obtained.

### Abbreviations

M-mode: Motion mode; B-mode: Brightness mode; MHz: Megahertz.

### Authors' contributions

SHS contributed to ultrasound and spirometry examinations, data analysis, study design, recruitment of participants, and writing of the manuscript. AL contributed to study design, recruitment of participants, and writing of the manuscript. CBL contributed to data analysis and writing of the manuscript. All authors read and approved the final manuscript.

### Author details

[1] Department of Respiratory Diseases and Allergy, Aarhus University Hospital, Nørrebrogade 44, 8000 Aarhus C, Denmark. [2] Department of Respiratory Medicine, Odense University Hospital, Odense, Denmark. [3] Department of Clinical Research, University of Southern Denmark, Odense, Denmark.

### Acknowledgements

Thanks to nurses at the Department of Respiratory Research, Aarhus University Hospital, for their help with spirometry setup.

### References

1. Nadel J, Murray J (2010) Textbook of respiratory medicine, 5th edn. Saunders Elsevier, Philadelphia
2. Lerolle N, Guérot E, Dimassi S et al (2009) Ultrasonographic diagnostic criterion for severe diaphragmatic dysfunction after cardiac surgery. Chest 135:401–407. https://doi.org/10.1378/chest.08-1531
3. Sarwal A, Walker FO, Cartwright MS (2013) Neuromuscular ultrasound for evaluation of the diaphragm. Muscle Nerve 47:319–329. https://doi.org/10.1002/mus.23671
4. Umbrello M, Mistraletti G, Galimberti A et al (2017) Drainage of pleural effusion improves diaphragmatic function in mechanically ventilated patients. Crit Care Resusc 19:64–70
5. Scheibe N, Sosnowski N, Pinkhasik A et al (2015) Sonographic evaluation of diaphragmatic dysfunction in COPD patients. Int J Chron Obstruct Pulmon Dis 10:1925–1930. https://doi.org/10.2147/COPD.S85659
6. Kang HW, Kim TO, Lee BR et al (2011) Influence of diaphragmatic mobility on hypercapnia in patients with chronic obstructive pulmonary disease. J Korean Med Sci 26:1209–1213. https://doi.org/10.3346/jkms.2011.26.9.1209
7. He L, Zhang W, Zhang J et al (2014) Diaphragmatic motion studied by M-mode ultrasonography in combined pulmonary fibrosis and emphysema. Lung 192:553–561. https://doi.org/10.1007/s00408-014-9594-5
8. Dubé B-P, Dres M (2016) Diaphragm dysfunction: diagnostic approaches and management strategies. J Clin Med 5:113. https://doi.org/10.3390/jcm5120113
9. Vivier E, Dessap AM, Dimassi S et al (2012) Diaphragm ultrasonography to estimate the work of breathing during non-invasive ventilation. Intensive Care Med 38:796–803. https://doi.org/10.1007/s00134-012-2547-7
10. Umbrello M, Formenti P, Longhi D et al (2015) Diaphragm ultrasound as indicator of respiratory effort in critically ill patients undergoing assisted mechanical ventilation: a pilot clinical study. Crit Care 19:161. https://doi.org/10.1186/s13054-015-0894-9
11. Parreira F, Machado R, Tomás T, Ribeiro R (2014) A reliable m-mode ultrasound protocol for the assessment of diaphragm motion. Chest 145:463A. https://doi.org/10.1378/chest.1822202
12. Boussuges A, Gole Y, Blanc P (2009) Diaphragmatic motion studied by M-mode ultrasonography. Chest 135:391–400. https://doi.org/10.1378/chest.08-1541
13. Houston JG, Angus RM, Cowan MD et al (1994) Ultrasound assessment of normal hemidiaphragmatic movement: relation to inspiratory volume. Thorax 49:500–503
14. Testa A, Soldati G, Giannuzzi R et al (2011) Ultrasound M-mode assessment of diaphragmatic kinetics by anterior transverse scanning in healthy subjects. Ultrasound Med Biol 37:44–52. https://doi.org/10.1016/j.ultrasmedbio.2010.10.004
15. Gethin-Jones TL, Noble VE, Morse CR (2010) Quantification of diaphragm function using ultrasound: evaluation of a novel technique. Ultrasound Med Biol 36:1965–1969. https://doi.org/10.1016/j.ultrasmedbio.2010.08.003
16. Cohen E, Mier A, Heywood P et al (1994) Excursion-volume relation of the right hemidiaphragm measured by ultrasonography and respiratory airflow measurements. Thorax 49:885–889
17. Epelman MM, Navarro OM, Daneman A, Miller SF (2005) M-mode sonography of diaphragmatic motion: description of technique and experience in 278 pediatric patients. Pediatr Radiol 35:661–667. https://doi.org/10.1007/s00247-005-1433-7

# 24

# Thoracic ultrasound evaluation and B-type natriuretic peptide value in elective cesarean section under spinal anesthesia

Luigi Vetrugno[1,2*], Teresa Dogareschi[2], Rossella Sassanelli[1], Daniele Orso[1], Ludmilla Seremet[3], Lisa Mattuzzi[1], Sara Scapol[1], Alessandra Spasiano[2], Angelo Cagnacci[4] and Tiziana Bove[1,2]

**Abstract**

**Background:** Pregnancy-induced changes in cardiovascular status make women more susceptible to pulmonary edema. During cesarean section, to counterbalance the effect of hypotension caused by spinal anesthesia, anesthesiologists must choose between two fundamental approaches to maintain the hemodynamic state—intravenous fluids or vasopressors—and this choice will depend upon their particular opinions and experience. We aim to assess for any correlations between thoracic ultrasound A- and B-line artifacts, brain natriuretic peptide (BNP) levels, and the amount of intraoperative fluids administered.

**Results:** From December 2016 to August 2018, at the University-Hospital of Udine, we enrolled 80 consecutive pregnant women undergoing cesarean section. We observed a statistically significant difference in the volume of fluids administered in the first 24 h ($p = 0.035$) between the patients presenting B-lines in at least one basal area of their thoracic ultrasound and patients with no evident B-lines (AUC 66.4%; IC 0.49–0.83). Dividing the population on whether their BNP levels were higher or less than 20 pg/mL, no statistically significant difference was revealed with regard to fluids administered in the first 24 h ($p = 0.537$).

**Conclusions:** Thoracic ultrasound is a non-invasive and easy-to-use tool for detecting fluid intolerance in pregnant women undergoing cesarean section. BNP levels were slow to rise following the cesarean section and did not show any clear correlation with fluid volumes administered.

**Keywords:** Thoracic ultrasound, Cesarean section, B-type natriuretic peptide

## Background

In the obstetric population, thoracic ultrasound (TUS) assessment and monitoring is a feasible and helpful diagnostic tool [1]. Importantly, in obstetric patients, the ultrasound exam is safe. The accuracy of TUS in revealing deviations from a healthy profile in pregnant women is very high: i.e., A-lines (indicative of an ordinary pattern), B-lines (indicative of an abnormal pattern), C-profiles (consolidation), A-lines without sliding (pneumothorax), etc. [2]. Furthermore, TUS expertise is easily attained following a concise training course for physicians and non-physicians alike [3]. In women with preeclampsia, pulmonary edema is associated with the appearance of B-lines, i.e., interstitial syndrome [4, 5]. Pregnancy causes an increase in the interstitial water compartment in multiple parts of the body, including the lungs [6, 7]. However, until now, despite the excellent diagnostic performance highlighted by the literature, TUS has never been used to evaluate this type of modification in pregnant women. During the cesarean section procedure, to counterbalance the effect of spinal anesthesia-induced hypotension, and depending on the knowledge and opinions of the individual anesthesiologist, the

*Correspondence: luigi.vetrugno@asuiud.sanita.fvg.it
[1] Anesthesia and Intensive Care Clinic, Department of Medicine, University of Udine, Via Colugna 50, 33100 Udine, Italy
Full list of author information is available at the end of the article

following hemodynamic strategies can be adopted: one based principally on the fluid administration and the other one addressed to vasopressor management [8–10]. In the present study, we hypothesized that changes in the TUS pattern and brain natriuretic peptide (BNP) level—a marker of congestive circulatory failure—could provide markers of fluid overload [11–13]. The aim of the present study was, therefore, to investigate whether a relationship exists between TUS, BNP, and the volume of intraoperative fluids administered (in the 24 h after cesarean section).

## Methods

This observational, single-center, retrospective study was carried out at the University-Hospital of Udine (Italy)—a level-3 maternity center performing approximately 300 cesarean sections per year. Ethical approval was provided by the Regional Ethics Committee of Friuli-Venezia-Giulia on 5th February 2019, ID #2637, for principal investigators Dr. V.L. and Dr. T.D.

Before performing the statistical analysis, the trial was registered at clinicaltrials.gov with NCT number 03851679 on 20th February 2019. Given the retrospective design of the present study, patient consent was waived, but the European Privacy Regulation 2016/679 on General Data Protection Regulation (GDPR) was respected. Only pregnant women aged 18 years or over undergoing elective cesarean section in the absence of hypertensive disorders at gestational age no less than 37 weeks were included in the study; all women presented a physical status of 2 according to the American Society of Anesthesiologists classification system. Exclusion criteria were: emergent cesarean section, a history of pre-existing respiratory or cardiac disease, twin pregnancy; refusal to participate in the study.

In the operating theater, non-invasive standard monitoring with heart rate, non-invasive arterial pressure, and peripheral oxygen saturation were used (Philips, IntelliVue MX 700, Milano, Italy). For subarachnoid anesthesia, the patient was placed on their left side and a 25 G Sprotte needle (Pajunk Sprotte 25G × 90 mm, Geisingen, Germany) inserted by the resident physician or the consultant anesthesiologist following a failed first attempt. Following cephalorachidian fluid spread, 2 mL hyperbaric bupivacaine 0.5% (10 mg in total) (Bupivacaine Fresenius Kabi 5 mg/mL, Verona, Italy) plus 0.1 mg morphine (Morfina Cloridrato 10 mg/1 mL Monico, Venezia, Italy), as long-term analgesia, were injected. Immediately afterward, the patient was returned to the supine position, and the uterus pushed to the left. Arterial hypotension was controlled using a 3 mL/kg fluid challenge of crystalloids (RA Baxter Viaflo 1000 mL, Monselice-Padua, Italy) or an ephedrine bolus (ephedrine 3 mg/mL, 10 mL Aguettant, Venezia, Italy). A bladder catheter was placed in the ward before coming into the theater. The surgeon then performed a Pfannenstiel skin incision with the layered opening of the abdomen and celiotomy. The bladder–uterine fold was opened and the bladder detached at the bottom. A transverse incision was made on the lower uterine segment and the uterine breach opened by digital divulsion followed by fetal extraction [14].

Patient venous access was obtained before entering the operating theater, and a blood sample taken for the first BNP dosage (*T0*). Postoperative BNP was measured at 6 (*T1*) and 24 h (*T2*) after surgery. Blood was collected in EDTA and lithium heparin vacutainer tubes, and sent immediately for analysis to the laboratory (through a specialized internal transport service) where BNP concentrations were assayed using a Bayer ADVIA Centaur-TM. Test values were not known in real-time, and the physician and patients were blind to their results.

Thoracic ultrasound was performed in a semi-recumbent position using a SonoSite machine (S-Fast, Ltd.-Alexander House, Wilbury Way, Hitchin, Herts, SG4 OAP, UK) with a convex or linear probe and the "eight-region technique" as defined by the "International Consensus Conference on Lung Ultrasound" [15]. The probe was placed perpendicular to the ribs to visualize the "bat sign", then translated into the oblique position along the intercostal spaces. A healthy lung was described as "A-Line with sliding"; an abnormal lung was described as "A-Line without sliding" (A'); a "B-Line" lung was one with three or more B-Lines per region; a coalescent B-Line was considered a "white lung"; and a "C-profile," i.e., consolidated parenchyma and anechoic space, indicated pleural effusion [15]. The exam was performed at *T0* (before cesarean section, immediately after obtaining the first BNP sample), at *T1* (6 h after cesarean section), and *T2* (24 h after surgery).

The perioperative data collected also included details regarding the duration of surgery; the spinal thermal level at discharge from the operating room, blood loss (mL); intraoperative diuresis (mL); and administered crystalloids (mL). Follow-up was planned until discharge.

The quantitative variables are presented as means and standard or median deviations plus the range according to their distribution. Qualitative variables are expressed as absolute and relative frequencies. The relative frequency and 95% confidence interval of patients with an altered TUS pattern is also shown. The quantitative variables of the positive TUS and negative TUS group are compared using the Mann–Whitney non-parametric test for independent samples, taking into account the distribution of the variables. The Chi-square test is used to estimate the association between qualitative variables. We also assessed the distribution of the relative increase in BNP ([logBNP2 − logBNP1]/BNP1) at the different time points (*T0*, *T1*, and *T2*) and applied ANOVA to assess for any statistically significant differences between the three groups. We used Hommel's method to correct for multiplicity [16].

All statistical analyses were carried out using SPSS Statistical Package version 22 (Armonk, NY: IBM Corp) and R-Cran ver. 3.4.2 language and environment for statistical computing (R Core Team; R Foundation for Statistical Computing, Vienna, Austria, http://www.R-project.org).

Our study was an observational retrospective study that intends to estimate the relative frequency of pregnant women with an elective cesarean section presenting sub-clinical changes in the TUS pattern in the peripartum period. Data of a total of approximately 80 patients were available. Having no previous information on the prevalence of pregnant women with elective cesarean section presenting sub-clinical changes in the TUS picture in the peripartum period and assuming that this prevalence settled at around 50% (cases with maximum variability), 80 patients would allow us to obtain an estimate of this prevalence with an accuracy of 10%, which for this study was considered acceptable from the clinical point of view.

## Results

From December 2016 to August 2018 at the University-Hospital of Udine, 84 pregnant women were approached to participate in the study. Of these, 80 were enrolled; in the remaining 4 cases, 3 had incomplete data, and in 1 case, the patient asked to leave the measurement after the first TUS evaluation. In all cases, patients underwent a cesarean section under spinal anesthesia. No further missing or lost data were encountered. Considering the sensitivity of TUS for the primary outcome of 50%, this sample size obtained an accuracy of 10%. The study population's characteristics are described in Table 1. Briefly, mean patient age was 34 years, mean BMI 28.5, and mean gestational age 38 weeks with no previous history of cardiac or respiratory disease. During the study period, 240 TUS were performed. The greatest number of actual TUS exams, defined as the presence of at least one basal area presenting three or more B lines (see "Methods" section), was observed 6 h after cesarean section, being observed in 10 patients (12.5%). By analyzing the distribution between the two groups of the sample population (i.e., positive TUS vs. negative TUS) using the Mann–Whitney test, we were able to identify a statistically significant difference in the amount of fluids administered in the first 24 h (740.50; SE 86.63; $p=0.035$) (Fig. 1). A receiver operating curve (ROC) was plotted for a total fluid balance at 24 h greater than 1000 mL and a positive TUS outcome. The best combination of sensitivity and

**Table 1 Descriptive statistics of the sample population (*n* patients = 80)**

| | Mean | St. dev. |
|---|---|---|
| Descriptive features | | |
| Age (years) | 34.10 | 5.71 |
| Gestational age | 38.66 | 0.67 |
| Number of pregnancies | 0.86 | 1.24 |
| Pre-pregnancy weight (kg) | 63.76 | 10.97 |
| Weight at the delivery (kg) | 76.68 | 11.22 |
| BMI pre-pregnancy | 23.70 | 4.43 |
| BMI at term | 28.49 | 4.53 |
| ΔBMI | 20.94 | 8.46 |
| Duration of delivery (min) | 57.60 | 14.73 |
| Max thermic level | 3.99 | 1.00 |
| Thermic level at the discharge | 5.26 | 1.24 |
| Duration of recovery (days) | 3.84 | 0.95 |
| Hemodynamic effects | | |
| Blood loss (mL) | 693.13 | 409.29 |
| Crystalloids (mL) | 1306.88 | 327.22 |
| Ephedrine (mg) | 13.82 | 9.35 |
| Neosynephrine (mcg) | 1.31 | 11.19 |
| Diuresis at 24 h (mL) | 1801.46 | 897.70 |
| Total amount of administered fluids in 24 h (mL) | 2665.94 | 962.41 |
| Total balance mL (mL) | 1478.23 | 1004.12 |

*BMI* body mass index

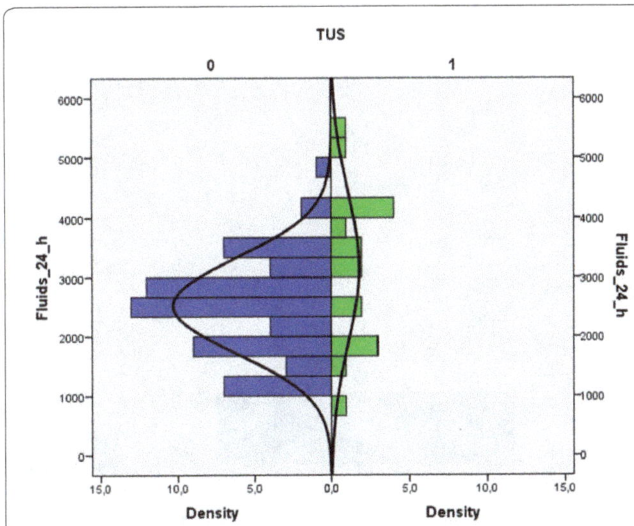


**Fig. 1** Distribution of the amount of fluids administered in the first 24 h after cesarean section, in the study population divided on the presence or absence of at least one area with B lines on thoracic ultrasound

specificity was for > 2500 mL fluids (sensitivity = 67% and specificity = 53%) with an area under the curve (AUC) of 66.4% [SE = 0.09; the 95% confidence interval (95% IC) ranged from 0.49 to 0.83]. We did not observe any correlation between the use of vasopressors and the amount of fluids (Fig. 2). Although the exact duration of each TUS exam was not recorded, in all cases, it required no more than just a few minutes to perform. During the study period, a total of 240 BNP tests were obtained. BNP values show a tendency to increase between time zero (*T0*) and 6 (*T1*) and 24 h (*T2*). As regards the relative increase between the three analysis times (*T0*-*T1*; *T1*-*T2* and *T0*-*T2* h), we found a statistically significant difference between the last two time comparisons (respective p-values: 0.437, 0.045 and 0.007). The BNP comparisons are shown in Fig. 3. When we divided the population based on a BNP value at 24 h (*T2*) greater than 20 pg/mL, we did not observe a statistically significant difference with regards to fluid balance in the first 24 h (Mann–Whitney test: 597.50; SE 93.90; $p = 0.537$). A statistically significant correlation was observed between the median BNP value at the time of delivery and 24 h (Chi-square = 4.09; $df = 1$; $p = 0.04$); while no correlations were observed between BNP and TUS, or between BNP and the volume of fluid administered (Table 2).

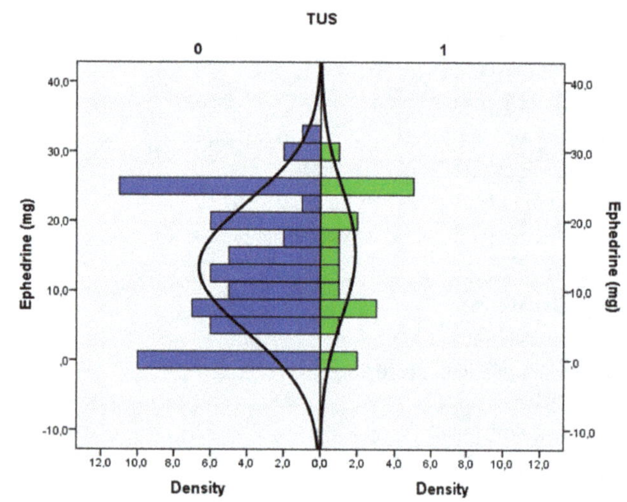


**Fig. 2** Distribution of the amount of ephedrine in the study population divided for the presence or absence of at least one area with B-lines

## Discussion

The main findings of our study are twofold: first, during the perioperative period of the cesarean section with subarachnoid anesthesia, the TUS pattern showed a parabolic representation with maximum expression 6 h after surgery; second, BNP levels followed a linear trend with maximum values at 24 h. Based on these results, the TUS result obtained does seem to correlate with the amount of fluids administered to the patients in the first 24 h. On the contrary, BNP values were seen to increase more gradually over time and did not demonstrate any clear correlation with the volume of fluids administered. These findings suggest that TUS is more sensitive than the BNP value for determining fluid intolerance in the population

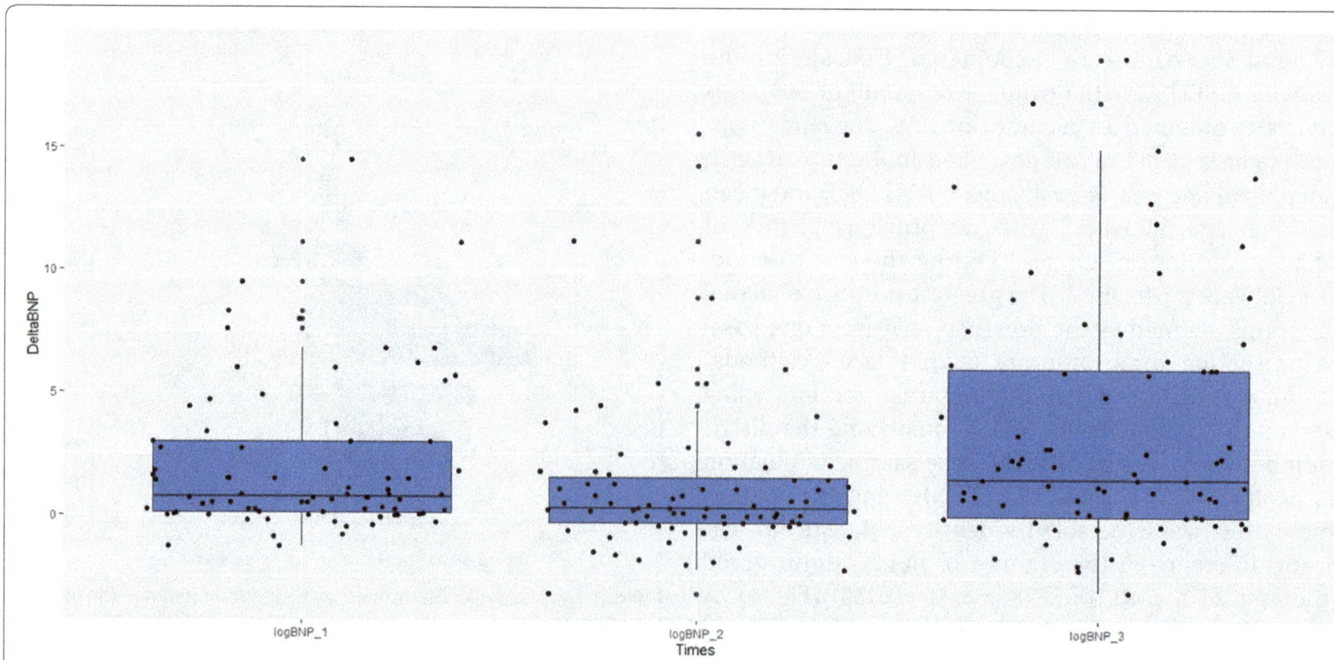


**Fig. 3** Comparison between the relative BNP increases between *T0*–*T6*; *T6*–*T24* and *T0*–*T24*

**Table 2 Correlation (Chi-square values) between BNP, TUS and amount of fluids in the first 24 h**

| | TUS | BNP at time 0 | BNP at 24 h | Fluids > 1000 mL |
|---|---|---|---|---|
| TUS | | 0.22 (*df* = 1; *p* = 0.64) | 0.48 (*df* = 1; *p* = 0.49) | 0.87 (*df* = 1; *p* = 0.35) |
| BNP at time 0 | 0.22 (*df* = 1; *p* = 0.64) | | *4.09 (df = 1; p = 0.04)* | 0.87 (*df* = 1; *p* = 0.35) |
| BNP at 24 h | 0.48 (*df* = 1; *p* = 0.49) | *4.09 (df = 1; p = 0.04)* | | 0.54 (*df* = 1; *p* = 0.46) |
| Fluids > 1000 mL | 0.87 (*df* = 1; *p* = 0.35) | 0.87 (*df* = 1; *p* = 0.35) | 0.54 (*df* = 1; *p* = 0.46) | |

*TUS* thoracic ultrasound, *BNP* brain natriuretic peptide

studied. However, pregnancy is accompanied by many different physiological changes in the metabolic, endocrine, respiratory and hemodynamic systems [6, 7, 17]. As the uterus becomes bigger, it compresses the abdominal vessels and reduces venous return to the heart; cardiac output and blood volume are both increased, and systemic vascular resistance and blood pressure are reduced, while thoracic hydrostatic pressure goes up [18]. Together, these changes can lead to an increase in vascular permeability and induce an interstitial syndrome in the lung that predisposes pregnant women to pulmonary edema, particularly during severe preeclampsia [4, 6, 7, 18].

Neuraxial anesthesia, as used in cesarean section, can induce hypotension by vasodilation, which is usually corrected with fluidic therapy and vasopressors [19]. Furthermore, due to the resolution of spinal anesthesia and fluid redistribution, obstetric patients have a greater risk of fluid overload [20]. Many studies have tried to address the management of hypotension during spinal anesthesia for cesarean section [21–23]. Given the morbidities associated with maternal hypotension, affecting both mother and child, a recent international expert consensus recommended the use of vasopressors to maintain systolic arterial pressure to $\geq$ 90% of baseline [24]. How this may reduce the administration of fluids and, therefore, at least potentially, reduce fluid overload is still a matter of debate. On the one hand, physicians must try to reduce hypotensive episodes, but on the other, the negative effects of excess fluids (especially crystalloids) are well documented [9, 10, 25].

In pregnant women, a different strategy is adopted to monitor fluid management: Burlingame et al. showed that in healthy women the levels of BNP, or its precursor N-terminal-pro-BNP, as well as left atrial and left ventricular volumes all increase within 48 h after partum and are associated with diastolic dysfunction [26]. Ortner et al. found an association between raised BNP levels and echocardiographic markers of impaired systolic and diastolic function with late-onset in severe preeclampsia women [27]. In our study, the kinetics of BNP does not seem to be particularly sensitive in detecting any fluidic overload, even though BNP levels showed an increase in the first 24 h after surgery. On the contrary, a previous study showed TUS to be highly sensitive in its quantification of extravascular lung water in critically ill patients [28].

In a recent observational study, Arbeid et al. demonstrated the efficacy and the feasibility of TUS as a diagnostic tool during pregnancy through their study of 150 parturients between the 36th and the 38th gestational week [29]. This study also showed that the most common ultrasound pattern in pregnant women is the A-profile. On the contrary, Krawczyc et al. reported that lung ultrasound (LUS) was abnormal in at least one region—showing three or more B-lines—in 21% of their population of women during labor [30]. Although this was a small study involving just 24 women with uncomplicated labor, it reminds us that a basal examination is of paramount importance for detecting changes during labor and for being able to identify the correct therapy. Zieleskiewicz et al. first demonstrated that TUS interstitial syndrome in preeclampsia women could be better detected using ultrasound than clinical signs [4] and that the accuracy of TUS in detecting interstitial edema at a pre-clinical stage allowed adequate fluid resuscitation in patients with a high risk of alveolar pulmonary edema [4, 5]. In our study, we provide evidence of a significant correlation between the volume of fluids given during the first 24 h post-cesarean section and the detection of at least one basal lung region showing more than three B lines. Considering the speed at which TUS results are obtained and the fairly good sense that this method demonstrates, TUS could prove to be a handy tool for the early detection of "fluid intolerance" in the post-partum period.

A particular strength of this study lies in the fact that our resident physicians in anesthesia extensively use TUS in the intensive care unit and complete a year-long internal course on its use before moving to the obstetrics department; thus, their proficiency level is particularly high [31]. A weakness, however, comes with the fact that it is a retrospective single-center observational study. This study is the first to show TUS as a potent tool in the detection of lung intolerance [32], paving the way for future opportunities in the application of TUS in the surgical setting. At present, this study does not achieve a very high degree of evidence, and last but not least, we describe B-pattern only in one basal lung zone [33]. Furthermore, we are aware that the correlation between the presence of at least one basal lung region with a B-pattern and the presence of an interstitial syndrome is not so close. Other conditions, such as position atelectasis, or diseases, can mimic this pattern. However, the periodic and sequential evaluations of our patients allowed us to exclude the above conditions in most cases. In any case, since it is a pilot study, further assessment in the same population must be carried out.

## Conclusions

In conclusion, our study shows that TUS abnormalities (B-lines) correlate in the first hours with the volume of fluids given during the perioperative period of cesarean section, whereas BNP levels were slow to increase and did not shown any clear correlation with administered fluid volumes. Thoracic ultrasound is a non-invasive and easy-to-use tool that holds great promise for the detection of fluid intolerance in pregnant women. A multi-center study is now warranted to confirm our results.

#### Abbreviations

TUS: Thoracic ultrasound; BNP: Brain natriuretic peptide; EDTA: Ethylene-diamine-tetra-acetic acid; ANOVA: Analysis of variance; BMI: Body mass index; ROC: Receiver operating characteristic; AUC: Area under the curve; SE: Standard error; IC: Interval of confidence.

#### Acknowledgements

None.

#### Authors' contributions

LV and TD conceptualized and designed the study. LS, RS, LM, and SS collected data, carried out the initial analyses and reviewed and revised the manuscript. DO carried out the initial analyses, drafted the initial manuscript, and reviewed and revised the manuscript. AS and AC reviewed and revised the manuscript. TB coordinated and supervised data collection and critically reviewed the manuscript. All authors read and approved the final manuscript.

#### Author details

[1] Anesthesia and Intensive Care Clinic, Department of Medicine, University of Udine, Via Colugna 50, 33100 Udine, Italy. [2] University-Hospital of S. M. Misericordia, Udine, Italy, 33100, P.le S. Maria della Misericordia n 15, Udine, Italy. [3] Hospital S. Vito al Tagliamento, Pordenone, Italy, Via della Vecchia Ceramica 1, 33170 Pordenone, Italy. [4] Gynecologic and Obstetric, Department of Medicine, University of Udine, Via Colugna 50, 33100 Udine, Italy.

#### References

1. Zieleskiewicz L, Bouvet L, Einav S, Duclos G, Leone M (2018) Diagnostic point-of-care ultrasound: applications in obstetric anaesthesia management. Anaesthesia 73:1265–1279
2. Lee A, Loughrey JPR (2017) The role of ultrasound in obstetric anesthesia. Best Pract Res Clin Anaesth 31:81–90
3. Rouby JJ, Arbelot C (2018) Training for lung ultrasound score measurement in critically ill patients. Am J Respir Crit Care Med. https://doi.org/10.1164/rccm.201802-0227le
4. Zieleskiewicz L, Contargyris C, Brun C, Touret M, Vellin A, Antonini F et al (2014) Lung ultrasound predicts interstitial syndrome and hemodynamic profile in parturients with severe preeclampsia. Anesthesiology 120:906–914
5. Pachman S, Koening S, Meirowitz N (2017) Detecting pulmonary edema in obstetric patients through point-of-care lung ultrasonography. J Obstet Gynec 129:525–529
6. Ouzounian JG, Elkayam U (2012) Physiologic changes of normal pregnancy and delivery. Cardiol Clin 30:317–319
7. Haemodynamic changes during labour (2017) continuous minimally invasive monitoring in 20 healthy parturients. Int J Obstet Anesth 31:74–83
8. Chooi C, Cox JJ, Lumb RS et al (2017) Techniques for preventing hypotension during spinal anaesthesia for cesarean section. Cochrane Database Syst Rev 8:CD002251
9. Chappell D, Jacob M, Hofmann-Kiefer K, Conzen P, Rehm M (2008) A rational approach to perioperative fluid management. Anesthesiology 109:723–740
10. Della Rocca G, Vetrugno L, Tripi G, Deana C, Barbariol F, Pompei L (2014) Liberal of restricted fluid administration: are we ready for a proposal of restricted intraoperative approach? BMC Anesthesiol 14:62
11. Burlingame JM, Yamasato K, Ahn HJ, Seto T, Tang WHW (2017) B-type natriuretic peptide and echocardiography reflect volume changes during pregnancy. J Perinat Med 45:577–583
12. Michinori M, Masato Y, Kaname U (2017) Factor influencing brain natriuretic peptide levels in healthy pregnant women. Int J Cardiol 228:749–753
13. Kumary M, Tang WH, Maroo AP (2014) Natriuretic peptide testing in high-risk pregnancy: a prevalence opportunity? Curr Heart Fail Resp 11:471–474
14. Stark M, Finkel AR (1994) Comparison between the Joel-Cohen and Pfannenstiel incisions in cesarean section. Eur J Obstet Gynecol Reprod Biol 53:121–122
15. Volpicelli G, Elbarbary M, Blaivas M et al (2012) International evidence-based recommendations for point-of-care lung ultrasound. Intensive Care Med 38:577–591
16. Vickerstaff V, Omar RZ, Ambler G (2019) Methods to adjust for multiple comparisons in the analysis and sample size calculation of randomised controlled trials with multiple primary outcomes. BMC Med Res Methodol 19:129
17. Lee W (1991) Cardiorespiratory alterations during normal pregnancy. Crit Care Clinic 7:763–775
18. Robson SC, Hunter S, Boys RJ, Dunlop W (1989) Serial study of factors influencing changes in cardiac output during human pregnancy. Am J Physiol 256:1060–1065
19. Morgan PJ, Halpern SH, Tarshis J (2001) The effects of increase of central blood volume before spinal anesthesia for cesarean delivery: a qualitative systematic review. Anesth Analg 92:997
20. Cyna AM, Andrew M, Emmett RS, Middleton P, Simmons SW (2006) Techniques for preventing hypotension during spinal anaesthesia for caesarean section. Cochrane Database Syst Rev 18:CD002251
21. Zieleskiewicz L, Noel A, Duclos G et al (2018) Can point-of-care ultrasound predict spinal hypotension during cesarean section? A prospective observational study. Anaesthesia 73:15–22
22. Mercier FJ, Bonnet MP, De la Dorie A et al (2007) Spinal anaesthesia for caesarean section: fluid loading, vasopressors and hypotension. Ann Fr Anesth Reanim 26:688–693
23. Heesen M, Kölhr S, Rossaint R, Straube S (2014) Prophylactic phenylephrine for cesarean section under spinal anaesthesia; a systematic review and meta-analysis. Anaesthesia 69:143–165
24. Kinsella SM, Carvalho B, Dyer RA et al (2018) Consensus Statement Collaborators International consensus statement on the management of hypotension with vasopressors during caesarean section under spinal anaesthesia. Anaesthesia 73(7):1–92
25. Della Rocca G, Vetrugno L (2016) Fluid therapy today: where are we? Turk J Anaesthesiol Reanim 44:233–235
26. Burlingame JM, Yamasato K, Ahn HJ, Seto T, Tang WH (2017) B-type natriuretic peptide and echocardiography reflect volume changes during pregnancy. J Perinat Med 45:577–583
27. Ortner CM, Krishnamoorthy V, Neethling E et al (2019) Point-of-Care Ultrasound Abnormalities in late-onset severe preeclampsia: prevalence and association with serum albumin and brain natriuretic peptide. Anesth Analg 128:1208–1216

28. Volpicelli G, Skuzak S, Boero E et al (2014) Lung ultrasound predicts well extravascular lung water but is limited usefulness in the prediction of wedge pressure. Anesthesiology 121:320–327
29. Arbeid E, Demi A, Brogi E et al (2017) Lung ultrasound pattern is normal during the last gestational weeks: an observational pilot study. Gynecol Obstet Invest 82:398–403
30. Krawczyk P, Jastrzębska A, Sałapa K, Szczeklik W, Andres J (2019) Abnormal lung ultrasound pattern during labor: a prospective cohort pilot study. J Clin Ultrasound 47:261–266
31. Vetrugno L, Volpicelli G, Barbariol F et al (2016) Phantom model and scoring system to assess ability in ultrasound-guided chest drain positioning. Crit Ultrasound J 8:1
32. Vetrugno L, Bove T, Guadagnin G, Orso D, Brussa A, Volpicelli G. Advances in lung ultrasound in critically ill patients. J Emerg Crit Care Med. http://dx.doi.org/10.21037/jeccm.2019.07.03 **(In press)**
33. Lichtenstein DA (2019) Current misconceptions in lung ultrasound: a short guide experts. Chest 156:21–25

# 25

# Eliciting renal tenderness by sonopalpation in diagnosing acute pyelonephritis

Jeremy S. Faust[1*] and James W. Tsung[2]

**Abstract**

Diagnosing acute pyelonephritis relies on the combination of historical, physical, and laboratory findings. Costovertebral angle tenderness is important, although its accuracy is unknown. Point-of-care ultrasound-guided palpation (sonopalpation) may aid clinicians in localizing pain to discrete anatomic structures in cases of suspected acute pyelonephritis lacking classic features. We describe three low-to-moderate pre-test probability cases wherein maximal tenderness was elicited by renal sonopalpation, aiding in the diagnosis of acute pyelonephritis. In a fourth case, absence of renal tenderness to sonopalpation in a patient exhibiting typical acute pyelonephritis features led to an alternate diagnosis. Therefore, renal sonopalpation may be useful in confirming or refuting suspected cases.

**Keywords:** Emergency medicine, Pyelonephritis, Point-of-care ultrasonography, Sonopalpation

## Background

No single finding is diagnostic of acute pyelonephritis. The decision to treat relies on a combination of history, physical examination, and laboratory findings. Establishing the diagnosis in part by eliciting costovertebral angle tenderness is a standard physical examination maneuver, first described in 1884 by American surgeon Murphy [1]. However, little data exist regarding its diagnostic accuracy [2]. Because body habitus of patients can vary greatly, it can be challenging to accurately determine the location of the costovertebral angle. The combination of ultrasound imaging and physical examination to localize pain and correlate it to a specific visualized anatomic structure has been termed "sonopalpation" and may achieve higher diagnostic accuracy than physical examination alone [3].

Point-of-care ultrasound has been shown to aid in source identification in patients with suspected sepsis [4]. However, the role of point-of-care ultrasound in identifying low-to-moderate pre-test probability cases of pyelonephritis has not been investigated. Doing so may lead to more accurate and rapid source identification in potentially septic patients, thereby promoting antibiotic stewardship.

In this study, we describe a series of three patients with acute pyelonephritis where costovertebral angle tenderness was equivocal, but sonopalpation definitively localized maximal pain and tenderness to the kidneys. In a fourth patient in which acute pyelonephritis was initially suspected, nontender kidney sonopalpation eventually led to an alternative diagnosis. In each of these cases, a second sonologist observer independently confirmed the presence or absence of renal tenderness to sonopalpation, with perfect inter-operator agreement.

## Main text

### Case 1

A 21-year-old woman with a past medical history of one uncomplicated urinary tract infection with a pan-sensitive urine culture presented to the emergency department (ED) with 2 days of new right-sided abdominal pain, noting some radiation to back. The patient had two episodes of nonbloody/nonbilious emesis the day before the encounter, but was able to tolerate liquids on day of the visit. The patient denied dysuria or other

*Correspondence: jsfaust@gmail.com
[1] Department of Emergency Medicine, Harvard Medical School, Brigham and Women's Hospital, 10 Vining Street, Neville House, Boston, MA 02115, USA
Full list of author information is available at the end of the article

urinary changes. Vital signs were notable for a temperature of 100.9 °F and a heart rate of 130 bpm. Examination elicited right upper quadrant tenderness and right lateral abdominal tenderness, but no rigidity or rebound tenderness. The patient was nontender elsewhere, including the suprapubic region. While performing a right upper quadrant point-of-care ultrasound to assess for biliary pathology, a negative sonographic Murphy sign was noted, while maximal tenderness was found directly over the ipsilateral kidney, in all orientations [5]. Tenderness increased with increasing pressure applied by the ultrasound probe. There were no other notable kidney abnormalities and the immediately adjacent areas were nontender to sonopalpation. Subsequent urinalysis testing was remarkable for nitrites and leukocyte esterase. The patient was successfully treated as an outpatient with cephalexin. At one month follow-up, the patient reported resolution of symptoms after the antibiotic course.

**Case 2**

A 19-year-old female with a history of recurrent but uncomplicated urinary tract infections presented to the ED with dysuria for 3–4 days and bilateral flank, back, and lateral abdominal pain, worse on the left. The patient noted nausea and one episode of vomiting at home. In the ED, the patient had normal vital signs but was uncomfortable and unable to tolerate oral pain medications. On physical examination, the patient was tender to palpation in the left mid-lateral abdomen, left lower back, and left costovertebral region. Point-of-care ultrasound delineated these non-specific findings and demonstrated maximal tenderness with direct sonopalpation over the left kidney (which demonstrated no hydronephrosis.) The patient was subsequently admitted for intravenous ceftriaxone, fluids, antiemetics, and pain control. Urinalysis revealed large leukocytes and a urine culture grew ampicillin-resistant but otherwise pan-sensitive *Escherichia coli*. Blood testing revealed no electrolyte abnormalities or leukocytosis, though an 80% neutrophil predominance was noted. A non-contrast computed tomography of the abdomen revealed no renal stones or perinephric stranding. A radiology suite ultrasound showed no hydronephrosis. The patient improved with antibiotic treatment and was discharged without complication on the 2nd day of hospitalization.

**Case 3**

A 37-year-old woman with no past medical history presented to the ED with a chief complaint of headache, body pain, and minimal dark vaginal discharge. In triage, she was febrile to 102.8 °F and tachycardic to 138 beats per minute and thus triggered a sepsis alert. She denied dysuria or pelvic pain. She also denied symptoms consistent with upper respiratory infections or gastrointestinal infections. She exhibited no altered mental status, neck pain, stiffness, or rash. On review of symptoms, she complained of mild right mid back pain. Her examination was unremarkable, including a normal pelvic examination. While she denied oliguria, the patient was initially unable to provide urine. A chest X-ray was normal. Initial lactate was normal at 1.8 mmol/L. Given no clear source of infection, imipenem-cilastatin was ordered. However, before the antibiotic was administered, a point-of-care ultrasound was performed demonstrating unequivocal and maximal tenderness to the right kidney on sonopalpation. At this point, the patient was able to produce a small amount of urine, and point-of-care urinalysis demonstrated 3+ blood and small leukocyte esterase. Given this, the diagnosis of pyelonephritis was made and ceftriaxone was administered instead of imipenem–cilastatin. Blood tests resulted as unremarkable, and urine culture and gonorrhea and chlamydia tests results were pending. The patient remained tachycardic in the 110 s for two more hours and her oral temperature improved to 99.8 °F. The patient was admitted to the ED observation unit for further doses of intravenous ceftriaxone where she improved dramatically over the subsequent 12 h and was discharged. She completed a course of oral antibiotics with excellent response. On follow-up, the urine culture grew *E. coli* and gonorrhea and chlamydia tests were negative.

**Case 4**

A 25-year-old obese woman with an intrauterine contraceptive device in place for two years presented to the ED with 7 days of dysuria and "colicky" nonradiating suprapubic pain which worsened one day earlier. She complained of a new fever and lower back pain in the past day, but no other infectious symptoms other than one year of occasional mild white vaginal discharge and trace vaginal spotting associated with the end of her menstruation. She stated a monogamous sexual relationship with no new partners. In triage, her temperature was 100.8 °F with otherwise unremarkable vital signs. On examination, she had moderate suprapubic tenderness. She also had tenderness in the right lower back. Because of obesity, costovertebral angle tenderness could not be definitively established. Subsequent point-of-care ultrasound demonstrated a maximal area of tenderness well inferior to the patient's right kidney, which was relatively superior and medial, in this patient. A bimanual pelvic examination was then performed, demonstrating mild cervical erythema and localized tenderness in the right adnexal region. An endocervical swab was obtained for gonococcal and chlamydia testing. Urinalysis revealed moderate leukocyte esterase. The patient was empirically treated for pelvic inflammatory disease with intramuscular ceftriaxone and oral doxycycline. She was also treated with oral cephalexin in the case of non-pyuric cystitis. The urine culture grew no organisms. The endocervical swab was positive for chlamydia. The patient was notified and advised to notify her partner. No complications were reported on a subsequent unrelated ED visit four months later.

## Discussion/conclusion

Sonopalpation is a well-established concept [3]. Its best-known application is the "sonographic Murphy sign," which has 63% sensitivity and 93.6% specificity for ruling-in acute cholecystitis [6]. Other diverse applications have been described, including pelvic inflammatory disease, appendicitis, sialolithiasis, breast cancer, and musculoskeletal disorders [7–12]. In this study, we describe the discovery of a new application for point-of-care sonopalpation: aiding in the diagnosis of pyelonephritis in cases of low-to-moderate pre-test probability cases that deviate from the classic clinical picture.

In our evaluations, sonopalpation was performed using a curvilinear probe. Renal tenderness was assigned only when a patient reported maximal tenderness to sonopalpation directly over the kidney, in comparison to less tender adjacent areas (negative controls.)

Our first case of acute pyelonephritis was discovered fortuitously while attempting to elicit a sonographic Murphy's sign in a patient with undifferentiated right upper abdominal pain and side pain. The sonographic Murphy sign was absent. However, the point of maximal tenderness was found to be directly over the right kidney. This in conjunction with subsequent urinalysis findings, presence of fever, and tachycardia confirmed the diagnosis of acute pyelonephritis. In the second case, pyelonephritis was suspected when renal sonopalpation was performed, but the patient's tenderness to standard examination techniques did not localize to the usual costovertebral angle area alone. Therefore, the finding of maximal point tenderness over the left kidney eliminated any diagnostic uncertainty. The third case represented the first instance in which point-of-care sonopalpation of the kidneys altered clinical impression resulting in improved antibiotic stewardship. Given recently lower thresholds to utilize broad-spectrum antibiotics for unexplained sepsis in accordance to clinical guidelines, this case may represent an important future use for renal sonopalpation. Our fourth case was the first instance in which non-tender sonopalpation of the kidney in suspected acute pyelonephritis caused us to change our initial diagnostic impression and led to alternate and important findings. This implies that renal sonopalpation may help clinicians reduce diagnostic error in patients whose physical examination may be less reliable, due to body habitus or atypical symptoms.

Taken together, these cases suggest that sonopalpation of the kidney may be a useful and reproducible finding in confirming or refuting the diagnosis of acute pyelonephritis. Kidney sonopalpation may potentially expedite ED care, especially in instances failing to reach an acceptable diagnostic threshold when relying on the tools currently in common use. For example, in the absence of a typical clinical picture combined with equivocal point-of-care urinalysis results (e.g., positive leukocyte esterase only), the resulting post-test probability of these factors may not surpass the treatment threshold for acute pyelonephritis. Positive renal tenderness to sonopalpation may therefore help confirm the diagnosis in such cases. However, these cases represent a very limited experience, and future studies are needed to establish test characteristics and inter-operator agreement of renal sonopalpation for diagnosing acute pyelonephritis as a part of point-of-care renal ultrasound evaluation.

#### Authors' contributions

JF conceived of the project and identified two cases of the four cases, in addition to several others not included in the manuscript. JT reviewed all images for quality and identified two of the four cases, in addition to several others not included in the manuscript. JF and JT wrote the manuscript in tandem and reviewed prior to submission. All authors read and approved the final manuscript.

#### Author details

[1] Department of Emergency Medicine, Harvard Medical School, Brigham and Women's Hospital, 10 Vining Street, Neville House, Boston, MA 02115, USA. [2] Department of Emergency Medicine and Division of Emergency Ultrasound, Icahn School of Medicine, Mount Sinai Hospital, New York, NY, USA.

#### Acknowledgements

Bret Nelson, Daniel Duque, and Jeremy Kim for technical assistance. Melanie Molina for manuscript preparation and editing.

#### References

1. Musana K, Yale SH (2005) John Benjamin Murphy (1857–1916). Clin Med Res 3(2):110–112
2. Eskelinen M, Ikonen J, Lipponen P (1998) Usefulness of history-taking, physical examination and diagnostic scoring in acute renal colic. Eur Urol 34:467–473
3. Riccabona M (2006) Modern pediatric ultrasound: potential applications and clinical significance: a review. Clin Imaging 30(2):77–86
4. Lichtenstein DA (2007) Point-of-care ultrasound: infection control in the intensive care unit. Crit Care Med 35(5 Suppl):S262–S267
5. YouTube. https://youtu.be/ytDLKTGJyBU. Accessed 1 Oct 2016
6. Ralls PW, Halls J, Lapin SA, Quinn MF, Morris UL, Boswell W (1982) Prospective evaluation of the sonographic Murphy sign in suspected acute cholecystitis. J Clin Ultrasound 10(3):113–115
7. Tayal VS, Crean CA, Norton HJ, Schulz CJ, Bacalis KN, Bliss S (2008) Prospective comparative trial of endovaginal sonographic bimanual examination versus traditional digital bimanual examination in nonpregnant women with lower abdominal pain with regard to body mass index classification. J Ultrasound Med 27(8):1171–1177
8. Lewiss RE, Saul T, Goldflam K (2012) Sonographic cervical motion tenderness a sign found in a patient with pelvic inflammatory disease. Crit Ultrasound J 4(1):20
9. Elikashvili I, Tay ET, Tsung JW (2014) The effect of point-of-care ultrasonography on emergency department length of stay and computed tomography utilization in children with suspected appendicitis. Acad Emeg Med 21(2):163–170

10. Patel NJ, Hashemi S, Joshi AS (2014) Sonopalpation: a novel application of ultrasound for detection of submandibular calculi. Otolarngol Head Neck Surg 15(5):770–775
11. Zuna I, Delorme S, Huber S, Danes J, Teubner J, Lorenz A, vanKaick G (1998) A multicenter study of diagnostic criteria in ultrasound mammography. Statistical pitfalls and ways out of the data jungle. Radiologe 38(5):355–363
12. Chang KV, Hung CY, Özçakar L (2015) Medial sesamoid bone avulsion but not plantar fasciitis: ultrasonographic diagnosis using sonopalpation. Pain Physician 18(1):E87–E88

# 26

# The FAST D protocol: a simple method to rule out traumatic vascular injuries of the lower extremities

Miguel Angel Montorfano[1,3*], Lisandro Miguel Montorfano[1], Federico Perez Quirante[1], Federico Rodríguez[1], Leonardo Vera[1] and Luca Neri[2]

**Abstract**

**Background:** The aim of this study is to assess the accuracy of a Fast Doppler protocol for the examination of an injured lower limb, namely 2-Point Fast Doppler (2PFD), in order to rapidly triage arterial lesions after penetrating trauma.

**Methods:** The presence of flow and the aspects of the Doppler waveform of the dorsalis pedis artery (DPA) and posterior tibial artery (PTA) of the injured lower limb (2PFD) were evaluated immediately before the execution of a standardized Color Duplex Doppler (SD) evaluation in 149 limbs of 140 patients with gunshot penetrating injuries. We considered 2PFD normal exams as the ones with triphasic patterns in both the DPA and PTA, and 2PFD pathologic exams as the ones with absent, biphasic, or monophasic flow patterns in the DPA and/or PTA. 2PFD data were then analyzed to assess accuracy variables, using SD results as matching test reference. According to the trauma center standard protocols, SD positive cases underwent also angiography and surgical exploration, whose findings were used to further match the 2PFD specificity.

**Results:** The 2PFD protocol showed a sensitivity of 100%, and a specificity of 100% compared with the SD, in the diagnostic workup of arterial injuries of the lower limbs after penetrating trauma. Furthermore, all the pathologic cases that resulted in all true positives (TP), compared with SD, were confirmed as TP also when matched with the angiography evaluation results.

**Conclusions:** The 2PFD protocol can rapidly identify arterial flow and differentiate between normal and pathologic spectral Doppler analyses in distal arteries. The presence of the normal triphasic flows in DPA and PTA is as sensitive as the standardized Color Doppler Duplex assessment of the entire limb in ruling out arterial lesions in lower-limb penetrating trauma. The absence of flow or the presence of a biphasic or monophasic pathologic flow in DPA and PTA is pathologic and should be always followed by further investigation. 2PFD is faster and easier to perform compared with the SD approach. It could become a new first-line screening technique, both in pre-hospital and hospital critical scenarios, particularly in contexts where advanced diagnostic performance is limited by time concerns or scarce resources.

**Keywords:** Doppler sonography, Critical ultrasound, Point-of-care ultrasound, Vascular injury, Lower extremity, Gunshot wounds, Trauma, FAST

*Correspondence: miguel.montorfano@winfocus.org
[1] Department of Ultrasound, Clemente Álvarez Emergency Hospital, Rosario, Argentina
Full list of author information is available at the end of the article

## Background

Gunshot wounds represent a major public health problem, with rising morbidity, mortality, and healthcare costs in many countries worldwide [1–7]. They are mainly caused by urban violence and account for the majority of penetrating vascular injuries in the civilian population. Many of these injuries are found in the lower limbs [8–10] (Fig. 1).

The primary evaluation and detection of significant vascular injury rests in the physical examination. The presence of the so-called "hard signs" (such as pulsatile external bleeding, expanding hematoma, absent distal pulses, cold/pale limb, palpable thrill, or audible bruit) mandates immediate intervention, particularly when the site of injury is obvious and the patient is hemodynamically unstable.

'Soft signs' of vascular injury (such as peripheral nerve deficit, history of moderate hemorrhage at scene, a reduced but palpable pulse, or an injury in proximity to a major artery) require instead further imaging investigation and observation, particularly when the site of vascular injury is less obvious (high-velocity weapons, multiple fragment injuries, and blunt trauma) and the patient is stable.

In stable patients without hard signs of vascular lesion, angiography of the lower extremities is considered the gold standard imaging method for the diagnosis of vascular injury after trauma. Yet, it is unavailable in certain scenarios, such as trauma scenes, mass casualty situations, and remote places.

Standardized Color Doppler Duplex ultrasound is a noninvasive examination combining B-mode and Doppler ultrasound widely available and can be used to obtain essential information for the diagnosis of these lesions [11–14]. Due to its highest sensitivity for limb artery injuries (Sn 95–97%), SD is presently considered a first-line examination for triaging such injuries, replacing conventional angiography in ruling out significant lesions. Although it may be less sensitive than angiography in the detection of clinically insignificant lesions such as small intimal defects or small vessel occlusions, it is as sensitive in detecting more significant lesions such as major intimal tears, pseudo-aneurysms, arteriovenous fistulas, thrombosis, and major vessel occlusions. SD is also considered highly specific (Sp 95–98%); however, when lesions are detected, angiography is also usually performed before any surgery, to better define the lesion itself and map the entire limb arterial and venous system. Nonetheless, the implementation of this technique on a large scale is limited by the fact that it is time consuming and quite operator-dependent.

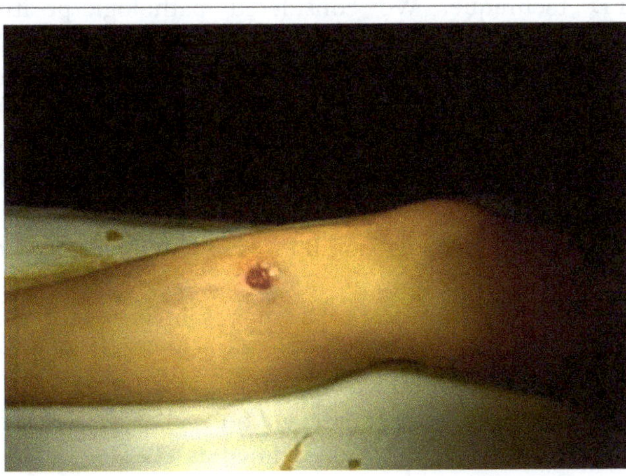

**Fig. 1** Gunshot injury

Point-of-care ultrasound (POCUS) has been used to deliver fast answers to focused life-threatening and/or goal-directed clinical questions. Over the last decade, it has been increasingly used across a large number of specialties and scenarios [15–17], as it can be delivered in a timely and accurate manner, also by nonimaging specialists, with portable and/or more accessible equipment.

To our knowledge, there are no reports in the literature regarding the use of focused Doppler ultrasound to detect vascular injuries after penetrating trauma of the lower extremities. The aim of this study is to assess the accuracy of a rapid Doppler ultrasound evaluation of two distal arteries of the lower limbs, such as TPA and DPA, in order to rule out or rule in vascular injuries after penetrating trauma.

## Methods

From February 2011 to December 2015, a prospective diagnostic test accuracy study was conducted at a level 1 trauma center in Rosario, Santa Fe, Argentina. The ultrasound department has a 4-year ultrasound residency program and performs over twenty-five thousand ultrasounds per year. The internal review board of the hospital approved this study and waived the requirement for informed consent.

All patients who presented with gunshot injuries in the lower limbs were considered for this study, with the exception of all the patients who were hemodynamically unstable and were taken directly to the operating room without further imaging diagnostic workout and those without follow-up.

As per standard of care, in this trauma center, a standardized full Color Doppler Duplex ultrasound of both limbs (SD) is routinely performed to all patients admitted for gunshot wounds of the extremities, who are hemodynamically stable, when there is clinical suspicion of vascular injury. For the purpose of this study, a two-point Doppler assessment of the TPA and DPA (2PFD) was immediately done before performing the SD.

All the studies were performed by two Board-certified medical doctors, specialists in ultrasound and Doppler (MM, VL). The official diagnosis was established in the hospitalization report. Both procedures were never performed by the same attending physician, and they were blinded to the previous results.

A specific data collection form was used. The 2PFD results were compared with the SD outcome data. All pathologic cases (SD+) underwent confirmatory computed tomography angiography or arteriography and went on to further surgical treatment.

**Ultrasound approach**

All Doppler ultrasound studies were performed with a broadband linear array transducer with a frequency range of 5–12 MHz (Toshiba Xario; Tokyo, Japan). Patients were scanned in a supine position. Transverse and longitudinal scans of the vessels were performed. The equipment was set with a depth of 2–3 cm to scan DPA and TPA, and with a depth of 5–6 cm to scan the proximal thigh (femoral artery, superficial femoral artery and deep femoral artery) depending on the body habitus of the patient. Two types of Doppler ultrasound modality were used. First, a color flow Doppler (CFD) imaging that showed the mean flow velocity distribution (displayed as a color-encoded map superimposed on the gray-scale B-mode tissue image), was used to recognize the arteries, both in transverse and longitudinal sections. Then, a spectral Doppler image showing the time-varying flow velocity distribution within a selected sample volume (PWD) was done only in longitudinal sections. To obtain reproducible information from PWD, the velocity scale was set between 10 and 60 cm per second, and a Doppler angle of insonation equal to or less than 60° was used.

According to the newly designed 2PFD protocol, we scanned two specific regions. First, the probe was placed posterior to medial malleolus of the tibia to evaluate the PTA flow (Fig. 2). Second, the probe was placed on the anterior part of the ankle to assess the flow of the DPA (Fig. 3). We considered normal (2PFD−) the presence of triphasic waveform with a narrow spectral width throughout the pulse cycle in both areas (Fig. 4). We defined as pathologic the absence of flow or the presence of biphasic or monophasic waveforms (2PFD+) in at least one of those arteries (Figs. 5, 6).

In the SD examination, we evaluated the entire arterial system of the injured lower limb, including the dorsalis pedis, posterior tibial, fibular, anterior tibial, popliteal, femoral, superficial femoral, deep femoral and iliac arteries.

## Results

Out of all the studied population assessed for gunshot injury at our institution from 2011 to 2015, 140 patients met the inclusion criteria. Out of these, 131 patients had an injury just in one limb and nine patients in both limbs, and thus, both 2PFD and SD examinations were performed over 149 injured lower limbs. Males represented the vast majority of our patient population (95%). Mean age was 27.15 years (STD = 10.64).

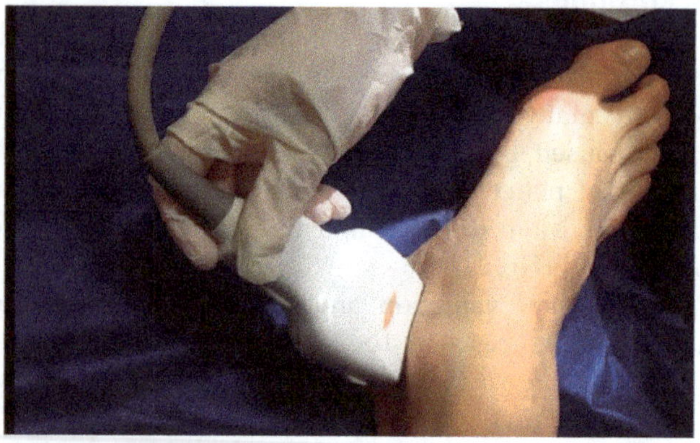

**Fig. 2** Posterior tibial artery scan

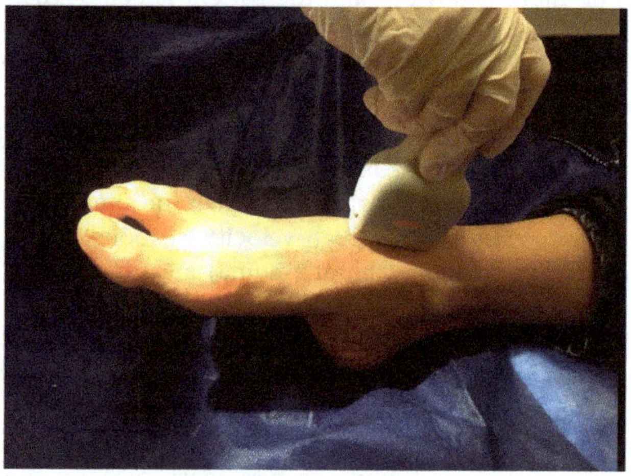

**Fig. 3** Dorsalis pedis artery scan

Injured lower limbs (149) were first screened with the 2PFD technique. We considered pathologic/positive exams (2PFD+), injured limbs with PDA and/or PTA presenting absent, biphasic or monophasic waveforms, and normal/negative exams (2PFD−) those ones with a triphasic flow pattern in both arteries. According to the results, the injured limbs were categorized into two groups: Group A ($n$ = 134 limbs) with nonpathologic results (2PFD−), and group B ($n$ = 15 limbs) with pathologic findings (2PFD+).

Distributions among groups are presented in Table 1.

After the 2PFD, all patients underwent a SD exam of the entire injured limb/s as a matching reference test.

The limbs where 2PFD detected normal triphasic blood flow both in DPA and PTA (defined as P2FD− and categorized as group A), in all cases showed also triphasic

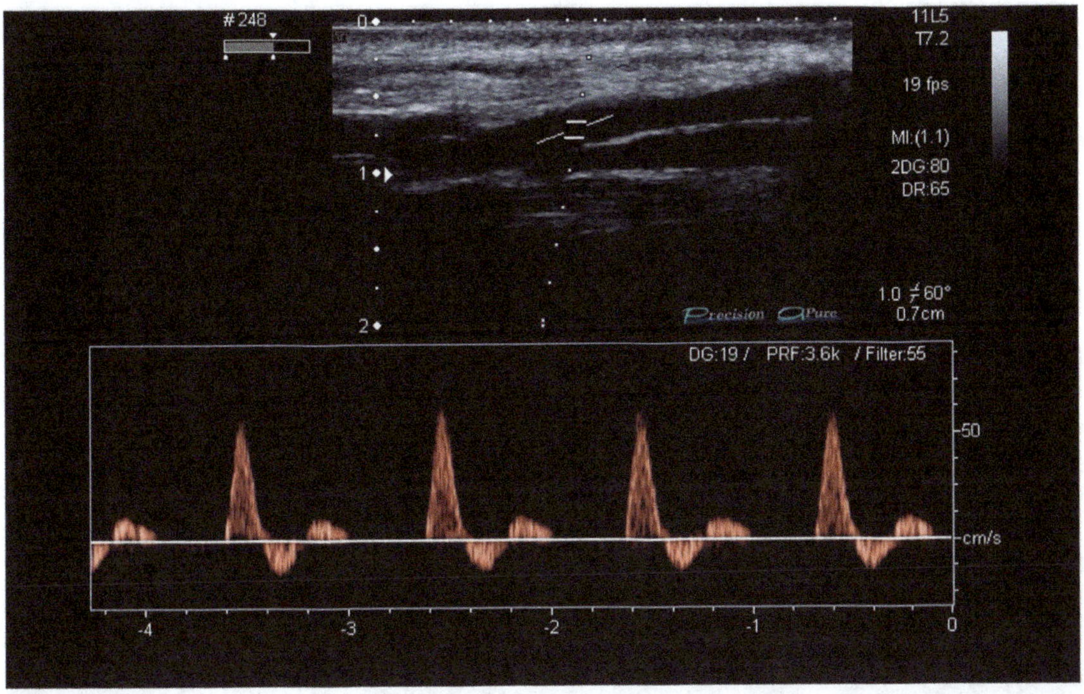


**Fig. 4** Triphasic Duplex waveform

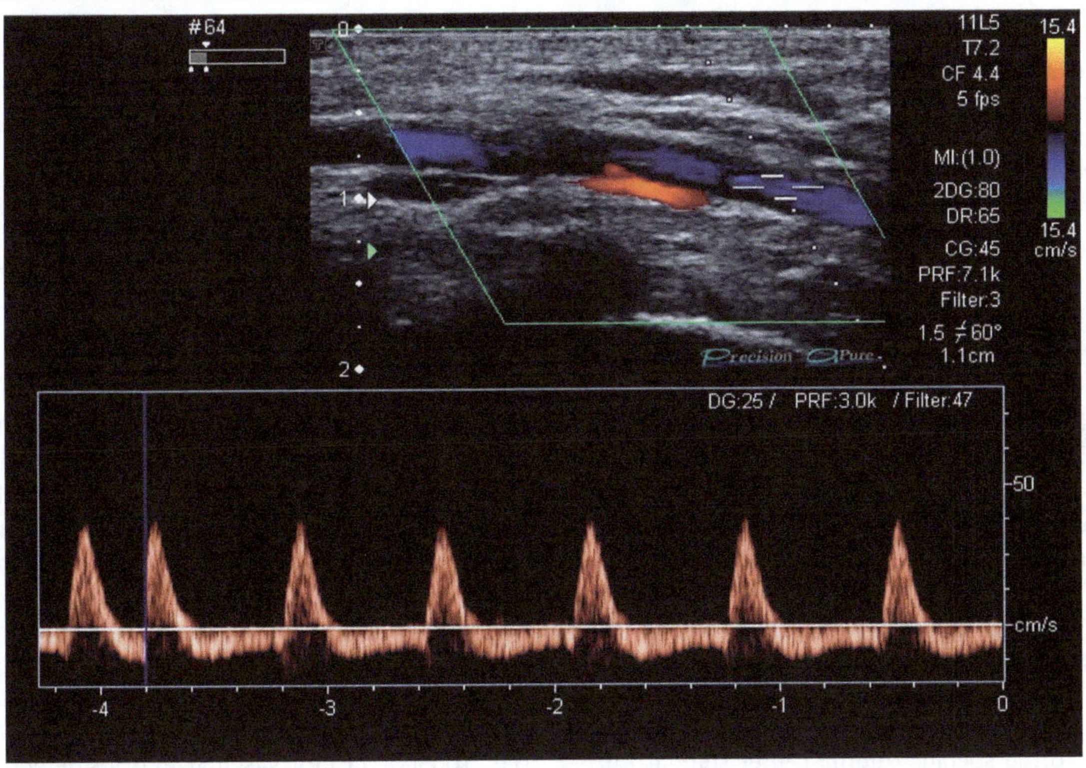


**Fig. 5** Biphasic Duplex waveform

nonpathologic patterns during the SD test. Thus, 100% of the 2PFD− results can be considered True Negatives (TN), matching perfectly with SD− reference results. Moreover, we found that the limbs where 2PFD detected the absence of flow or the presence of biphasic or monophasic flow in the DPA and/or PTA (defined as 2PFD+,

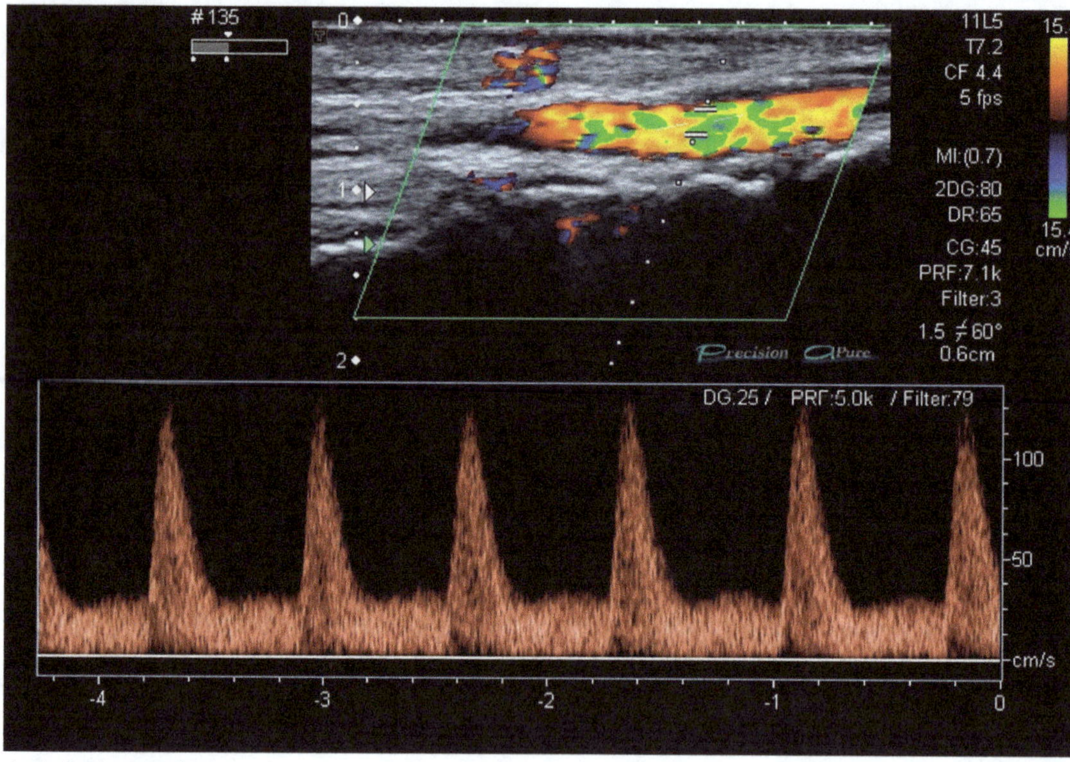


**Fig. 6** Monophasic Duplex waveform

**Table 1 Population distribution**

| | Overall patients, $N = 140$ | Normal, $N = 125$ | Pathologic, $N = 15$ |
|---|---|---|---|
| One-limb injuries | 94% (131) | 93% (116) | 100% (15) |
| Two-limb injuries | 6% (9) | 7% (9) | 0% (0) |
| Sex: male | 95% (133) | 94% (118) | 100% (15) |
| Age (years) | 27.15 (STD = 10.64) | 27.41 (STD = 10.92) | 24.87 (STD = 7.43) |

Numbers after percents are frequencies

*STD* standard deviation

and categorized as group B), showed pathologic findings in all cases during the SD exam (SD+). Then also 100% of the 2PFD+ results have to be considered True Positives (TP), compared with SD+.

Within this specific sample of patients, we thus found that the 2PFD was 100% sensitive and 100% specific, and has 100% positive predicted value, compared with the reference results of the SD technique, respectively, in ruling out and ruling in vascular injuries of the lower limbs after penetrating trauma.

According to the specific trauma center standard protocol, all the 15 SD+ patients/limbs (who were also 2PFD+), were further evaluated by angiographic techniques. Thirteen patients underwent computed tomography angiography and two underwent arteriography. In all cases, these studies confirmed the suspicion of arterial injury, as suggested both by the 2PFD and SD+, so that all the patients underwent surgical intervention. Comprehensive SD and surgical exploration finally reported, out of the 15 patients/limbs, a similar anatomic-pathologic type of diagnosis: 7 pseudo-aneurysms (47%), 5 direct injuries to the artery (33%), 2 arteriovenous fistulas (13%), and 1 artery compressing hematoma (7%). As collateral finding of the study, we can then highlight that using angiography and surgical exploration as reference exams, both 2PFD and SD proved to be 100% specific (i.e., 100% of TP) for vascular injuries detection; furthermore, SD proved to be 100% specific also for the evaluation of the type of injury.

With regard to the general distribution of entrance wounds along the lower limb, out of a total of 156 injuries throughout the 149 legs in 140 patients (seven patients had two gunshots in the same leg), we found 57% on the thigh (*n* 90), 26% on the leg (*n* 41), 7% on the knee (*n* 12), 4% on the inguinal region (*n* 6), 3% on the popliteal region (*n* 4), and 3% in the gluteal region (*n* 3). Further distribution is presented on Table 2. Regarding the specific distribution of entrance wounds among Doppler positive cases, 40% (6) were found on the thigh, 40% (6) on the leg, 13.3% (2) on the popliteal region, and 6.6% (1) in the gluteal region. All the pathologic cases had only one gunshot in the injured leg.

We only found exit wounds in 31% (*n* 49) of cases. Among the patients where we found an exit wound, 47% was through the thigh (*n* 23), 29% was through the lower leg (*n* 14), 8% was through the knee (*n* 4), 2% was through the inguinal region (*n* 1), 4% was through the popliteal region, and 10% were through the gluteal region (*n* 5). Regarding the specific distribution of exit wounds along the limb with positive Doppler exam, only 6.6% (*n* 1) were found in the thigh and 13.3% (*n* 2) in the leg. The rest of the pathologic cases did not have exit wounds.

## Discussion

Gunshot injuries are a substantial cause of vascular damage in the civilian population worldwide. Furthermore, they are associated with high morbidity and mortality [3–7]. Arterial limb injuries can result in extremity amputation or become a life-threatening scenario which demands immediate attention.

Angiography and surgical exploration have been defined in the literature as the gold standard approaches when the clinical suspicion for vascular injury is high [18]. Angiography is sometimes limited in critical scenarios or remote locations. Surgical exploration carries severe limitations as it is very resource dependent, and it is not always widely available for all patients. In catastrophe sites, for example, the physician has to carry out a triage assessment and decide who is in the most-urgent need of transportation to the operating room.

Less-invasive methods such as arterial pressure indexes and standardized Color Doppler Duplex ultrasound can be considered as valuable alternatives for the triage assessment. Burg et al. [19] reported an ankle-brachial index (ABI) of 0.9 or less as a sensitive test for the identification of vascular injury of the lower extremities. However, the palpation of the peripheral pulses can be difficult in some patients due to vasoconstriction, hypovolemia, and pain. SD exam of the extremities allows for diagnosis of vascular lesions with a high sensitivity. Knudson et al. [20] stated that SD exam was equal in sensitivity compared with angiography in detecting vascular injury with the advantage of being noninvasive. The pulsed Doppler spectral analysis recorded from a peripheral lower extremity artery has the feature of a triphasic waveform with a narrow spectral width throughout the pulse cycle, indicating red blood cells moving at a similar speed and direction in a nondisturbed or laminar flow pattern [21]. Any lesion, including arteriovenous fistulas, traumatic thrombotic arterial obstructions, pseudo-aneurisms, or external hematomas compressing the arteries, will impact distal flow, presenting abnormal patterns, such as monophasic, biphasic, or absent flow. Nevertheless, SD has also limitations, as it can be time consuming, and a properly trained radiologist is not always present in the emergency setting to perform the study (e.g.,, peripheral and/or resource-scarce hospitals, extra-hospital, or disaster scenarios).

Point-of-care ultrasound is a novel tool being increasingly used not only by the emergency physician but also by clinicians in several other specialties [15–17]. In the trauma setting, it allows physicians to make faster diagnostic and therapeutic decisions. A large volume of the literature describes how point-of-care ultrasound can be used to diagnose and manage a broad spectrum of conditions in critically ill patients [22–24]. In trauma patients, the evaluation of the extremities using focused ultrasound is limited nowadays to the diagnosis of fractures, soft tissues injuries, and the presence of foreign bodies [25, 26]. Yet, to our knowledge, this is the first report in the literature that describes how to rapidly rule out/in vascular injuries in patients who suffered from penetrating trauma of the lower extremities, by means of a 2-point Doppler technique.

The 2PFD protocol allows physicians to rapidly asses the presence or the absence of flow in two distal arteries of the lower limb, PDA, and PTA. Once this first assessment is done and flow is detected, the physician evaluates the waveform pattern (triphasic or biphasic/monophasic flow). In the absence of vascular injury, the spectral

**Table 2 Entrance wounds distribution**

| | Thigh | Lower leg | Knee | Inguinal region | Popliteal region | Gluteal region |
|---|---|---|---|---|---|---|
| Group A, $N = 141$ | 59% (84) | 25% (35) | 8% (12) | 4% (6) | 2% (2) | 2% (2) |
| Group B, $N = 15$ | 40% (6) | 40% (6) | 0% (0) | 0% (0) | 13% (2) | 7% (1) |
| Total, $N = 156$ | 57% (90) | 26% (41) | 7% (12) | 4%(6) | 3% (4) | 2% (3) |

Numbers after percents are frequencies

Doppler analysis normally shows a triphasic waveform over each cardiac cycle, representing the blood acceleration during systole: an early diastolic flow reversal caused by the closure of the aortic valve; and a late anterograde diastolic flow related with the elasticity of the arterial wall, peripheral resistance, and transmural gradient. In the presence of any kind of vascular damage or external compression (i.e., large hematoma), the physician could find no flow or the presence of either a monophasic or biphasic waveform pattern.

The 2PFD protocol has the advantage of being noninvasive and a rapid test, requiring no more than 2 min and probably easier to learn by nonimaging specialist, although learning curve analysis of this technique is a subject matter of further investigation.

The 2P Fast Doppler imaging technique can present yet some limitations. The absence of flow or a monophasic/biphasic Doppler Duplex pattern in distal arteries can be detected not only in acutely injured arteries, but also as result of chronic conditions, such as proximal diabetic angiopathy, severe atherosclerosis, or aging. This can cause misinterpretation of the results. As the 2PFD cannot differentiate if the pathologic flow is caused by an acute or a chronic lesion in positive cases, further investigation is always required. In our series, there were no diabetic patients, and the average age was 27 years (24.8 among the pathologic cases). Probably for this reason, there were no false positives related to these comorbidities in this study. As such comorbidities are generally related to older patients, the latter ones may represent a targeted population for more thorough examination.

In targeted patient populations, such as the "injured nondiabetic young patients" of our study, due to the low prevalence, or even the absence of concurrent chronic lesions (i.e., low or no false positives for vascular injuries), 2PFD could be used also as a triage tool to "rule in" acute cases with high specificity equal to SD (Sp 100%).

On another note, if the injured artery has no distal extension (i.e., profunda femoris artery = PFA), and there are no hematomas compressing other arteries, there will be no distal repercussion [27]. In this particular case, the FAST Doppler protocol would not show any abnormal distal pattern, leading to potentially false negative results. We did not have any PFA injuries in our study so this limitation did not affect the sensitivity of our findings. To overcome this limitation, when a penetrating injury of the supero-internal part of the thigh is present, further workup may still be warranted, and physicians would have to explore the thigh with point-of-care ultrasound and SD to identify if large hematomas, pseudoaneurysms, or arteriovenous fistulas are present in each particular case [28]. In our hospital, we always explore the region injured by gunshot wounds in order to search not only for vascular lesions but also for bone fractures and soft tissue lesions.

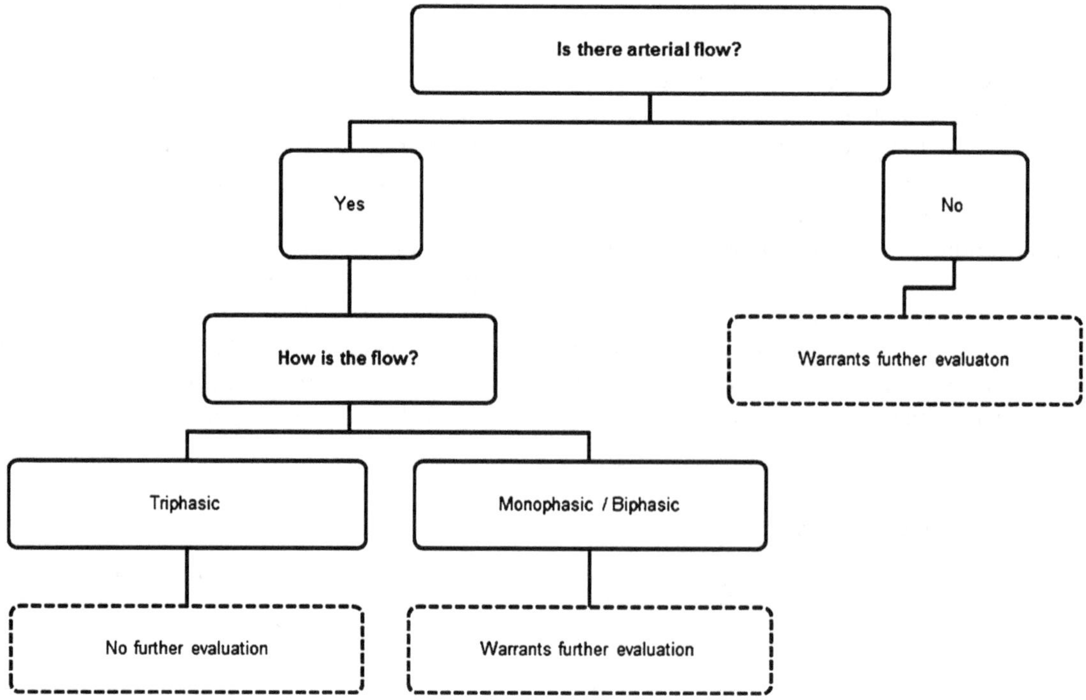


**Fig. 7** Fast D Protocol

In our study population, the 2PFD protocol has proven to be a triage technique as sensitive as SD (Sn 100%). In fact, our data show that the detection of triphasic waveforms can be a highly sensitive method in ruling out vascular injuries of the lower extremities after penetrating trauma.

The absence of flow or the presence of a biphasic or monophasic pathologic flows in PDA and/or PTA must be considered pathologic and should be always followed by further investigation, such as SD, angiography, or surgical exploration, to confirm the proximal lesion, and define its type, extension, and distribution (Fig. 7).

## Conclusions

The 2-PFD protocol is a focused goal-directed Doppler procedure that could be used both in pre-hospital and hospital critical settings, as a triage tool capable to "rule out" arterial injuries in lower-limb penetrating trauma, with the highest sensitivity comparable with standard Doppler examination and angiography.

In particular clusters of patients, where the prevalence of chronic vascular lesions is negligible (e.g., nondiabetic young subjects), this focused technique could be also considered a reliable tool to "rule in" acute lesions with high specificity.

However, as the 2PFD cannot differentiate if the pathologic flow is cause by an acute or a chronic lesion, in positive cases, further immediate investigation and observation is always required.

In the future, if such an accuracy will be confirmed, the 2PFD protocol could become part of a broader FAST Doppler integrated protocol for the primary assessment of the trauma patient, particularly in contexts where the diagnostic and management performance is limited by time concerns (unstable and/or multi-injured patients, mass casualties, combat, or other risky settings) or scarce resources (poor technology and/or competences, and remote/rural/austere settings), enhancing the decision-making process and allowing for better allocation of resources and improved patient care [29].

### Authors' contributions

MAM: main hypothesis, Doppler Ultrasounds, spreadsheet design, data collection, manuscript writing and final review, and providing figures. LMM: data collection, data analysis, manuscript writing, and edition. FPR: data analysis, and manuscript writing. FR: data collection. LV: Doppler Ultrasounds. LN: data analysis, manuscript review and edition, and advisory input. All authors read and approved the final manuscript.


### Author details

[1] Department of Ultrasound, Clemente Álvarez Emergency Hospital, Rosario, Argentina. [2] AREU EMS Public Regional Company, Niguarda Ca' Granda Hospital, Milan, Italy. [3] Present Address: Av. Pellegrini 3205, 2000 Rosario, Santa Fe, Argentina.



### Acknowledgements

Not applicable.


### References


1. Bonnie RJ, Fulco CE, Liverman CT (1999) Reducing the burden of injury: advancing prevention and treatment. National Academy Press, Washington
2. Livingston DH, Lavery RF, Lopreiato MC, Lavery DF, Passannante MR (2014) Unrelenting violence: an analysis of 6,322 gunshot wound patients at a level I trauma center. J Trauma Acute Care Surg 76(1):2–9 **(discussion 9–11)**
3. Thomas MO, Giwa SO, Adekoya-Cole TO (2005) Arterial injuries in civilian practice in Lagos, Nigeria. Niger J Clin Pract. 8(2):65–68
4. Franz RW, Shah KJ, Halaharvi D et al (2011) A 5-year review of management of lower extremity arterial injuries at an urban level I trauma center. J Vasc Surg 53(6):1604–1610
5. Jaha L, Andreevska T, Rudari H, Ademi B, Ismaili-Jaha V (2012) A decade of civilian vascular trauma in Kosovo. World J Emerg Surg 7(1):24
6. Davies MJ, Wells C, Squires PA, Hodgetts TJ, Lecky FE (2012) Civilian firearm injury and death in England and Wales. Emerg Med J 29:10–14
7. Perkins ZB, De'Ath HD, Aylwin C, Brohi K, Walsh M, Tai NR (2012) Epidemiology and outcome of vascular trauma at a British major Trauma Centre. Eur J Vasc Endovasc Surg 44(2):203–209
8. Dorlac WC, DeBakey ME, Holcomb JB (2005) Mortality from isolated civilian penetrating extremity injury. J Trauma 59:217–222
9. Cheek RC, Pope JC, Smith HF, Britt LG, Pate JW (1975) Diagnosis and management of major vascular injuries: a review of 200 operative cases. Am Surg 41:755–760
10. Ockert S, Winkler M, Richter A, Palma P, Post S (2002) Vascular injuries after extremity trauma. ZentralblChir 127:689–693 **(German)**
11. Schwartz M, Weaver F, Yellin A, Ralls P (1993) The utility of color flow Doppler examination in penetrating extremity arterial trauma. Am Surg 59(6):375–378
12. Bergstein JM, Blair JF, Edwards J et al (1992) Pitfalls in the use of color-flow duplex ultrasound for screening of suspected arterial injuries in penetrated extremities. J Trauma 33:395–402
13. Schoder M, Prokof M, Lammer J (2002) Traumatic injuries: imaging and intervention of large arterial trauma. Eur Radiol 12:1617–1631
14. Gaitini D et al (2008) Sonographic evaluation of vascular injuries. J Ultrasound Med 27:95–107
15. Levin DC, Rao VM, Parker L, Frangos AJ (2011) Noncardiac point-of-care ultrasound by non radiologist physicians: how widespread is it? J Am Coll Radiol 8(11):772–775
16. Volpicelli G, Lamorte A, Tullio M et al (2013) Point-of-care multiorgan ultrasonography for the evaluation of undifferentiated hypotension in the emergency department. Intensive Care Med 39(7):1290–1298
17. Dip F1, Nguyen D1, Sasson M1, Menzo EL1, Szomstein S1, Rosenthal R2 (2016) The relationship between intracranial pressure and obesity: an ultrasonographic evaluation of the optic nerve. Surg Endosc 30(6):2321–2325
18. Volgas DA, Stannard JP, Alonso JE (2005) Current orthopaedic treatment of ballistic injuries. Injury 36(3):380–386
19. Burg A, Nachum G, Salai M et al (2009) Treating civilian gunshot wounds to the extremities in a level 1 trauma center: our experience and recommendations. Israel Med Assoc J 11(9):546–551
20. Knudson MM, Lewis FR, Atkinson K, Neuhaus A (1993) The role of duplex ultrasound arterial imaging in patients with penetrating extremity trauma. Arch Surg 128(9):1033–1037 **(discussion 1037–1038)**
21. Hodgkiss-Harlow KD, Bandyk DF (2013) Interpretation of arterial duplex testing of lower-extremity arteries and interventions. Semin Vasc Surg 26(2–3):95–104
22. Volpicelli G (2014) Lung ultrasound for pneumothorax: elementary considerations. Am J Emerg Med 32(12):1545
23. Williams SR, Perera P, Gharahbaghian L (2014) The FAST and E-FAST in 2013: trauma ultrasonography: overview, practical techniques, controversies, and new frontiers. Crit Care Clin 30(1):119–150
24. Blanco P, Aguiar FM, Blaivas M (2015) Rapid Ultrasound in Shock (RUSH) velocity-time integral: a proposal to expand the RUSH protocol. J Ultrasound Med 34(9):1691–1700
25. Blaivas M (2012) Update on point of care ultrasound in the care of the critically ill patient. World J Crit Care Med 1(4):102–105
26. Lyon M, Blaivas M (2003) Evaluation of extremity trauma with sonography. J Ultrasound Med 22(6):625–630

27. Pilson HTP, Halvorson J, Teasdall RD, Eben AC (2012) Missed profunda artery injuries in two patients with penetrating lower extremity trauma: a case report. Injury Extra 43(1):6–8
28. Montorfano MA, Pla F, Vera L, Cardillo O, Geniere Nigra S, Montorfano LM (2017) Point-of-care ultrasound and Doppler ultrasound evaluation of vascular injuries in penetrating and blunt trauma. Crit Ultrasound J 9:5. doi:10.1186/s13089-017-0060-5
29. Neri L, Storti E, Lichtenstein D (2007) Toward an ultrasound curriculum for critical care medicine. Crit Care Med 35(5):290–304

# Correlation of carotid blood flow and corrected carotid flow time with invasive cardiac output measurements

Irene W. Y. Ma[1,2*], Joshua D. Caplin[3], Aftab Azad[1,4], Christina Wilson[1], Michael A. Fifer[3], Aranya Bagchi[5], Andrew S. Liteplo[1] and Vicki E. Noble[1,6]

**Abstract**

**Background:** Non-invasive measures that can accurately estimate cardiac output may help identify volume-responsive patients. This study seeks to compare two non-invasive measures (corrected carotid flow time and carotid blood flow) and their correlations with invasive reference measurements of cardiac output. Consenting adult patients ($n = 51$) at Massachusetts General Hospital cardiac catheterization laboratory undergoing right heart catheterization between February and April 2016 were included. Carotid ultrasound images were obtained concurrently with cardiac output measurements, obtained by the thermodilution method in the absence of severe tricuspid regurgitation and by the Fick oxygen method otherwise. Corrected carotid flow time was calculated as systole time/$\sqrt{}$cycle time. Carotid blood flow was calculated as $\pi \times$ (carotid diameter)$^2$/4 $\times$ velocity time integral $\times$ heart rate. Measurements were obtained using a single carotid waveform and an average of three carotid waveforms for both measures.

**Results:** Single waveform measurements of corrected flow time did not correlate with cardiac output ($\rho = 0.25$, 95% CI −0.03 to 0.49, $p = 0.08$), but an average of three waveforms correlated significantly, although weakly ($\rho = 0.29$, 95% CI 0.02–0.53, $p = 0.046$). Carotid blood flow measurements correlated moderately with cardiac output regardless of if single waveform or an average of three waveforms were used: $\rho = 0.44$, 95% CI 0.18–0.63, $p = 0.004$, and $\rho = 0.41$, 95% CI 0.16–0.62, $p = 0.004$, respectively.

**Conclusions:** Carotid blood flow may be a better marker of cardiac output and less subject to measurements issues than corrected carotid flow time.

**Keywords:** Cardiac output, Carotid ultrasound, Carotid flow time, Carotid blood flow

## Background

To be able to identify patients who are fluid responsive is important in the management of those who are acutely ill. At present, there is no non-invasive method that can reliably and accurately identify fluid responsiveness. As such, in patients with undifferentiated shock, treatment often involves empiric fluid administration, in the hopes that volume expansion will increase preload, which will then serve to increase cardiac output (CO). However, for patients on the flat portion of the Starling curve, aggressive fluid administration results in no appreciable increase in CO and may be detrimental [1–3]. Thus, the ability to identify where each patient is on his/her Starling curve can help identify patients who would benefit from additional fluid (fluid responsive) and those who would not (fluid unresponsive). Unfortunately, traditional measures of preload such as central venous pressure have not consistently been shown to be helpful in identifying volume responsiveness [4, 5]. The use of pulse pressure variation shows promise in ventilated patients, but requires the insertion of an arterial line [5]. As such, there remains a pressing need to be able to identify fluid responsiveness non-invasively at the bedside.

Fluid responsiveness is typically defined as an increase in CO by 10–15% in response to fluid administration [6].

*Correspondence: ima@ucalgary.ca
[2] Division of General Internal Medicine, Department of Medicine, University of Calgary, 3330 Hospital Dr NW, Calgary, AB T2N 4N1, Canada
Full list of author information is available at the end of the article

To avoid excess fluid administration, an increase of CO in response to maneuvers such as the passive leg raise (PLR) is considered indicative of fluid responsiveness [7]. PLR is typically performed with the patient either in the supine or semirecumbent position, followed by repeat measurements with the patient's legs passively raised at 30–45° [7]. This maneuver is considered to result in an auto-bolus of fluid of approximately 300 mL in volume [8]. The benefit of the PLR is that its hemodynamic effects are rapidly reversible, since no fluid administration actually takes place.

Cardiac output, however, has been challenging to measure at the bedside. The traditional reference standard for measuring CO requires the insertion of a pulmonary artery catheter [5, 9] which is invasive, associated with a risk for serious complications [10], and its use may offer no clinical benefits [11–15]. Newer non-invasive devices using bioreactance parameters have mixed evidence in their accuracy and reliability [16–20], and require a dedicated machine that may not be readily available. Lastly, estimations of CO using echocardiography have been suggested as a bedside measure. However, its use may not be feasible due to high training requirements [21].

In the quest to identify feasible, non-invasive, and reproducible bedside estimates of CO, carotid Doppler imaging shows promise. In particular, two carotid measurements have emerged as candidate markers of CO: corrected carotid flow time (CFT) and carotid blood flow (CBF). CFT is the carotid systole time, with heart rate correction applied. This measure is easy to perform and may correlate with intravascular volume [22]. CBF is the integral of blood volume that is ejected through the carotid artery with each cardiac cycle. This measure has been shown to be feasible to perform at the bedside [23, 24].

Studies to date have shown that corrected CFT increases in response to fluid administration or consumption [25, 26], and decreases in response to volume removal in dialysis [22] and blood donation [27]. However, none of these studies correlated corrected CFT with CO. CBF has been less extensively studied. However, in one study of 34 patients, a change in CBF in response to PLR was found to correlate significantly with a change in stroke volume index, measured by bioreactance [28].

Despite these promising studies, neither measure has been correlated directly with a commonly used invasive reference standard for measuring CO via the pulmonary artery catheter. As such, this study seeks to compare corrected CFT and CBF with invasive measures of CO.

## Methods

All adult patients at Massachusetts General Hospital cardiac catheterization laboratory undergoing right heart catheterization between February and April 2016 were invited to participate. Non-consenting patients, patients on mechanical ventilation, and those unable to tolerate a passive leg raise (PLR) maneuver were excluded (e.g., unable to lie supine or had pain with PLR).

Carotid ultrasound images were obtained concurrently with CO measures with the patient in the supine position. A PLR was then performed by elevating the legs using a standardized 30° foam wedge (RayShield® AADCO Medical Inc., Vermont). Repeat carotid ultrasound images and concurrent CO measurements were then obtained within 1 min after PLR, as maximal blood flow changes were felt to be observed within 1 min [8, 29].

Carotid ultrasound images were obtained by an emergency ultrasound fellow (I.M.). Images were obtained using a linear-array (15–4 MHz) transducer on a bedside ultrasound system (uSmart® Terason 3200T, Burlington, MA). The carotid vascular preset was used (pulse repetition frequency 5.0 kHz, wall filter 75 Hz). The common carotid artery was scanned in transverse and longitudinal planes. Spectral Doppler tracings were then obtained by placing a 0.5 mm sample gate through the center of vessel, within 2–3 cm proximal to the carotid bulb in the longitudinal plane, in accordance to standard guidelines [30]. The angle correction cursor was placed parallel to the direction of blood flow. Images with insonation angles >60° were excluded because of resultant inaccuracies of flow and velocity measurements at such angles [31].

### Carotid measurements

Corrected CFT was calculated as systole time/$\sqrt{}$cycle time [27]. Systole time was measured from the start of systolic upstroke to the start of the dicrotic notch, while cycle time was the duration of the cycle (Fig. 1a).

CBF was calculated as

$$\text{blood flow} = \pi \times (\text{carotid diameter})^2/4 \times \text{VTI} \times \text{heart rate},$$

where VTI indicates velocity time integral [28]. VTI of the Doppler signal was measured using manual tracings (Fig. 1b). Intimal-to-intimal carotid diameter was measured at the level of the sample gate (Fig. 1b).

All carotid measurements (systole time, cycle time, VTI, diameter) were measured on a single waveform by one investigator (I.M.) in order to calculate corrected CFT and CBF. Average corrected CFT and average CBF were then calculated using a mean of three waveforms. To establish interrater reliability on obtaining measurements, all measurements on obtained images were then repeated by a second independent investigator (C.W. or A.A., both with similar training to I.M.), who was blinded to all CO and carotid measurements. Results from the second investigator were used only to provide interrater reliability estimates.

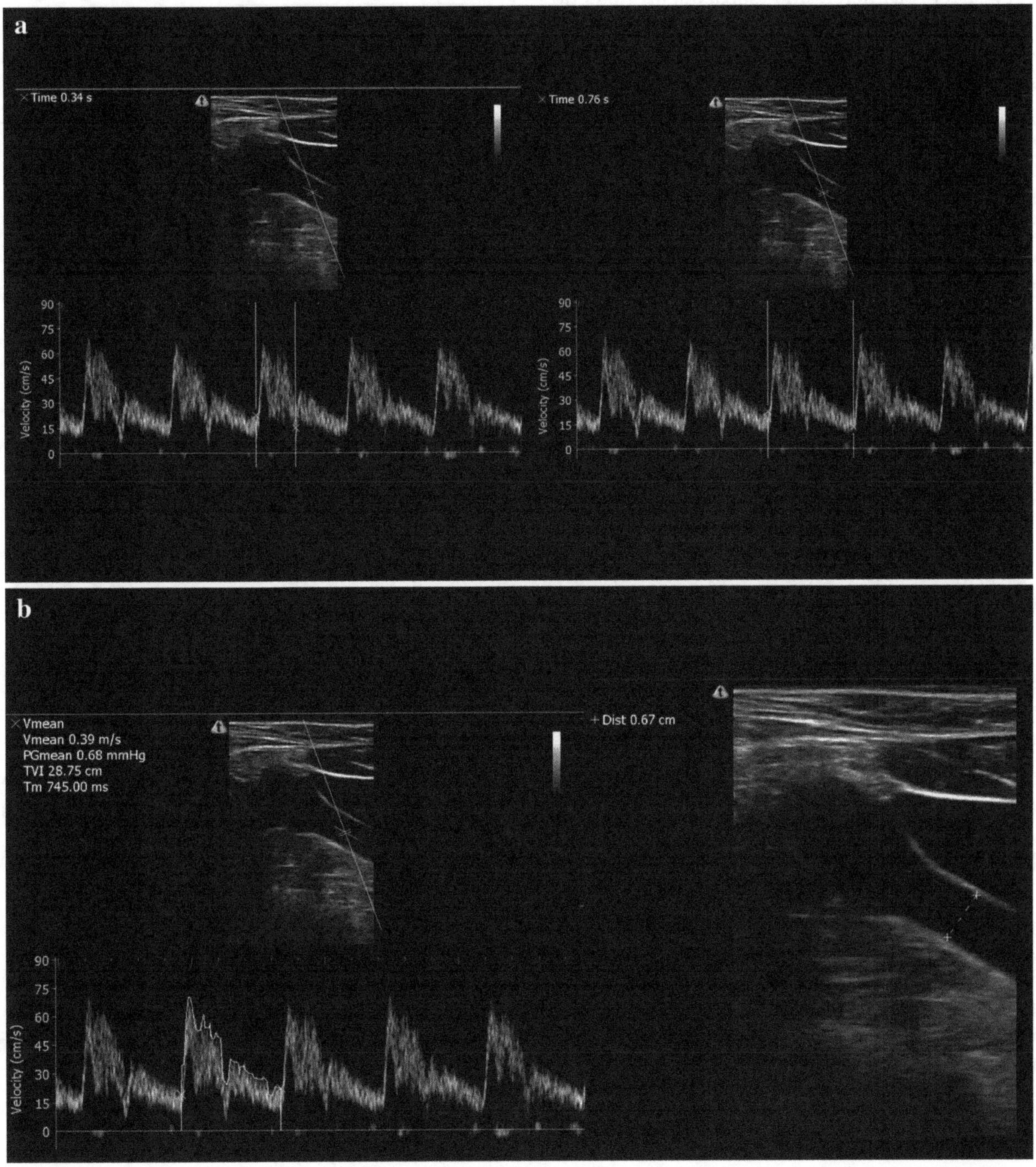


**Fig. 1** **a** Carotid systole time, as measured from the start of the systolic upstroke to the start of the dicrotic notch (*left*). Carotid cycle time, as measured from start of one systolic upstroke to the next (*right*). **b** Velocity time integral tracing of the spectral Doppler signal (*left*). Carotid diameter (*right*)

Image acceptability was rated independently by two trained raters (C.W., A.A.), using five domains (internal reliability acceptable, Cronbach's alpha = 0.84): correction angle parallel to vessel, sample gate in the center of the vessel, sufficient gain, vessel was non-oblique, and measurements made within 2–3 cm proximal to carotid bulb (see Additional file 1). All domains were rated using a 5-point Likert scale, where 1 = poor quality and 5 = excellent quality, with overall image quality rated as a summary measure, based on global expert opinion.

Cardiac output measurements were obtained by thermodilution method in the absence of severe tricuspid regurgitation, by an injection of 10 mL of sterile 0.9% saline injection into the proximal lumen of the pulmonary artery catheter and subsequent detection of the temperature change at the distal thermistor [32]. Fick oxygen method was used in the presence of severe tricuspid regurgitation [33]. The Fick method involved simultaneous arterial and mixed venous blood sample measurement, and cardiac output was determined based upon the ratio between estimated oxygen consumption and arteriovenous oxygen gradient [34]. Post hoc analyses of correlation measures were performed in subgroups of patients in and not in atrial fibrillation at the time of the procedure.

This study was approved by the Partners Human Research Committee Institution Review Board.

### Statistical analysis

On the basis of Marik et al.'s prior study on estimates of stroke volume indices correlations with carotid blood flow [28], we estimated that 26 patients would have 90% power to detect a correlation of 0.59 ($\alpha = 0.05$). However, as interim analyses revealed a lower than 0.59 correlation in our study sample. A repeat sample size calculation suggested that an estimated 48 patients would be needed to detect a correlation of 0.45 ($\alpha = 0.05$, power = 0.9).

Pre- and post-PLR measurements were compared using paired $t$ tests and Wilcoxon signed-rank tests, as appropriate. Correlations between CO and carotid parameters were made using Spearman's rho, a non-parametric correlation coefficient. Confidence intervals around Spearman's rho were based on Fisher's r to z transformation [35]. Correlation coefficients of 0.10–0.29 were considered weak, 0.30–0.49 as moderate, and 0.50–1.00 as strong [36]. All $p$ values were adjusted for multiple comparisons using the Benjamini–Hochberg procedure [37], which allows the false discovery rate to be controlled at the 0.05 level.

All analyses were performed using SAS 9.4 (SAS Institute Inc. Cary, NC) and SPSS version 24 (IBM Corp. Armonk, NY).

## Results

Of the 67 eligible patients, 51 patients (76%) were included in the final analysis (Fig. 2; Table 1). The majority of patients had cardiac output measurements done using thermodilution ($n = 44$; 86%). Five patients were excluded because of angles of insonation of >60°. Of the included 51 patients, median angle of insonation was 60°, with a range of 38–60°. Overall image quality of the included patients was rated as above-average quality [mean score 4.1 ± standard deviation (SD) 0.6] based on global expert opinion. As there were no differences in CO, corrected CFT, or CBF between pre- and post-PLR maneuver (Table 2), only baseline measures (i.e., pre-PLR) will be further discussed. Interrater reliability for corrected CFT and CBF measurements on obtained images was excellent [intraclass correlation coefficient (ICC) 0.90, 95% CI 0.82–0.94; ICC 0.96, 95% CI 0.58–0.99, respectively].

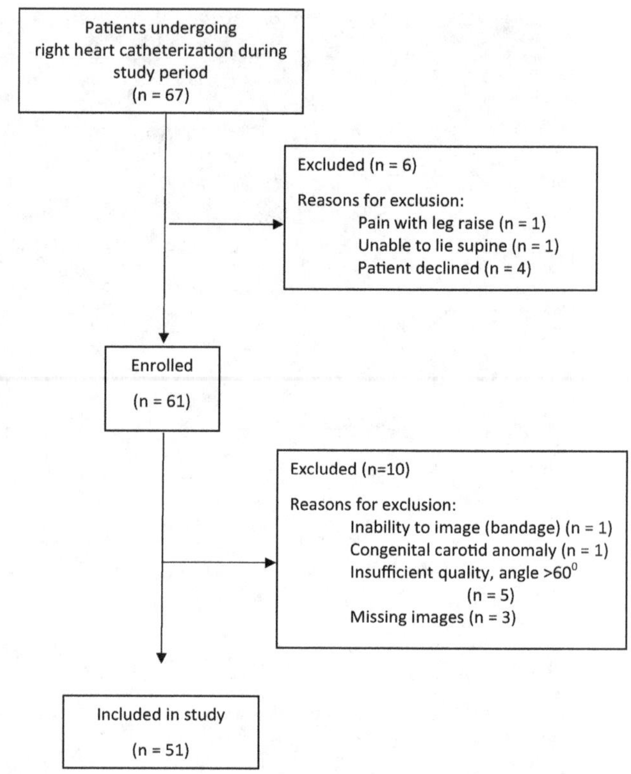


**Fig. 2** Flow chart of number of patients enrolled in the study and included in the analyses

### Corrected carotid flow time (CFT)

Single waveform measurements of corrected CFT did not correlate with CO measurements [$\rho = 0.25$, 95% confidence interval (CI) −0.03 to 0.49, adjusted $p = 0.08$]. Corrected CFT measurements using three waveforms correlated significantly, but weakly, with CO ($\rho = 0.29$, 95% CI 0.02–0.53, adjusted $p = 0.046$).

### Carotid blood flow (CBF)

Single waveform CBF correlated moderately and significantly with CO [$\rho = 0.44$, 95% CI 0.18–0.63, adjusted $p = 0.004$). CBF measurements using three waveforms also moderately and significantly correlated with CO ($\rho = 0.41$, 95% CI 0.16–0.62, adjusted $p = 0.004$).

### Subgroup analysis

In a subgroup of patients not in atrial fibrillation at the time of the procedure ($n = 45$), single waveform measurements of corrected CFT did not correlate with CO ($\rho = 0.26$, 95% CI −0.04 to 0.51, adjusted $p = 0.17$). For patients in atrial fibrillation at the time of the procedure

**Table 1 Baseline characteristics of 51 patients included in the study**

| Baseline characteristics | Number (%) |
|---|---|
| Mean age in years ± standard deviation | 59.6 ± 16.3 |
| Gender | |
| Male | 39 (76) |
| Female | 12 (24) |
| Body mass index (kg/m$^2$) ± standard deviation | 26.3 ± 5.9 |
| History of | |
| Diabetes mellitus | 13 (25) |
| Hypertension | 26 (51) |
| Dyslipidemia | 22 (43) |
| Coronary artery disease | 17 (33) |
| Prior angioplasty and/stent placement | 7 (14) |
| Prior coronary bypass surgery | 4 (8) |
| Stroke or transient ischemic attacks | 11 (22) |
| Atrial fibrillation | 13 (25) |
| Moderate or severe aortic insufficiency | 1 (2) |
| Moderate or severe aortic stenosis | 5 (10) |
| Indication for right heart catheterization | |
| Diagnostic right heart catheterization only | 24 (47) |
| Cardiac biopsy | 27 (53) |
| Cardiac output measurement method | |
| Thermodilution | 44 (86) |
| Fick oxygen method | 7 (14) |
| Vascular access | |
| Internal jugular | 40 (78) |
| Forearm (cephalic or basilic) | 5 (10) |
| Femoral | 6 (12) |

($n$ = 6), single waveform corrected CFT measurements did not correlate with CO ($\rho$ = 0.09, 95% CI −0.78 to 0.84, adjusted $p$ = 0.88). In patients not in atrial fibrillation ($n$ = 45), corrected CFT measurements using three waveforms correlated moderately and significantly with CO ($\rho$ = 0.33, 95% CI 0.04–0.56, adjusted $p$ = 0.03). In patients in atrial fibrillation ($n$ = 6), corrected CFT measurements using three waveforms did not correlate with CO ($\rho$ = −0.14, 95% CI −0.86 to 0.76, adjusted $p$ = 0.92).

Single waveform measurements of CBF correlated moderately and significantly with CO in patients not in atrial fibrillation at the time of the procedure ($\rho$ = 0.42, 95% CI 0.15–0.64, adjusted $p$ = 0.03). For the six patients in atrial fibrillation, single waveform measurements did not correlate with CO ($\rho$ = 0.66, 95% CI −0.33 to 0.96, adjusted $p$ = 0.28). In patients not in atrial fibrillation ($n$ = 45), CBF measurements using three waveforms correlated moderately and significantly with CO ($\rho$ = 0.40, 95% CI 0.12–0.62, adjusted $p$ = 0.02). For the six patients in atrial fibrillation at the time of the procedure, CBF measurements using three waveforms did not correlate with CO ($\rho$ = 0.60, 95% CI −0.41 to 0.95, adjusted $p$ = 0.31).

### Self-report feasibility

Overall, reported ease of carotid diameter measurement was high (mean score 4.1 ± SD 0.8, where 1 = very difficult and 5 = very easy). Reported ease of measuring VTI tracings was moderate (mean score 3.5 ± SD 0.8). Ease of systole time was moderate (3.7 ± SD 0.8) and high for cycle time (4.2 ± SD 0.7).

## Discussion

In this study of 51 adult patients undergoing invasive right heart catheterization and simultaneous carotid ultrasound, CBF correlated moderately and significantly with CO. This relationship was present whether a single waveform or an average of three waveforms was used. Corrected CFT, on the other hand, when measured using only a single waveform, as per the method used by prior studies [22, 25–27], demonstrated no correlation with CO. Only by measuring three waveforms was corrected carotid flow time's correlation with CO significant. However, the strength of this relationship was weak. Altogether, our findings suggest CBF may be a better surrogate marker for CO and that CBF measurements may be less subject to measurements issues than corrected CFT.

The ability to estimate CO in an accurate, reliable, and feasible manner is an important part of determining patients' volume responsiveness. Carotid ultrasound is

**Table 2 Baseline mean cardiac output and median carotid ultrasound parameters (corrected flow time and blood flow) pre- and post-passive leg raise**

| Parameter | Pre-passive leg raise median (interquartile range) | Post-passive leg raise median (interquartile range) | $p$ value |
|---|---|---|---|
| Mean cardiac output ± standard deviation (SD) (L/min) | 5.15 ± 1.58 | 5.19 ± 1.58 | 0.69 |
| Corrected flow time (single waveform in milliseconds) | 331.7 (308.6–357.8) | 344.2 (321.6–360.6) | 0.06 |
| Corrected flow time (average of three waveforms in milliseconds) | 335.2 (311.0–359.3) | 339.6 (322.1–368.9) | 0.13 |
| Blood flow (single waveform in mL/min) | 576.3 (389.5–806.9) | 551.77 (441.5–763.5) | 0.45 |
| Blood flow (average of three waveforms in mL/min) | 555.4 (422.1–766.6) | 558.3 (452.7–741.6) | 0.45 |

a promising tool for two reasons. First, unlike the traditional reference standard of CO measurement from a pulmonary artery catheter [5, 9], carotid ultrasound imaging is non-invasive and readily available in many centers. Second, as evidenced by reported ease of measurements in our study, and confirmed by prior studies [23, 24], carotid ultrasound is easy to perform. This is in contrast to echocardiographic measures of CO [21], which requires more extensive training [38], as its accuracy is dependent on scan techniques and patient factors such as obesity and availability of sonographic windows [39].

In deciding whether to use corrected CFT or CBF as an estimate of CO, one should consider the following factors: (1) strength of the correlation with reference standard, (2) contextual factors that may limit its accuracy, (3) reliability, (4) feasibility, and (5) sensitivity in detecting CO changes. We argue that CBF is superior for the first two factors, and that both CBF and corrected CFT demonstrated high interrater reliability and feasibility.

To our knowledge, ours is the first study to compare both carotid ultrasound measures with invasive measures of CO. Our study demonstrates that CBF correlates stronger than corrected CFT with CO and is less sensitive to measurements errors. We hypothesize that two sources of errors may be contributing to measurement errors in corrected CFT: cardiac arrhythmia and underlying cardiac conditions.

With respect to the cardiac arrhythmia hypothesis, we noted that corrected CFT measurements based on averaging three waveforms yielded a higher and significant correlation, compared to measurements based only on one waveform. The potential of respiratory contribution to the variations in cycle time and systole time (sinus arrhythmia) may contribute to this finding. The hypothesis regarding the contribution of arrhythmias to inaccurate measurements was further supported by findings from our subgroup analysis, whereby the correlation of corrected CFT with CO became significant in a subgroup of patients not in atrial fibrillation at the time of the procedure, and only if an average of three waveforms were used. Correlations were lower in general for patients in atrial fibrillation compared with those not in atrial fibrillation, whether a single waveform or three waveforms were used. Indeed, prior studies evaluating corrected carotid flow time excluded patients with atrial fibrillation [22, 25–27]. In our subgroup analysis of patients in atrial fibrillation, we were unable to detect significant correlations with cardiac output measurement regardless of whether CBF or corrected CFT was used, and regardless of whether a single waveform or an average of three waveforms was used. However, our small sample size ($n = 6$) is likely too small to demonstrate a significant correlation. Future studies should evaluate the use of these parameters in patients in atrial fibrillation. Until such studies are performed, it may be prudent to continue to exclude patients with significant cardiac arrhythmia when attempting to use carotid measurements as surrogates for CO.

With respect to the cardiac condition hypothesis, it is noteworthy that measurements of systole time require the identification of the start of the dicrotic notch. Valvular diseases are known to affect carotid tracings, which may render the dicrotic notch more difficult to appreciate [40–42]. Indeed, in our study, self-report ease of measuring cycle time was higher than for systole time, which may be a reflection of the difficulty in identifying the dicrotic notch in certain cases. Carotid blood flow, on the other hand, utilizes more clinical parameters (diameter, VTI, and heart rate) that may be less subject to the changes of any single parameter and may therefore more accurately estimate for the volumetric flow of blood through the carotid. For example, adaptation to a lower VTI may be accommodated by a larger carotid diameter and/or a faster heart rate. Therefore, accounting for these additional parameters may result in an overall more accurate estimate.

There are a number of limitations in our study. First, this is a single-centered study. Second, we are able to report only interrater reliability for image interpretation and not for image acquisition (a single sonographer performed all the scanning). Image acquisition by untrained sonographers may potentially result in unacceptable interrater reliability. Future studies should examine image acquisition interrater reliability and the role of training. Third, as our patients were largely euvolemic, PLR maneuvers resulted in no demonstrable changes in any of our measured parameters. Therefore, we cannot comment on the sensitivity of carotid measurements to changes imposed by dynamic maneuvers. Further, our use of a 30° foam wedge rather than the more commonly used 45° leg lift [7] may have further limited our ability to induce significant changes pre- and post-PLR. In addition, although it has been argued that the maximal blood flow changes occur within one minute [8, 29], the majority of studies evaluating PLR use a longer time frame [7]. The optimal timing remains unclear. Fourth, our subgroup analysis of patients in and not in atrial fibrillation was performed in a post hoc manner. Results from these analyses should be considered as hypothesis generating only. Fifth, our carotid VTI measurements were performed manually. Therefore, measurement errors may be present. However, measurement errors would be expected to dilute correlation coefficients towards the null [43]. Because many machines are equipped with automatic VTI tracings, correlation coefficients for CBF measured in an automated manner may yield higher correlations than those reported in our study. Sixth, we do not have information on the history of carotid disease. Therefore, we are unable to determine the impact of carotid disease on the accuracy of our carotid ultrasound measurements. Last but not least, the majority of our patients underwent the thermodilution method for cardiac output estimation. While its use is commonly accepted as the practical gold standard, its use is not without limitations, especially in the presence of significant tricuspid regurgitation, intracardiac shunts, or concurrent intravenous infusions [9, 44, 45].

## Conclusions

Our study demonstrates that compared to corrected CFT, CBF demonstrated stronger and more consistent correlation with CO. Its use for assessing volume responsiveness should be further evaluated.

## Additional file

**Additional file 1.** Carotid artery doppler quality assessment tool (CADQAD).

### Abbreviations

CBF: carotid blood flow; CFT: carotid flow time; CO: cardiac output; CI: confidence interval; ICC: intraclass correlation coefficient; PLR: passive leg raise; SD: standard deviation; VTI: velocity time integral.

### Authors' contributions

IWYM contributed to conception and design, acquisition of data, analysis, interpretation of data, and drafting and revision of article. JDC, AA, CW, and MAF contributed to acquisition of data and interpretation of data and revision of article. AB and ASL contributed to conception and design, interpretation of data, and revision of article. VEN contributed to conception and design, acquisition of data, interpretation of data, and drafting and revision of article. All authors have provided final approval of the version submitted. All authors read and approved the final manuscript.

### Author details

[1] Division of Emergency Ultrasound, Department of Emergency Medicine, Massachusetts General Hospital, 326 Cambridge Street, Suite 410, Boston, MA 02114, USA. [2] Division of General Internal Medicine, Department of Medicine, University of Calgary, 3330 Hospital Dr NW, Calgary, AB T2N 4N1, Canada. [3] Cardiology Division, Department of Medicine, Massachusetts General Hospital, 15 Parkman Street #800, Boston, MA 02114, USA. [4] Department of Emergency Medicine, Hamad Medical Corporation, PO Box 3050, Doha, Qatar. [5] Department of Anaesthesia, Massachusetts General Hospital, 55 Fruit Street, Boston, MA 02114, USA. [6] Department of Emergency Medicine, University Hospitals, Cleveland Medical Center, Case Western Reserve University, 11100 Euclid Ave, Cleveland, OH 44106, USA.

### Acknowledgements

The authors would like to thank all the colleagues and patients at the Massachusetts General Hospital cardiac catheterization laboratory for their collaboration and participation in this work.

### References

1. Kelm DJ, Perrin JT, Cartin-Ceba R, Gajic O, Schenck L, Kennedy CC (2015) Fluid overload in patients with severe sepsis and septic shock treated with early-goal directed therapy is associated with increased acute need for fluid-related medical interventions and hospital death. Shock 43:68–73
2. Boyd JH, Forbes J, Nakada TA, Walley KR, Russell JA (2011) Fluid resuscitation in septic shock: a positive fluid balance and elevated central venous pressure are associated with increased mortality. Crit Care Med 39:259–265
3. Acheampong A, Vincent J-L (2015) A positive fluid balance is an independent prognostic factor in patients with sepsis. Crit Care 19:251
4. Marik PE, Cavallazzi R (2013) Does the central venous pressure predict fluid responsiveness? An updated meta-analysis and a plea for some common sense. Crit Care Med 41:1774–1781
5. Bentzer P, Griesdale DE, Boyd J, MacLean K, Sirounis D, Ayas NT (2016) Will this hemodynamically unstable patient respond to a bolus of intravenous fluids? JAMA 316:1298–1309
6. Bendjelid K, Romand JA (2012) Fluid responsiveness in mechanically ventilated patients: a review of indices used in intensive care. Intensive Care Med 29:352–360
7. Cavallaro F, Sandroni C, Marano C, La Torre G, Mannocci A, De Waure C, Bello G, Maviglia R, Antonelli M (2012) Diagnostic accuracy of passive leg raising for prediction of fluid responsiveness in adults: systematic review and meta-analysis of clinical studies. Intensive Care Med 36(9):1476–1483
8. Monnet X, Teboul JL (2015) Passive leg raising: five rules, not a drop of fluid! Crit Care 19:18
9. Pugsley J, Lerner AB (2010) Cardiac output monitoring: is there a gold standard and how do the newer technologies compare? Semin Cardiothorac Vasc Anesth 14:274–282
10. Dee Boyd K, Thomas SJ, Gold J, Boyd AD (1983) A prospective study of complications of pulmonary artery catheterizations in 500 consecutive patients. Chest 84:245–249
11. Harvey S, Harrison DA, Singer M, Ashcroft J, Jones CM, Elbourne D, Brampton W, Williams D, Young D, Rowan K (2005) Assessment of the clinical effectiveness of pulmonary artery catheters in management of patients in intensive care (PAC-Man): a randomised controlled trial. Lancet 366:472–477
12. Sandham JD, Hull RD, Brant RF, Knox L, Pineo GF, Doig CJ, Laporta DP, Viner S, Passerini L, Devitt H, Kirby A, Jacka M (2003) A Randomized, controlled trial of the use of pulmonary-artery catheters in high-risk surgical patients. N Engl J Med 348:5–14
13. Richard C, Warszawski J, Anguel N, Deye N, Combes A, Barnoud D, Boulain T, Lefort Y, Fartoukh M, Baud F (2003) Early use of the pulmonary artery catheter and outcomes in patients with shock and acute respiratory distress syndrome: a randomized controlled trial. JAMA 290:2713–2720
14. Shah MR, Hasselblad V, Stevenson LW, Binanay C, O'Connor CM, Sopko G, Califf RM (2005) Impact of the pulmonary artery catheter in critically ill patients: meta-analysis of randomized clinical trials. JAMA 294:1664–1670
15. Wheeler A, Bernard G, Thompson B, Schoenfeld D, Wiedemann H, DeBoisblanc B, Connors A Jr, Hite R, Harabin A (2006) Pulmonary-artery versus central venous catheter to guide treatment of acute lung injury. N Engl J Med 354:2213–2224
16. Benomar B, Ouattara A, Estagnasie P, Brusset A, Squara P (2010) Fluid responsiveness predicted by noninvasive bioreactance-based passive leg raise test. Intensive Care Med 36:1875–1881
17. Fagnoul D, Vincent J-L, Backer D (2012) Cardiac output measurements using the bioreactance technique in critically ill patients. Crit Care 16:460
18. Raval NY, Squara P, Cleman M, Yalamanchili K, Winklmaier M, Burkhoff D (2008) Multicenter evaluation of noninvasive cardiac output measurement by bioreactance technique. J Clin Monit Comput 22:113–119
19. Squara P, Denjean D, Estagnasie P, Brusset A, Dib JC, Dubois C (2007) Noninvasive cardiac output monitoring (NICOM): a clinical validation. Intensive Care Med 33:1191–1194
20. Kupersztych-Hagege E, Teboul JL, Artigas A, Talbot A, Sabatier C, Richard C, Monnet X (2013) Bioreactance is not reliable for estimating cardiac output and the effects of passive leg raising in critically ill patients. Br J Anaesth 111:961–966
21. Gunst M, Ghaemmaghami V, Sperry J, Robinson M, O'Keeffe T, Friese R, Frankel H (2008) Accuracy of cardiac function and volume status estimates using the bedside echocardiographic assessment in trauma/critical care. J Trauma 65:509–516
22. Hossein-Nejad H, Mohammadinejad P, Lessan-Pezeshki M, Davarani SS, Banaie M (2015) Carotid artery corrected flow time measurement via bedside ultrasonography in monitoring volume status. J Crit Care 30:1199–1203
23. Stolz LA, Mosier JM, Gross AM, Douglas MJ, Blaivas M, Adhikari S (2015) Can emergency physicians perform common carotid Doppler flow measurements to assess volume responsiveness? W J Emerg Med 16:255–259

24. Adedipe AA, Fly DL, Schwitz SD, Jorgenson DB, Duric H, Sayre MR, Nichol G (2015) Carotid Doppler blood flow measurement during cardiopulmonary resuscitation is feasible: a first in man study. Resuscitation 96:121–125
25. Blehar DJ, Glazier S, Gaspari RJ (2014) Correlation of corrected flow time in the carotid artery with changes in intravascular volume status. J Crit Care 29:486–488
26. Shokoohi H, Berry GW, Shahkolahi M, King J, Salimian M, Poshtmashad A, Pourmand A (2016) The diagnostic utility of sonographic carotid flow time in determining volume responsiveness. J Crit Care 38:231–235
27. Mackenzie DC, Khan NA, Blehar D, Glazier S, Chang Y, Stowell CP, Noble VE, Liteplo AS (2015) Carotid flow time changes with volume status in acute blood loss. Ann Emerg Med 66:277–282
28. Marik PE, Levitov A, Young A, Andrews L (2013) The use of bioreactance and carotid doppler to determine volume responsiveness and blood flow redistribution following passive leg raising in hemodynamically unstable patients. Chest 143:364–370
29. Monnet X, Rienzo M, Osman D, Anguel N, Richard C, Pinsky MR, Teboul JL (2006) Passive leg raising predicts fluid responsiveness in the critically ill. Crit Care Med 34:1402–1407
30. American College of Radiology (2016) ACR-AIUM-SRU practice parameter for the performance of an ultrasound examination of the extracranial cerebrovascular system. http://www.acr.org/~/media/5d63a45f7a54417c93cd58f109f0fdd2.pdf. Accessed 5 Apr 2017
31. Tola M, Yurdakul M (2006) Effect of Doppler angle in diagnosis of internal carotid artery stenosis. J Ultrasound Med 25:1187–1192
32. Ganz W, Donoso R, Marcus HS, Forrester JS, Swan HJ (1971) A new technique for measurement of cardiac output by thermodilution in man. Am J Cardiol 27:392–396
33. Callan P, Clark AL (2016) Right heart catheterisation: indications and interpretation. Heart 102:147–157
34. Wilkinson JL (2001) Haemodynamic calculations in the catheter laboratory. Heart 85:113–120
35. Shen D, Lu Z (2006) Computation of correlation coefficient and its confidence interval in SAS. http://www2.sas.com/proceedings/sugi31/170-31.pdf. Accessed 5 Apr 2017
36. Cohen J (1988) Statistical power analysis for the behavioral sciences. Academic Press, New York
37. Benjamini Y, Hochberg Y (1995) Controlling the false discovery rate: a practical and powerful approach to multiple testing. J R Stat Soc B Methodol 57:289–300
38. Garcia X, Mateu L, Maynar J, Mercadal J, Ochagavía A, Ferrandiz A (2011) Estimating cardiac output. Utility in the clinical practice. Available invasive and non-invasive monitoring. Med Intensiva 35:552–561
39. Nicolosi GL, Pungercic E, Cervesato E, Pavan D, Modena L, Moro E, Dall'Aglio V, Zanuttini D (1988) Feasibility and variability of six methods for the echocardiographic and Doppler determination of cardiac output. Br Heart J 59:299–303
40. Madhwal S, Yesenko S, Kim ESH, Park M, Begelman SM, Gornik HL (2014) Manifestations of cardiac disease in carotid Duplex ultrasound examination. JACC 7:200–203
41. O'Boyle MK, Vibhakar NI, Chung J, Keen WD, Gosink BB (1996) Duplex sonography of the carotid arteries in patients with isolated aortic stenosis: imaging findings and relation to severity of stenosis. AJR Am J Roentgenol 166:197–202
42. Kallman C, Gosink B, Gardner D (1991) Carotid duplex sonography: bisferious pulse contour in patients with aortic valvular disease. AJR Am J Roentgenol 157:403–407
43. Kelsey JL, Whittemore AS, Evans AS, Thompson WD (1996) Methods in observational epidemiology. Oxford University Press Inc, New York
44. Lee AJ, Cohn JH (2011) Ranasinghe JS (2011) Cardiac output assessed by invasive and minimally invasive techniques. Anesthesiol Res Pract 17:475151
45. Marino PL (2014) The ICU Bok, 4th edn. Lippincott Williams & Wilkins, Philadelphia

# Phantom model and scoring system to assess ability in ultrasound-guided chest drain positioning

Luigi Vetrugno[1], Giovanni Volpicelli[2], Federico Barbariol[1*], Ilaria Toretti[1], Livia Pompei[1], Francesco Forfori[3] and Giorgio Della Rocca[1]

**Abstract**

**Background:** Chest tube positioning is an invasive procedure associated with potentially serious injuries. In the last few years, we have been running a project directed at developing a practical simulator of a surgical procedure taught on our medical training program. The phantom model reconstructs the pleural anatomy, visible by lung ultrasound, used for the assessed performance of the Seldinger technique. The aim of the present study was to investigate the validity of this simulation technology for assessing residents in anesthesia and intensive care medicine; specifically, their skill in positioning a US-guided chest tube drain was tested using the simulator device. The second aim of the paper was to evaluate the learning curve of our residents over their 5-year study course and validate the phantom scoring system.

**Methods:** This was a prospective, single-blinded observational study. Participants were recruited from residents in anesthesia and intensive care medicine and divided into two groups: 'Novice' and 'Expert,' based on the course year attended (years 1, 2, and 3 vs. years 4 and 5, respectively). We asked them to position a chest tube drain in a phantom model, guided by ultrasound, to drain a simulated pleural effusion. Each subject performed two tests that simulated pleural effusions of 4 and 2 cm, respectively. Every step of the maneuver was constantly monitored and the performance scored by the investigators. We then performed a Spearman correlation analysis to evaluate the effect of experience level on the performance of the two groups of residents.

**Results:** Thirty-one residents were included in this study: 20 in the Novice group and 11 in the Expert group. The mean performance rating score was 0.75 ± 4.38 for the Novice Group and 5.91 ± 3.75 for the Expert group ($p = 0.0026$). The Spearman correlation analysis examining the relationship between year of residency and performance rating score confirmed a positive correlation ($r = 0.58$, $p = 0.0006$). Post-test trend analysis revealed a statistically significant linear trend for skill growth across time, i.e., course year ($p = 0.0022$).

**Conclusions:** Our simulated procedure using a phantom model of lung anatomy can accurately and reliably be used to assess the skill levels of operators in their ability to drain pleural effusion.

**Keywords:** Chest tube, Chest drainage, Learning, Training, Simulator, Simulation technology

## Background

Percutaneous pleural drain positioning is the third most technical procedure performed in the intensive care unit (ICU) after vascular catheterization and tracheal intubation. Pleural drain positioning can constitute a crucial maneuver for the treatment of critically ill patients [1–3]; for example, it has the potential to improve respiratory function, thereby avoiding intubation in spontaneous breathing patients or leading to earlier weaning in patients under mechanical ventilation. Because of its paramount clinical utility, chest tube positioning has

*Correspondence: barbariol.federico@gmail.com
[1] Anesthesia and Intensive Care Medicine-Department of Medical and Biological Sciences, University of Udine, P.le S. M. della Misericordia 15, 33100 Udine, Italy
Full list of author information is available at the end of the article

become an incumbent skill for many specialists, such as general surgeons, intensivists, pulmonologists, and emergency medicine specialists [4, 5]. However, pleural drainage is burdened by substantial risks and can result in potentially serious harm if not performed accurately [6, 7]. Even if small-bore tubes are inserted using the Seldinger technique, the procedure is not without risk due to the many major vascular and visceral structures that lay in close proximity to the usual insertion sites and the course of the chest tubes [8]. According to some studies, the complication rate of this procedure ranges from 21 to 30 % [9–11].

Meanwhile, the growing use of point-of-care ultrasound (US) has led to an improvement in the bedside diagnosis and fluid quantification of pleural effusion, and US guidance has proved to increase the success rate of chest tube insertion and the safety of the procedure [12, 13]. International guidelines now recommend US to guide all pleural drainage procedures [14]. This has led to the need for the novice not only to acquire the traditional skills necessary for the Seldinger technique but also to achieve an appropriate level of pulmonary US knowledge. Despite these institutional recommendations, a survey performed at 101 acute hospitals in the UK showed that formal training in the subject matter is not yet sufficiently widespread [6]. In 2010, the British Thoracic Society (BTS) updated its guidelines, recommending that all clinicians performing a chest drain insertion should be appropriately trained and/or supervised [14]. Training should include a theoretical component covering the procedure, pleural anatomy and the risks involved, and a practical component involving a manikin as well as supervised clinical practice. The first aim of our study was to test a new model for assessing the skills of our residents training in anesthesia and intensive care medicine (divided into Novices and Experts) in positioning a US-guided chest tube drain using a simulator device. The second aim was to evaluate the learning curve of our residents over the 5 years of their medical training program and validate the phantom scoring system.

## Methods

### Study setting

This was a prospective, single-blinded observational study for the evaluation of chest drain placement in a US-compatible simulator. Verbal consent was obtained from each participant, and each performance was recorded anonymously. Study subjects were blinded to the purpose of the study and to the parameters that were recorded and scored. Authorization for the study, which did not involve any patients, was given by the Ethical Committee of the Azienda Ospedaliero-Universitaria of Udine. The study was performed in the Department of Anesthesia and Intensive Care Medicine, in the School of Medicine and Residency of the University of Udine, Udine, Italy. Study participants were recruited from residents in anesthesia and intensive care medicine and then divided into two groups: the 'Novice' group including residents attending the 1st, 2nd, and 3rd years of the 5-year program and the 'Expert' group including residents attending the 4th and 5th years. Our school of residency has an active ultrasound education program that runs throughout the course of the 5 years of residency. As suggested by the American College of Chest Physicians [15], the program is divided into general critical care ultrasonography (GCCUS; which includes vascular and lung US) and critical care echocardiography (CCE). During this training period, residents are required to acquire all of the abovementioned technical skills and are gradually introduced to clinical practice under supervision.

### Phantom model and technique

We used the simulator 'Ultrasound Thoracentesis Model THM-30' (SIMULAB, Seattle, USA). This simulator features a partial torso with anatomical landmarks such as skin texture, ribs, and a fluid reservoir. Needles and catheters can be inserted and fluid withdrawn (Fig. 1). The simulated lung can be seen as an echogenic structure, and it is equipped with an inflating mechanism that modulates the size of the pleural effusion. It includes a reconstruction of the chest wall tissues, the 6th, 7th, 8th, and 9th ribs with intercostal spaces, the pleural cavity with a normal lung and an atelectatic lung, the diaphragm, and the sub-diaphragmatic spleen. The open configuration of the model (Fig. 2) allows the instructor to provide feedback on procedural concepts, offering students the possibility of visualizing the catheter depth and placement once inserted into the pleural cavity and enabling instructors to evaluate student performance. A positive fluid outflow offers useful positive feedback when pleural effusions are correctly drained.

Each resident was asked to position the needle tip carefully through the phantom manikin, using continuous US guidance to target the pleural effusion. Residents then inserted a Seldinger guidewire into the pleural space, on to which a dilator and then a catheter were subsequently passed to drain the pleural effusion. For this purpose, a 5-Fr pediatric Pneumopericardial Drainage Set (Cook Medical, Bloomington, USA) was used. Two successive tests were performed by each subject: in the first, we simulated a 4 cm pleural effusion (corresponding to about 800 mL) to drain; in the second, the effusion was 2 cm (about 400 mL). No time pressure was put on the study subjects, and they were free to utilize the ultrasound approach they desired. Every step of the manoeuver was constantly observed by the investigators through the

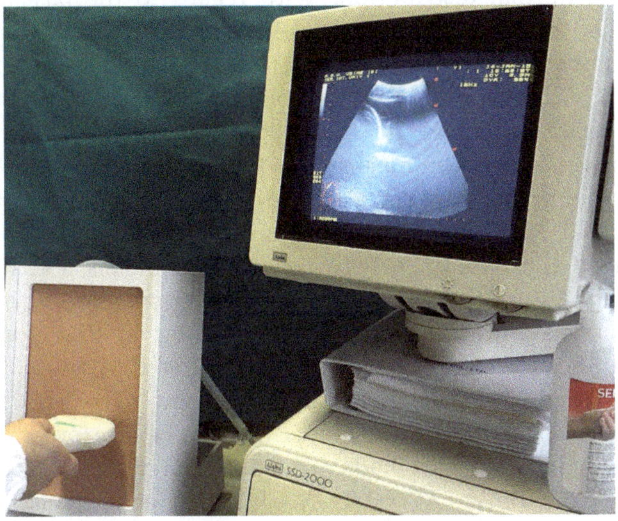

**Fig. 1** The thoracentesis simulator 'Ultrasound Thoracentesis Model THM-30' developed by SIMULAB, Seattle, USA. It features a partial torso with anatomical landmarks, such as skin texture, ribs, and a fluid reservoir. Its simulated lung is seen as an echogenic structure with an inflating mechanism to adjust the size of the pleural effusion

opening of the cephalic part of the phantom, and checked for injuries, technical errors, and/or difficulties.

### Scoring system

A 9-item Case Report Form (Additional file 1: CRF) was designed for the investigators' evaluation of each resident. Each skill or action was scored dichotomously (correct or incorrect). This CRF was then used in a pilot examination of two chief medical residents (FB, IT) in order to estimate the checklist's reliability and validity. Two assessors scored each resident's performances: the senior sonographer for our Department (LV) and a trained resident (IT). After each test, the two investigators discussed the case, with the aim of reaching a common assessment. In the case of disagreements, the lowest score was kept.

The specific data collected were the following:

previous experience: year of residency, number of previous chest drains positioned, and type of US technique used.

actual performance: success in pleural drainage (at 2 and 4 cm), development of pneumothorax (at 2 and 4 cm), dilator trauma, rib trauma, difficulties (at 2 and 4 cm) with catheter manipulation or placement, and difficulties with the use of US.

Using these data, we calculated a global numerical performance rating score (PRS, ranging from −10 to +10) for the assessment of each subject's overall performance

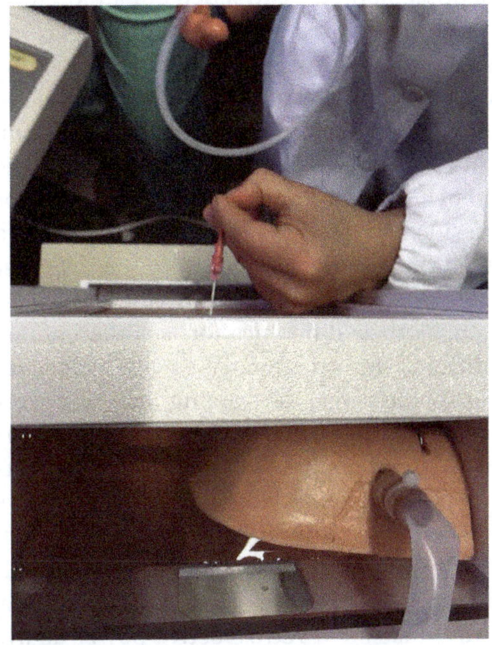

**Fig. 2** The open top of the Ultrasound Thoracentesis Model. The model's open top allows the instructor to provide feedback on procedural concepts, offering students the possibility to visualize the catheter depth and placement once inserted into the pleural cavity. This characteristic was used by the investigators to evaluate the performance of each subject

and ability; all subsequent statistical analyses were performed using these score values. The PRS was calculated as follows:

evidence of pneumothorax at 4 cm effusion pleural drainage: −3 points. No pneumothorax: +2 points;
evidence of procedural difficulties at 4 cm effusion pleural drainage: −3 points. No difficulties: +2 points;
evidence of pneumothorax at 2 cm effusion pleural drainage: −2 points. No pneumothorax: +3 points;
evidence of procedural difficulties at 2 cm effusion pleural drainage: −2 points. No difficulties: +3 points;

See Additional file 1 for the CRF and PRS calculation. CRF was reviewed for completeness and consistency by authors VL and IT, who frequently perform and supervise thoracentesis.

### Statistical analysis

The data collected for the two groups were first tested for normality using the D'Agostino-Pearson omnibus normality test; descriptive statistics (mean and standard deviation for quantitative variables, and absolute and relative frequencies for qualitative variables) were subsequently calculated for each group. To test for a difference between the two groups with respect to the performance score, we implemented a two-sided unpaired $t$ test as well as an $F$ test to compare variances and to control whether the $t$ test assumptions were met. Our second aim was to assess how performance of the maneuver developed over the 5 years of residency. To this end, we performed a Spearman rank correlation analysis to evaluate the effect of experience level, examining the relationship between year of residency and PRS. We also performed a Pearson correlation (using true values), to see if its result was comparable to that obtained with the Spearman rank correlation, as their difference (or lack thereof) will provide additional information. We subdivided residents according to their year of training and compared their PRS by one-way analysis of variance (ANOVA) and then performed a trend analysis using an ANOVA post-test to test the hypothesis that skill development follows a linear trend according to number of years of experience (i.e., year of residency). Sample size was not calculated before the study given the absence of available comparable data in literature; instead, a retrospective power analysis was implemented. Our goal was to achieve a power of 80 % for a 0.05 significance level (alpha error) using a two-tailed unpaired $t$ test.

Statistical analyses were performed using a specifically designed Microsoft Excel 2010 spreadsheet (Microsoft, Redmond, Washington) and GraphPad Prism, version 6.01 for Windows (GraphPad Software, San Diego, USA).

## Results

Thirty-one residents with different skill levels in US-guided techniques and different amounts of previous experience were enrolled in this study. Twenty subjects were assigned to the 'Novice' group and 11 to the 'Expert' group. The distribution of the study subjects by residency year and the mean performance rating scores per year are shown in Table 1.

Each resident made two successive attempts at the procedure (making a total number of 62 test attempts for the study group). All of the residents were able to complete the procedure. Data from the two groups were first tested for normality and were found to be well approximated by a normal distribution. With regard to the baseline skills for the two groups, the mean performance rating score was 0.75 ± 4.38 for the Novice Group and 5.91 ± 3.75 for the Expert group ($p = 0.0026$; $F$ test to compare variances, $p = 0.6329$; Table 1; Fig. 3), with a difference between means of 5.16 (95 % CI 1.956–8.362). These results confirm a statistically different stratification of participants according to their experience level. Given the difference between the two means and the sample size of our two groups and their standard deviation, the power of the study was higher than 88 % for a significance level (alpha error) of 0.05 with a two-tailed unpaired $t$ test, exceeding our a priori power goal of 80 %. Regarding the development of this skill over the 5 years of residency, we performed correlation analyses to evaluate the effect of year of residency. The Spearman correlation analysis examining the relationship between year of residency and PRS confirmed a positive correlation ($r = 0.58$, $p = 0.0006$, 95 % confidence interval 0.2799–0.7820; Table 2), thus proving that higher scores were obtained by residents with greater levels of experience (i.e., years of residency). Correlation analysis was repeated using the Pearson test, and the same results were obtained, further consolidating these results (Pearson $r = 0.56$, $p = 0.001$, 95 % confidence interval 0.2571–0.7633; Table 2). Finally,

**Table 1 Distribution of study subjects by residency year and mean performance rating scores**

| Year | N (%) | PRS (SD) | Group | N (%) | PRS (SD) |
|---|---|---|---|---|---|
| 1 | 4 (12.9) | −1.25 (2.5) | Novice | 20 (64.5) | 0.75 (4.38) |
| 2 | 8 (25.8) | 0.00 (2.67) | | | |
| 3 | 8 (25.8) | 2.50 (5.98) | | | |
| 4 | 5 (16.1) | 6.00 (4.18) | Expert | 11 (35.5) | 5.91 (3.75) |
| 5 | 6 (19.4) | 5.83 (3.76) | | | |
| Total | 31 (100) | $p = 0.025$ | | 31 (100) | $p = 0.0026$ |

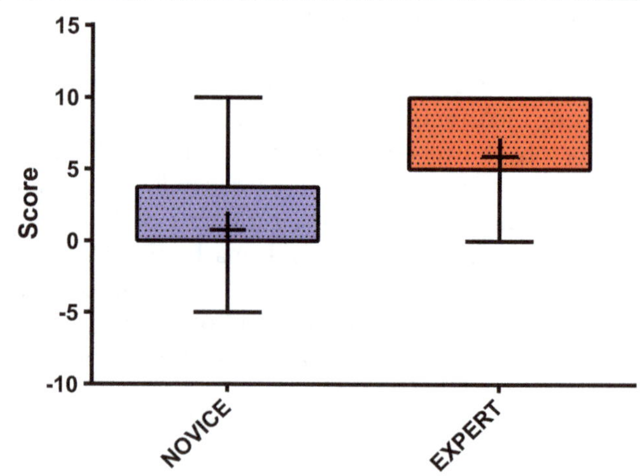


**Fig. 3** Performance rating score for the Novice and Expert groups. The *colored boxes* extend from the 25th to 75th percentiles. The *whiskers* indicate the minimum and maximum values. The *plus signs* indicate the mean value. $p = 0.0026$

**Table 2 Correlation analysis examining the relationship between year of residency and performance rating score**

| Spearman | 0.58 ($p = 0.0006$) |
|---|---|
| Pearson | 0.56 ($p = 0.001$) |
| ANOVA post-test linear trend analysis | $p = 0.0022$ |

residents were re-divided according to year of residency and the mean PRSs compared using one-way ANOVA (Table 1; Fig. 4). Once again, a statistically significant different distribution of the mean score was obtained across years ($p = 0.025$). Trend analysis was then performed using an ANOVA post-test and confirmed our hypothesis that a linear trend exists between PRS magnitude and year of residency ($p = 0.0022$—see Fig. 4).

Potential complications resulting from each attempt were also assessed using the phantom dummy (Table 3); the main complication suffered concerns the occurrence of dilator trauma, caused by inserting the dilator too far beyond the pleura, which threatens to cause damage to the lung parenchyma. Dilator trauma occurred in 14.5 % of tests, especially in the Novice group. Other less frequent complications were the development of pneumothorax (defined as accidental puncture of the lung parenchyma; in this case of the phantom lung) in 4.8 % of cases, and the development of rib trauma (1.6 %). No statistically significant differences were found on analyzing the distribution of every single complication or the overall rate of complications between the two groups.

## Discussion

The main achievement of this study is to show that the phantom model with the scoring system developed by the authors is useful to assess skills in US pleural puncture and drainage positioning. Another important finding of this study is that residents clearly showed a rapid progression in their proficiency in US-guided pleural drain positioning in a phantom model. This learning curve appears to progress steadily over the 5-year residency course (Fig. 4), with significant improvements evident in the first 3 years, and a plateau from the 4th year onward.

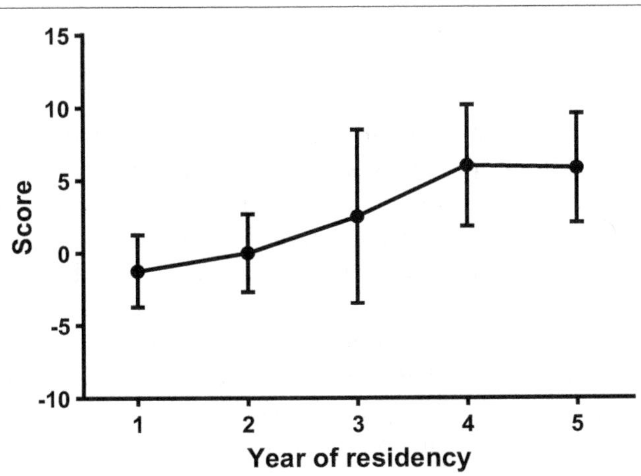


**Fig. 4** Mean performance rating score in residents subdivided by year. *Error bars* represent standard deviations. The development of residents' skills in pleural effusion ultrasound and chest drain positioning appears to progress steadily with increasing years of residency, reaching a plateau in the last 2 years. $p = 0.025$

**Table 3 Main complications occurred**

| Group | Novice, *n* (%) | Expert, *n* (%) | Total, *n* (%) |
|---|---|---|---|
| Number of tests | 40 | 22 | 62 |
| Complications | | | |
| PNX (at 2 cm only) | 2 (5) | 1 (4.5) | 3 (4.8) |
| Rib trauma | 0 (0) | 1 (4.5) | 1 (1.6) |
| Dilator trauma | 6 (15) | 3 (13.6) | 9 (14.5) |

In order to increase patient safety, our institution has designed and implemented a teaching program in which residents are gradually given more responsibility in performing US-guided maneuvers: the first procedures performed by residents are vein and arterial cannulations, followed by loco-regional anesthesia, paracentesis, and finally lung and pleural procedures. Along this learning journey, the use of simulation technology for practicing chest tube positioning provides an important stepping stone before a resident moves on to real patients under a qualified supervision.

Salamonsen et al. [16] assessed 22 physicians (eight novices, seven intermediates and seven advanced) performing thoracic ultrasound on a pleural effusion phantom. These authors found the mean scores for the novice, intermediate, and advanced groups to be 49.3, 73.0, and 91.5, respectively, in a 100-point scale, with a significant difference between groups ($p < 0.0001$). The authors concluded that their phantom procedure could be used to determine the 'adequacy' of thoracic ultrasound training before the physician moves into clinical practice, and/or as a tool that provides a way of documenting ongoing procedural competence. Scoring systems for assessing technical competence have already been profitably used and validated in echocardiography too [17, 18].

Wayne et al. [19] reported the use of a thoracentesis model in a structured educational program, giving trainees the opportunity for deliberate practice with feedback, which resulted in consistent improvements in residents' skills. In agreement with our data, most of their study subjects (who were internal medicine residents) demonstrated poor clinical skill in thoracentesis procedures at the baseline level. It could be argued that some inexperienced participants may have a natural affinity for this procedural task and would be able to develop the required proficiency more rapidly than other more experienced trainees. This was only partially found to be true in our study; we observed a continual growth in US-guided procedure skills with increasing years of residency—comparable to a 'snowball effect.' Our teaching program begins with theoretical classes on the basic principles, followed their application in real clinical practice, according to the residency year. For instance, the residents acquire US skills for guided central venous catheterization in their 1st and 2nd years and for nerve blocks in their 2nd and 3rd years. The nature of this curriculum may underlie the linear growth of skill acquisition in thoracic ultrasound and chest tube positioning.

Our study is unique in its field because it combines an assessment of the skills required for lung ultrasound examination with testing for proficiency in performing the Seldinger technique.

The UK National Patient Safety Agency, in the aftermath of 12 deaths and 15 incidents of serious harm following chest drainage procedures over a three-year period (2005–2008), published a warning report [20] which showed that the vast majority of complications were the result of inexperience, inadequate training, and/or poor technical skills; this has since been confirmed by other studies [21, 22]. It is probable that these complications could have been avoided if US guidance had been used. Another important aspect reported by this UK Agency was the lack of familiarity with the Seldinger technique for chest drain insertion and the excessive insertion of the dilator.

In our study, this latter procedural error was indeed the main complication encountered, occurring in 6 out of 40 tests in the novice group (15 %) and in 3 out of 22 tests in the expert group (13.6 %); the overall incidence was 14.5 %. A dilator should never be inserted by more than one centimeter, as recommended by the BTS guidelines [14]. We also observed 3 cases of pneumothorax, all of which occurred when the pleural effusion was 2 cm (2 cases in the Novice group and 1 in the Expert group), while no cases of pneumothorax were observed when the pleural effusion was 4 cm. The most obvious explanation for this is the larger safety margin when the extent of pleural effusion is greater. Finally, a single case of a broken needle also occurred, caused by impact against a phantom rib. According to our teaching program, residents in their 4th and 5th years should achieve the necessary levels of proficiency in lung ultrasound to distinguish all the thoracic anatomic structures and to identify pleural effusion. This is critical for guaranteeing basic levels of competence and safety in thoracic procedures. In our opinion, thoracic ultrasound should be practiced daily in the ICU to ensure the progressive improvement of these fundamental skills.

## Limitations

This study has a number of limitations. First, it was conducted in a single teaching hospital in a selected population of trainee physicians (residents in anesthesia and intensive care medicine). For this reason, our results cannot be extended to other academic institutions. The phantom model that we used is a thoracentesis model adapted to pleural chest drainage performed using small 5-French pediatric pig-tail catheters. This device is not commonly used as a chest drain and presents some limitations. For example, penetration of the phantom's gel layers becomes more difficult after a failed first attempt, because the catheter gradually warms up and loses its rigidity, which makes all further attempts more difficult. Another limitation of our study is that the investigators rated the residents' performances according to their own overall impression of each subject's ability, without the application of any objective assessment criteria. We did, however, try to limit any potential bias by combining a double evaluation on the same performance, released by two independent investigators, one of whom was the senior sonographer of our department.

Simulation technology could be used to document the progression of technical proficiency during residency training and to determine the adequacy of a doctor's mastery of the procedure for chest drainage before their introduction into clinical practice. However, working on a simulator manikin is less technically challenging and stressful compared with performing the same procedure on real patients. A physician's expertise must include the ability to communicate with the patient, to adapt techniques to different body habitus and to tailor the procedure to specific situations. None of these can be currently trained using simulator technology. Simulation-based training provides a relaxed environment where technical skills can be practiced, but it cannot completely substitute the real clinical setting. Finally, another limitation of our model is that a phantom simulator cannot test for the occurrence of a hemothorax.

## Conclusion

Our phantom model and scoring system provide a reliable method for the assessment of procedural competences in ultrasound and pleural drain positioning. Traditionally, the teaching model for medical education has primarily been based on direct experiential learning in the clinical environment. However, a more contemporary concept of training should also include theoretical components as well as the opportunity for the simulated practice of supervised procedures using suitable technology before proceeding on to real patients.

## Additional file

**Additional file 1.** A 9-item Case Report Form.

#### Abbreviations

ANOVA: analysis of variance; BTS: British Thoracic Society; CCE: critical care echocardiography; GCCUS: general critical care ultrasonography; ICU: intensive care unit; NPSA: National Patient Safety Agency; PRS: performance rating score; US: ultrasound.

#### Authors' contributions

LV and GDR planned the study and drafted the manuscript. FB and IT collected data, helped develop the bibliography, and drafted the manuscript. GV, LP, and FF helped draft and edit the manuscript. All the authors have read and approved the final manuscript.

#### Author details

[1] Anesthesia and Intensive Care Medicine-Department of Medical and Biological Sciences, University of Udine, P.le S. M. della Misericordia 15, 33100 Udine, Italy. [2] Department of Emergency Medicine, San Luigi Gonzaga University Hospital, Turin, Italy. [3] Anesthesia and Intensive Care Medicine IV, Pisa University Hospital, Pisa, Italy.

#### Acknowledgements

No funds were received for the manuscript's preparation.

#### References

1. Goligher EC, Leis JA, Fowler RA, Pinto R, Adhikari NK, Ferguson ND (2011) Utility and safety of draining pleural effusions in mechanically ventilated patients: a systematic review and meta-analysis. Crit Care 15(1):R46
2. Nishida O, Arenallo R, Cheng DCH, DeMajo W, Kawanagh BP (1999) Gas exchange and hemodynamics in experimental pleural effusion. Crit Care Med 27:583–587
3. Razazi K, Thille AW, Carteaux G, Beji O, Brun-Buisson C, Brochard L, Mekontso Dessap A (2014) Effects of pleural effusion drainage on oxygenation, respiratory mechanics, and hemodynamics in mechanically ventilated patients. Ann Am Thorac Soc 11(7):1018–1024
4. Ramoska EA, Sacchetti AD, Warden TM (1988) Credentialing of emergency medicine physicians: support for delineation of privileges in invasive procedures. Am J Emerg Med 6:278–281
5. Sanders AB, Criss E, Witzke D (1986) Core content survey of undergraduate education in emergency medicine. Ann Emerg Med 15:6–11
6. Harris A, O'Driscoll BR, Turkington PM (2010) Survey of major complications of intercostal chest drain insertion in the UK. Postgrad Med J 86:68–72
7. Kwiatt M, Tarbox A, Seamon MJ, Swaroop M, Cipolla J, Allen C et al (2014) Thoracostomy tubes: a comprehensive review of complications and related topics. Int J Crit Illn Inj Sci 4(2):143–155
8. Gilbert TB, McGrath BJ, Soberman M (1993) Chest tubes: indications, placement, management and complications. J Intensive Care Med 8:73–86
9. Etoch SW, Bar-Natan MF, Miller FB, Richardson JD (1995) Tube thoracostomy. Factors related to complications. Arch Surg 130(5):521–525
10. Bailey RC (2000) Complications of tube thoracostomy in trauma. J Acid Emerg Med 17(2):111–114
11. Deneuville M (2002) Morbidity of percutaneous tube thoracostomy in trauma patients. Eur J Cardiothorac Surg 22(5):673–678
12. Wrightson JM, Fysh E, Maskell NA, Lee YC (2010) Risk reduction in pleural procedures: sonography, simulation and supervision. Curr Opin Pulm Med 16:340–350
13. See KC, Ong V, Teoh CM, Ooi OC, Widjaja LS, Mujumdar S et al (2014) Bedside pleural procedures by pulmonologists and non-pulmonologists: a 3-year safety audit. Respirology 19(3):396–402
14. Havelock T, Teoh R, Laws D, Gleeson F, BTS Pleural Disease Guideline Group (2010) Pleural procedures and thoracic ultrasound: British Thoracic Society pleural disease guideline. Thorax 65(Suppl 2):61–76
15. Mayo PH, Beaulieu Y, Doelken P, Feller-Kopman D, Harrod C, Kaplan A et al (2009) American College of Chest Physicians/La Société de Réanimation de Langue Française statement on competence in critical care ultrasonography. Chest 135(4):1050–1060
16. Salamonsen M, McGrath D, Steiler G, Ware R, Colt H, Fielding D (2013) A new instrument to assess physician skill at thoracic ultrasound, including pleural effusion markup. Chest 144(3):930–934
17. Jozwiak M, Monnet X, Cinotti R, Bontemps F, Reignier J, Belliard G (2014) Prospective assessment of a score for assessing basic critical-care transthoracic echocardiography skills in ventilated critically ill patients. Ann Intensive Care 27(4):12
18. Charron C, Prat G, Caille V, Belliard G, Lefèvre M, Aegerter P, Boles JM, Jardin F, Vieillard-Baron A (2007) Validation of a skills assessment scoring system for transesophageal echocardiographic monitoring of hemodynamics. Intensive Care Med 33(10):1712–1718
19. Wayne DB, Barsuk JH, O'Leary KJ, Fudala MJ, McGaghie WC (2008) Mastery learning of thoracentesis skills by internal medicine residents using simulation technology and deliberate practice. J Hosp Med 3(1):48–54
20. National Patient Safety Agency (2008) Risks of chest drain insertion. NSPA/2008/RRR003. http://www.npsa.nhs.uk/corporate/news/npsa-warns-of-risks-associated-with-chest-drains/
21. Diacon AH, Brutsche MH, Solèr M (2003) Accuracy of pleural puncture sites: a prospective comparison of clinical examination with ultrasound. Chest 123(2):436–441
22. Cavanna L, Mordenti P, Bertè R, Palladino MA, Biasini C, Anselmi E et al (2014) Ultrasound guidance reduces pneumothorax rate and improves safety of thoracentesis in malignant pleural effusion: report on 445 consecutive patients with advanced cancer. World J Surg Oncol 2(12):139

29

# The relationship between single and two-dimensional indices of left ventricular size using hemodynamic transesophageal echocardiography in trauma and burn patients

Duraid Younan[1], T. Mark Beasley[2,5], David C. Pigott[3*], C. Blayke Gibson[3], John P. Gullett[3], Jeffrey Richey[1], Jean-Francois Pittet[4] and Ahmed Zaky[4]

**Abstract**

**Background:** Conventional echocardiographic technique for assessment of volume status and cardiac contractility utilizes left ventricular end-diastolic area (LVEDA) and fractional area of change (FAC), respectively. Our goal was to find a technically reliable yet faster technique to evaluate volume status and contractility by measuring left ventricular end-diastolic diameter (LVEDD) and fractional shortening (FS) in a cohort of mechanically ventilated trauma and burn patients using hemodynamic transesophageal echocardiographic (hTEE) monitoring.

**Methods:** Retrospective chart review performed at trauma/burn intensive care unit (TBICU). Data on 88 mechanically ventilated surgical intensive care patients cared for between July 2013 and July 2015 were reviewed. Initial measurements of LVEDA, left ventricular end-systolic area (LVESA) and FAC were collected. Post-processing left ventricular end-systolic (LVESD) and end-diastolic diameters (LVEDD) were measured and fractional shortening (FS) was calculated. Two orthogonal measurements of LV diameter were obtained in transverse (Tr) and posteroanterior (PA) orientation.

**Results:** There was a significant correlation between transverse and posteroanterior left ventricular diameter measurements in both systole and diastole. In systole, $r = 0.92$, $p < 0.01$ for LVESD-Tr (mean 23.47 mm, SD $\pm$ 6.77) and LVESD-PA (mean 24.84 mm, SD = 8.23). In diastole, $r = 0.80$, $p < 0.01$ for LVEDD-Tr (mean 37.60 mm, SD $\pm$ 6.45), and LVEDD-PA diameters (mean 42.24 mm, SD $\pm$ 7.97). Left ventricular area (LVEDA) also significantly correlated with left ventricular diameter LVEDD-Tr ($r = 0.84$, $p < 0.01$) and LVEDD-PA ($r = 0.90$, $p < 0.01$). Both transverse and PA measurements of fractional shortening were significantly ($p < 0.0001$) and similarly correlated with systolic function as measured by FAC. Bland–Altman analyses also indicated that the assessment of fractional shortening using left ventricular posteroanterior diameter measurement shows agreement with FAC.

**Conclusions:** Left ventricular diameter measurements are a reliable and technically feasible alternative to left ventricular area measurements in the assessment of cardiac filling and systolic function.

**Keywords:** Transesophageal echocardiography, Left ventricular area, Left ventricular diameter, Resuscitation, Critical care, Ultrasonography, Trauma

*Correspondence: dpigott@uabmc.edu
[3] Department of Emergency Medicine, University of Alabama at Birmingham, Birmingham, AL, USA
Full list of author information is available at the end of the article

## Background

Historically, the assessment of volume status and cardiac function with the goal of achieving appropriate resuscitation targets has been an area of ongoing interest to intensivists worldwide. The pulmonary artery catheter has long been used in the intensive care unit (ICU) to evaluate volume status, cardiac function, and to guide resuscitation. Recently, multiple studies have questioned the benefits of pulmonary artery catheter use and increased the awareness of associated complications, resulting in a decline in its use [1, 2].

Recently, the debate between static and dynamic indices of volume responsiveness was resolved in favor of the latter with multiple studies demonstrating that central venous pressure lacks predictability as a measure of volume responsiveness [3] compared with stroke volume and pulse pressure variation [4]. It is important to mention, however, that the validity of dynamic indices is limited by the presence of spontaneous respiration, dysrhythmia, or vasopressor use [5].

Over the last few years, the use of bedside ultrasonography and echocardiography has expanded both in trauma and ICU settings; surgeons, intensivists, and emergency care physicians have developed training protocols to facilitate the ability to detect free fluid in the abdomen with high sensitivity and specificity [6]. The BEAT exam (Bedside Echocardiographic Assessment in Trauma/Critical Care) is an example of a bedside hemodynamic evaluation protocol that has been developed to assess stroke volume, the presence of pericardial or pleural effusion, ventricular function, size, and volume status [7].

Monoplane hemodynamic transesophageal echocardiography (hTEE; ImaCor, Inc., Garden City, NY) is a relatively new diagnostic tool, allowing the intensivist to directly assess both the contractility and filling status of both the right and left ventricles at the bedside in real-time. Unlike conventional transesophageal echocardiography (TEE) probes, the hTEE probe is smaller (5.5 mm in diameter), disposable, and can remain in place for up to 72 h, permitting continuous visual quantitative estimation of cardiac contractility and cardiac filling. The probe can be placed safely [8] in intubated patients by intensivists with a basic level of hTEE training without the need for formal training in conventional TEE [9]. Additionally, hTEE is only capable of displaying three echocardiographic windows compared with 28 views in the case of conventional TEE. The diagnostic yield of hTEE was shown to be non-inferior to thermodilution in the postoperative care of cardiac surgical patients [10]. In fact, information recovered from hTEE led to changes in the plan of care for those patients compared to those evaluated solely with thermodilution [8, 10]. In addition, hTEE was proven useful in weaning from ventriculoarterial extracorporeal membrane oxygenation (VA ECMO) [11], and has led to changes in intensive care management in patients with left ventricular assist devices [12]. To date, however, no validation studies have been performed to compare hTEE with conventional multiplane TEE.

Echocardiographically estimated fractional area of change (FAC) calculated as the percentage change between left ventricular end-systolic and end-diastolic areas (LVESA and LVEDA, respectively) has been used as a surrogate marker for left ventricular ejection fraction (and thus, systolic function). Similarly, LV preload can also be assessed using LVEDA with consistent accuracy [13]. Despite their obvious appeal, LV area-based measurements are time-consuming and challenging to obtain due to technical issues associated with chamber border detection. These measurements become even more challenging during periods of hemodynamic instability. Additionally, hTEE is incapable of measuring ejection fraction (EF) because it lacks the echocardiographic windows necessary to measure EF such as the midesophageal 2-chamber view. This limitation becomes more evident in current-generation hTEE systems that lack software capable of calculating end-systolic and end-diastolic volumes and hence performing automatic ejection fraction calculation. The current hTEE systems are only capable of calculating end-diastolic and end-systolic areas, requiring multiple manual steps for LV FAC calculation compared with conventional TEE systems that are capable of volumetric EF calculation.

In this study, the authors used hTEE to obtain LV diameter measurements to estimate left ventricular systolic function (using left ventricular fractional shortening), and filling status (using left ventricular end-diastolic diameter) as a technically feasible, less time-consuming alternative to area-based measurements.

## Methods

This is a retrospective chart review performed at the trauma and burn intensive care unit (TBICU) at the University of Alabama at Birmingham. After Institutional Review Board (IRB) approval, medical records and hTEE video clips of patients admitted to our TBICU between July 1, 2013 and July 1, 2015 were reviewed. Inclusion criteria were all mechanically ventilated trauma and burn patients admitted to our TBICU during the study period who underwent hTEE exam to evaluate volume status and hemodynamic stability, or with persistent hypotension (systolic blood pressure < 90 mmHg after a 1 L fluid bolus). Patients with poor-quality echocardiographic windows or with known or recognized wall motion abnormalities as agreed upon by two hTEE-trained examiners (DY and JR) or with incomplete data were excluded from the study.

hTEE exams were performed by an intensivist, resident staff, or a trained mid-level provider (physician assistant). We used all echocardiographic views available by hTEE to perform our evaluation of cardiac function and filling. We did not endorse a specific protocol for resuscitation. Personnel who performed the hTEE measurements were all previously trained in performing focused transthoracic echocardiography (TTE). Personnel who performed the hTEE measurements also attended a dedicated 6-hour hTEE training session. A total of ten hTEE exams performed independently were deemed sufficient to achieve competence. Exams were performed using monoplane hTEE (ImaCor ClariTEE, ImaCor, Inc., Garden City, NY). hTEE cineloops were stored and analyzed on the Imacor Zura imaging system (Imacor, Inc., Garden City, NY). The hTEE system used in this study was not equipped with automated border detection technology.

We obtained two perpendicular LV diameter measurements from video clips of the standard transgastric mid-papillary short-axis view. Diameter 1 (transverse–Tr) was obtained by measuring between the papillary muscles from the lateral wall to the septal wall in a transverse orientation (i.e., from 3 to 9 o'clock) while Diameter 2 (postero-anterior–PA) was obtained by measuring from the inferior wall to the anterior wall (corresponding to an inner diameter drawn between the mid-inferior and mid-anterior segments in the standard 17-segment echocardiographic model) [14], medial to the papillary muscles in a top-to-bottom orientation (i.e., from 12 to 6 o'clock) (Figs. 1, 2).

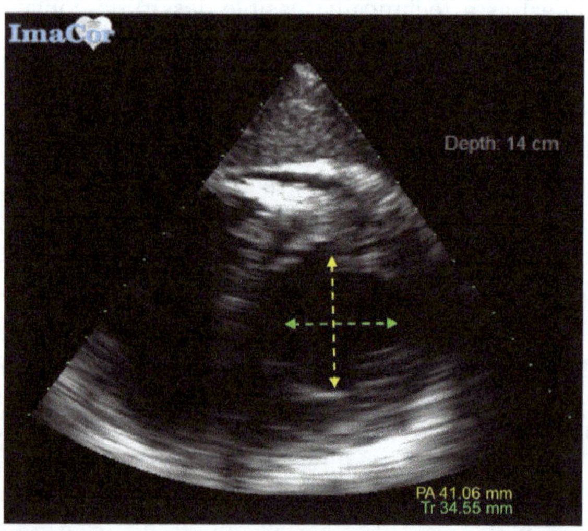


**Fig. 1** Transesophageal echocardiographic view demonstrating transverse and posteroanterior measurements of left ventricle in end-diastole

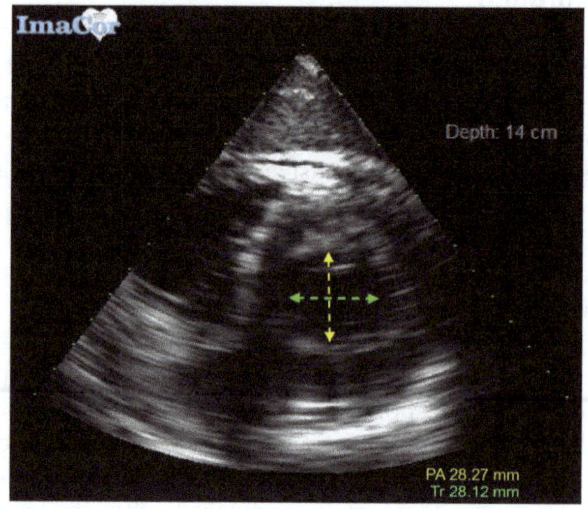


**Fig. 2** Transesophageal echocardiographic view demonstrating transverse and posteroanterior measurements of left ventricle in end-systole

Maximum end-diastolic diameters were determined by electrocardiography and echocardiography. All measurements were agreed upon by two hTEE-trained examiners (DY and JR). Evaluation of cardiac filling and contractility were obtained by using LVEDA and LVESA (Figs. 3, 4) measurements to calculate LV FAC, according to the following formula: FAC = (LVEDA − LVESA)/LVEDA. Transesophageal four-chamber views were not utilized in this study.

Left ventricular endocardial fractional shortening (FS), a surrogate marker for LV systolic function, was calculated using the formula, FS = (LVEDD − LVESD)/LVEDD, corresponding to the FAC formula based on LVEDA and LVESA measurements.

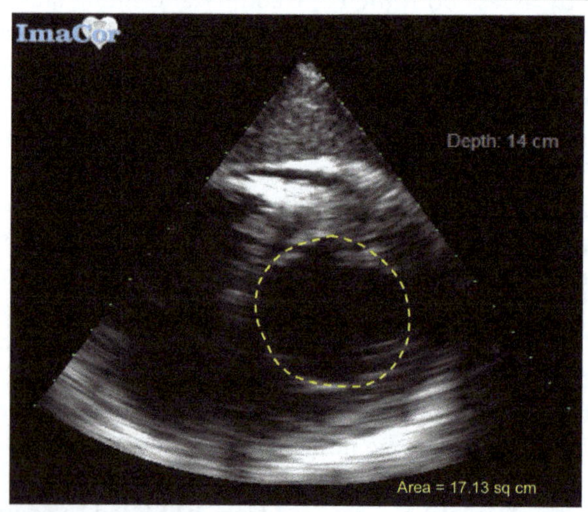


**Fig. 3** Transesophageal echocardiographic view demonstrating area tracing of left ventricle in end-diastole

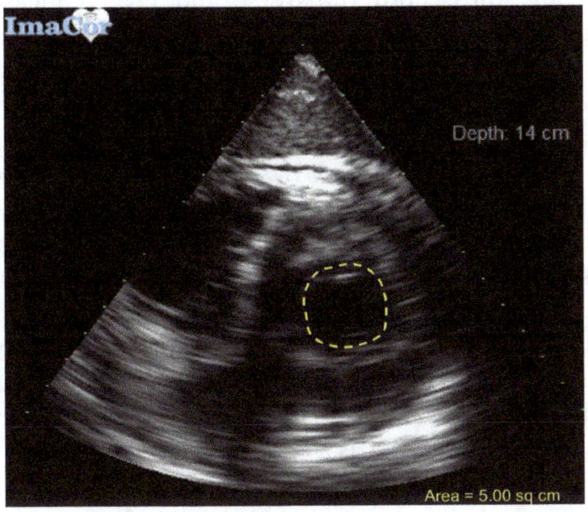


**Fig. 4** Transesophageal echocardiographic view demonstrating area tracing of left ventricle in end-systole

**Table 1 Patient demographics, $N = 88$**

| | (M ± SD) |
|---|---|
| Age (years) | 49.7 ± 20.7 |
| IVF (liters) | 6.7 ± 5.5 |
| Lactic acid (mg/dL) | 2.1 ± 1.6 |
| HCT (%) | 27.0 ± 5.1 |
| Time from admission to procedure (days) | 7.3 ± 8.5 |
| ICU stay (days) | 26.8 ± 19.1 |
| ISS | 23.4 ± 12.1 |
| Race | *N* (%) |
| White | 53 (60.2%) |
| Black | 29 (33.0%) |
| Other | 7 (6.8%) |
| Gender *N* (%) | |
| Male | 68 (77.3%) |
| Female | 20 (23.7%) |
| Injury type *N* (%) | |
| Trauma-blunt | 50 (56.8%) |
| Trauma-penetrating | 14 (15.9%) |
| Burn | 24 (27.3%) |
| Indication for test *N* (%) | |
| Sepsis | 26 (29.9%) |
| Trauma/burn volume assessment | 56 (63.3%) |
| Spinal cord injury (SCI) | 1 (1.1%) |
| ARDS | 4 (4.6%) |
| Cardiogenic shock | 1 (1.1%) |

### Statistical analysis

Pearson correlations were used to assess the relationships between area- and diameter-based measurements and FAC and FS ratios. With a sample size of approximately 100, we had 80% statistical power to detect correlation coefficients of $r = 0.277$ ($r^2 = 0.073$) or larger at a 5% level. The relationship between area- and diameter-based measurements and FAC were also examined using the Bland–Altman technique, which compares the difference in two measures to their mean. Specifically, the bias in measurement is reflected in the mean difference in measures, which was tested with a paired *t* test. Given the strong correlations among these measures, we had 80% statistical power to detect a difference of 0.16 standard deviation units at a 5% significance level. The covariance (correlation) between the difference in the mean is used to assess agreement, in that a significant correlation indicates poor agreement. The limits of agreement are defined as bias ± 1.96 (standard deviation of bias). All statistical analyses were performed using SAS 9.3 (SAS Institute, Inc., Cary, NC).

## Results

A total of 107 echocardiographic studies were performed during the study period. Eight patients had incomplete data and were excluded from the study, resulting in a total of 88 patients with 99 measurements.

Table 1 shows patient demographics. Patients were predominantly white, male with a mean Injury Severity Score (ISS) of 23.4 ± 12.1. The mean LVEDD-Tr was 37.60 mm (SD ± 6.45), whereas the mean LVEDD-PA was 42.24 mm (SD ± 7.97). A paired *t* test indicated that this difference in means was significant ($p < 0.0001$). There was a significant correlation between LVEDD-Tr and LVEDD-PA diameters ($r = 0.80$, $p < 0.0001$). The intraclass correlation coefficient (ICC) for LVEDD measures was 0.83.

The mean LVESD-Tr was 23.47 mm (SD ± 6.77); the mean LVESD-PA was 24.84 mm (SD ± 8.23); however, a paired *t* test indicated that this difference in means was significant (t (98) = 4.10, $p < 0.0001$). Pearson correlation indicated that the transverse and PA LVESD measures were significantly correlated ($r = 0.92$, $p < 0.0001$). The ICC for these LVESD measures was 0.93.

We also compared area-based (LVEDA) with diameter-based measurements (both transverse and PA LVEDD) as surrogates for LV preload. The LVEDA significantly correlated with LVEDD-Tr ($r = 0.84$, $p < 0.0001$) and LVEDD-PA ($r = 0.90$, $p < 0.0001$). Similarly, LVESA significantly correlated with LVESD-Tr ($r = 0.90$, $p < 0.0001$) and LVESD-PA ($r = 0.92$, $p < 0.0001$), respectively, suggesting that diameter-based and area-based measurements provide a similar assessment of LV preload.

We compared area-based FAC with diameter-based FS in both PA and transverse planes to evaluate contractility. Table 2 shows that both transverse- and PA-measured FS are significantly and similarly correlated to FAC

**Table 2 Mean ± standard deviations for FAC, FS and Pearson correlations for FAC with FS (both transverse and PA)**

| $N = 99$ | M ± SD | Correlation with FAC | Bland–Altman correlation |
|---|---|---|---|
| FAC | 58.08 ± 16.45 | | |
| FS transverse | 37.74 ± 13.29 | $r = 0.85$ $p < 0.0001$ | $r = 0.38$ $p = 0.0001$ |
| FS PA | 41.16 ± 15.29 | $r = 0.85$ $p < 0.0001$ | $r = 0.14$ $p = 0.1707$ |

FAC = (LVEDA − LVESA)/LVEDA; FS = (LVEDD − LVESD)/LVEDD
$p$ values for all correlations are $p < 0.0001$

($p < 0.0001$), indicating that each of these measurements has the potential to serve as proxy measure for contractility. The Bland–Altman technique tests the relationship between the mean of the two measures (e.g., FS and FAC) and their difference. A statistically significant relationship between the mean and the difference indicates that the two measures are not in close agreement. The results in Table 2 indicate a lack of agreement between FS-Tr and FAC. FS-PA, however, does show reasonable agreement with FAC, suggesting that it may be a feasible technique for estimating LV systolic function. There were no complications of probe placement in any of the patients included in this study.

## Discussion

This study demonstrates a correlation between area-based and diameter-based measurements of left ventricular contractility and preload. Despite this correlation, hTEE-based posterior–anterior and transverse measurements used in diameter-based calculations significantly differed in a cohort of mechanically ventilated trauma and burn patients. This difference may be explained by ventricular shape and geometry.

Our study is in line with previous studies that have used end-diastolic diameter as a surrogate marker for preload and in the assessment of contractility. Inoue et al. [15] in a cohort of 166 patients on hemodialysis found LVEDD to be an independent predictor of mortality. Our study differed from Inoue in that it was conducted on surgical patients and was not designed to study outcomes. Indovina et al. [16]. found that LVEDD better discriminates between patients with depressed and normal LV systolic function (based on ejection fraction) compared with LV end-diastolic volume measured by blood pool-gated radioisotopic angiography. The authors in that study used the end-diastolic transverse diameter. LVEDD was also found to be an independent predictor of recovery of left ventricular function after therapy in patients with dilated cardiomyopathy [17]. From the above-mentioned studies, it is reasonable to conclude that LVEDD has utility in the assessment of LV preload and contractility.

In our study, both transverse and PA FS measurements correlated with area-based FAC measurements. The higher correlation of transverse diameter compared with PA diameter with FAC measurements can likely be explained by the relatively easier and hence more consistent measurements of LV end-diastolic transverse diameter compared with LV end-diastolic PA diameter. It is important to note that both PA and transverse diameters are linear measurements and may vary from area measurement based on LV geometry in health and in disease. Equally important, LV geometry should only be measured in the context of accurate and adequate image acquisition, since imaging errors such as foreshortening may be misinterpreted as a change in LV geometry.

Additionally, diameter-based measurements, due to their linear nature, may not be applicable for patients with regional wall motion abnormalities such as the elderly or those with known ischemic heart disease. It is also important to note that the use of either area or diameter measurement does not preclude other methods of assessment and that the purpose of this study is to highlight a more feasible way of assessing cardiac filling and contractility for clinicians who are not formally trained in echocardiography. Whether a difference in clinical outcomes can be detected by either measurement remains to be determined in future studies.

As of now, there is no consensus on a formal training protocol for the use of hTEE as compared with conventional TEE. As a result, trainees are exposed most commonly to training protocols performed by the company representatives or by a trained echocardiographer at the bedside. Although hTEE training protocols provide significant utility, they may vary between institutions and currently lack accreditation. Likewise, hTEE-guided resuscitation protocols also vary between institutions and have not yet been validated in multicenter trials. A consensus on the appropriate level of mastery for basic hTEE use and goal-directed, hTEE-guided therapies is an important topic for future exploration in adequately powered studies.

## Limitations

Our study suffers from several limitations. First, diameters are linear rather than volume measurements. As such, they are more prone to missing LV pathology not incorporated in the area of measurement. It should be noted, however, that our study demonstrated a significant agreement between LV diameter and area. Second, an LV with greater mass may require higher filling pressures to manifest a change in diameter compared with an LV with smaller mass. Finally, our study suffers from the limitations of retrospective studies such as missing data, lack of a gold standard against which our measurements were made, reliance on qualitative rather than quantitative agreements between hTEE-trained individuals, and the absence of concomitant conventional transthoracic echocardiography to rule out cardiac abnormalities undetected by hTEE. However, we would like to emphasize that the goal of this paper was to test the correlation between two TEE-based methods of assessing cardiac filling and contractility. We did not attempt to explore the adequacy of either measurement in terms of outcomes or in terms of comparison to a gold standard.

## Conclusions

Further prospective, adequately powered studies are required to compare diameter-based measurements with previously validated volumetric measurements of left ventricular preload and contractility using a more standardized level of operator training. Similarly, the utility of diameter-based echocardiographic assessment for the evaluation of volume responsiveness and to guide resuscitation must be validated before its role in the resuscitation of critically ill or injured patients can be clearly established.

In conclusion, left ventricular diameter-based measurements are reliable, less technically challenging alternatives to area-based measurements in the assessment of cardiac filling and LV contractility. More studies are needed to compare the use of diameter-based measurements to left ventricular volumes as a gold standard for assessing left ventricular systolic function and preload. More studies are needed to examine the feasibility of performing LVEDD by less-experienced caregivers.

### Abbreviations

LV: left ventricle; LVEDA: left ventricular end-diastolic area; FAC: fractional area of change; LVEDD: left ventricular end-diastolic diameter; FS: fractional shortening; LVEDS: left ventricular end-systolic diameter; hTEE: hemodynamic transesophageal echocardiography; LVESA: left ventricular end-systolic area; LVEDD-Tr: left ventricular end-diastolic diameter, transverse; LVEDD-PA: left ventricular end-diastolic diameter, posteroanterior; ICU: intensive care unit; BEAT: Bedside Echocardiographic Assessment in Trauma/Critical Care; TEE: transesophageal echocardiography; ICC: intraclass correlation coefficient.

### Authors' contributions

DY contributed to conception and design, interpretation of data, and drafting and revision of article. TMB contributed to data analysis. DCP, CBG, JPG, and JFP contributed to interpretation of data, drafting, and revision of article. JR contributed to data acquisition, drafting, and revision of article. AZ contributed to conception and design, methodology, interpretation of data, and drafting and revision of article. All authors have provided final approval of the version submitted. All authors read and approved the final manuscript.

### Author details

[1] Department of Surgery, Division of Acute Care Surgery, University of Alabama at Birmingham, Birmingham, AL, USA. [2] Department of Biostatistics, University of Alabama at Birmingham, Birmingham, AL, USA. [3] Department of Emergency Medicine, University of Alabama at Birmingham, Birmingham, AL, USA. [4] Department of Anesthesiology and Perioperative Medicine, University of Alabama at Birmingham, Birmingham, AL, USA. [5] Birmingham/Atlanta VA Geriatric Research, Education, & Clinical Center, Department of Veteran's Affairs, Birmingham, AL, USA.

### Acknowledgements

Special thanks to the sonographer who performed the image measurements (area and diameter), an employee of ImaCor, Inc. (Garden City, NY).

### References

1. Chiang Y, Hosseinian L, Rhee A, Itagaki S, Cavallaro P, Chikwe J (2015) Questionable benefit of the pulmonary artery catheter after cardiac surgery in high-risk patients. J Cardiothorac Vasc Anesth 29:76–81
2. Tenaa B, Gomar C, Roux C, Fontanals J, Jimenez MJ, Rovira I et al (2008) Serious mechanical complications associated with pulmonary artery catheters in cardiovascular and thoracic surgery. Rev Esp Anestesiol Reanim 55:487–492
3. Marik PE, Baram M, Vahid B (2008) Does central venous pressure predict fluid responsiveness? A systematic review of the literature and the tale of seven mares. Chest 134:172–178
4. Wiesenack C, Fiegl C, Keyser A, Prasser C, Keyl C (2005) Assessment of fluid responsiveness in mechanically ventilated cardiac surgical patients. Eur J Anaesthesiol 22:658–665
5. Reuter DA, Felbinger TW, Schmidt C, Kilger E, Goedje O, Lamm P et al (2002) Stroke volume variations for assessment of cardiac responsiveness to volume loading in mechanically ventilated patients after cardiac surgery. Intensive Care Med 28:392–398
6. Rozycki GS, Ochsner MG, Jaffin JH, Champion HR (1993) Prospective evaluation of surgeons' use of ultrasound in the evaluation of trauma patients. J Trauma 34:516–526 **(discussion 526–517)**
7. Gunst M, Sperry J, Ghaemmaghami V, O'keeffe T, Friese R, Frankel H (2008) Bedside echocardiographic assessment for trauma/critical care: the BEAT exam. J Am Coll Surg 207:e1–e3
8. Sarosiek K, Kang CY, Johnson CM, Pitcher H, Hirose H, Cavarocchi NC (2014) Perioperative use of the imacor hemodynamic transesophageal echocardiography probe in cardiac surgery patients: initial experience. ASAIO J 60(5):553–558
9. Fletcher N, Geisen M, Meeran H, Spray D, Cecconi M (2015) Initial clinical experience with a miniaturized transesophageal echocardiography probe in a cardiac intensive care unit. J Cardiothorac Vasc Anesth 29(3):582–587
10. Treskatsch S, Balzer F, Knebel F et al (2015) Feasibility and influence of hTEE monitoring on postoperative management in cardiac surgery patients. Int J Cardiovasc Imaging 31(7):1327–1335
11. Cavarocchi NC, Pitcher HT, Yang Q et al (2013) Weaning of extracorporeal membrane oxygenation using continuous hemodynamic transesophageal echocardiography. J Thorac Cardiovasc Surg 146(6):1474–1479
12. Haglund NA, Maltais S, Bick JS et al (2014) Hemodynamic transesophageal echocardiography after left ventricular assist device implantation. J Cardiothorac Vasc Anesth 28(5):1184–1190
13. Preisman S, Kogan S, Berkenstadt H, Perel A (2005) Predicting fluid responsiveness in patients undergoing cardiac surgery: functional haemodynamic parameters including the Respiratory Systolic Variation Test and static preload indicators. Br J Anaesth 95:746–755
14. Cerqueira MD, Weissman NJ, Dilsizian V et al (2002) Standardized myocardial segmentation and nomenclature for tomographic imaging of the heart. A statement for healthcare professionals from the Cardiac Imaging Committee of the Council on Clinical Cardiology of the American Heart Association. Circulation 105(4):539–542
15. Inoue T, Ogawa T, Iwabuchi Y, Otsuka K, Nitta K (2012) Left ventricular end-diastolic diameter is an independent predictor of mortality in hemodialysis patients. Ther Apheresis Dial 16:134–141
16. Indovina A (2000) Evaluation of heart dysfunction using non-invasive methods. A comparison between left ventricular end diastolic volume measured using blood pool gated radioisotope angiography and left ventricular transverse end diastolic diameter measured using two dimensional echocardiography. Minerva Cardioangiol 48:149–154
17. Zou C, Wu X, Zhou Q, Zhang Y, Lyu R, Zhang J (2014) Frequency and predictors of recovery of normal left ventricular ejection fraction and end-diastolic diameter in patients with dilated cardiomyopathy. Zhonghua xin xue guan bing za zhi 42:851–855

# 30

# Transient systolic anterior motion with junctional rhythm after mitral valve repair in the intensive care unit

Yusuke Seino*, Nobuo Sato, Kimiya Fukui, Junya Ishikawa, Masahi Nakagawa and Takeshi Nomura

**Abstract**

Systolic anterior motion (SAM) after mitral valve repair (MVR) can adversely affect hemodynamics due to exacerbation of left ventricular outflow tract obstruction and mitral regurgitation. Intraoperative transient SAM after MVR can usually be managed with hemodynamic maneuvers under continuous monitoring by transesophageal echocardiography (TEE). However, during postoperative intensive care management, transient SAM is seldom diagnosed and the start of treatment may be delayed. We present a case of transient SAM after MVR with abrupt deterioration due to junctional rhythm in the intensive care unit (ICU). TEE revealed that conversion from normal sinus rhythm into junctional rhythm induced the exacerbation of SAM. TEE was useful for identifying the etiology of unstable hemodynamics after cardiac surgery in the ICU, similar to its use in the operating room.

**Keywords:** Systolic anterior motion, Left ventricular outflow tract obstruction, Mitral valve repair, Transesophageal echocardiography

## Background

Systolic anterior motion (SAM) after mitral valve repair (MVR) can adversely affect hemodynamics due to exacerbation of left ventricular outflow tract obstruction (LVOTO) and mitral regurgitation (MR) [1]. Although some mechanisms are understood, the effect of junctional rhythm on SAM, LVOTO, and MR remains unclear [1, 2]. Intraoperative transient SAM is usually diagnosed with transesophageal echocardiography (TEE), and should immediately be treated with hemodynamic agents under TEE monitoring. However, transient SAM in the ICU due to junctional rhythm without signs of ischemia can be difficult to diagnose. Even in this case, SAM cannot be thought of as the cause of hemodynamic disorder. Only TEE observation after an event can assist in the choice of treatment.

*Correspondence: yu-seino@twmu.ac.jp
Department of Intensive Care Medicine, Tokyo Women's Medical University, 8-1, Kawada-cho, Shinjuku-ku, Tokyo, Japan

## Case presentation

A 55-year-old man with severe MR and middle scallop prolapse due to torn chordae underwent MVR. Preoperative LV ejection fraction, tricuspid annular plane systolic excursion and right ventricular fractional area change were 62%, 26 mm and 44%, respectively. MVR was performed with folding middle scallop and annuloplasty with a 30-mm Physio II annuloplasty ring (Edwards Lifesciences LLC, Irvine, CA, USA). MR was well controlled. Despite difficulty weaning from cardiopulmonary bypass and some persistent surgical bleeding, he was hemodynamically stabilized on admission to the ICU without evidence of SAM and LVOTO.

He became hemodynamically unstable on the first postoperative day, with parameters as follows: heart rate 87 beats/min (bpm), sinus rhythm, arterial pressure 80/48 mmHg, pulmonary artery pressure 28/20 mmHg, central venous pressure 17 mmHg, cardiac index 1.7 L/min/m$^2$, right ventricular stroke work index (RVSWI) 1.6 g/m$^2$/beat, and mixed venous oxygen saturation ($SvO_2$) 54%.

Transthoracic echocardiography (TTE) was performed to investigate the cause of hemodynamic deterioration;

however, adequate images could not be obtained. TEE was then performed and showed right ventricular (RV) dysfunction without SAM and LVOTO. We decided to increase the dose of inotrope (adrenaline) to improve RV function and the hemodynamics stabilized.

Severe hypotension developed on the second postoperative day. Hemodynamic parameters were as follows: heart rate 90 bpm, arterial pressure 50/42 mmHg, pulmonary artery pressure 28/20 mmHg, central venous pressure 13 mmHg, cardiac index 1.6 L/min/m$^2$, RVSWI 2.4 g/m$^2$/beat, and $SvO_2$ 48%. The ventilator settings were as follows: pressure assist-control ventilation, respiratory rate 14 breaths/min, peak inspiratory pressure 16 $cmH_2O$, inspiration time 1.6 s, positive end-expiratory pressure 10 $cmH_2O$, and fraction of inspiratory oxygen 0.6.

Although the dose of dopamine, dobutamine and adrenaline was greatly increased to 5.4 μg/kg/min, 5.4 μg/kg/min and 0.05 μg/kg/min, respectively, and intra-aortic balloon pumping was started, hemodynamic parameters did not show improvement. No pulmonary vasodilator was used because of avoiding hypotension.

Repeat TEE revealed the hyperdynamic left ventricle (LV) without any regional wall motion abnormality, as well as LVOTO and severe MR (vena contracta 8 mm) due to SAM (Fig. 1; Additional file 1). In addition, RV dysfunction was still presented. We immediately reduced the inotrope dose and started vasopressors (vasopressin 2 unit/h) with volume loading (acetate Ringer 500 mL and 5% albumin 250 mL). SAM, LVOTO, and MR rapidly resolved and hemodynamic parameters stabilized. However, when normal sinus rhythm converted into junctional rhythm, SAM, LVOTO and severe MR recurred and hemodynamic parameters again became unstable (Figs. 2, 3; Additional files 2, 3, 4). TEE showed that conversion from normal sinus rhythm into junctional rhythm worsened the severity of SAM, LVOTO, and MR. The electrocardiogram showed junctional rhythm alternating with sinus rhythm, repeated at short intervals. We found that the rhythm change had a significant effect on the emergence of SAM and hemodynamic deterioration. Temporary atrial pacing was used to stabilize the heart rhythm. After starting atrial pacing, the hemodynamics stabilized and SAM, LVOTO, and MR did not recur (Fig. 4). He discharged from ICU on the 22nd postoperative day and from the hospital on the 43rd postoperative day.

## Conclusions

We identified two important clinical issues. Junctional rhythm can cause deterioration of SAM, LVOTO, and MR, and atrial pacing can improve hemodynamics in unstable normal sinus rhythm. TEE is useful for the identification of causes of unstable hemodynamics after cardiac surgery in the ICU as well as in the operating room.

First, junctional rhythm can cause deterioration of SAM, LVOTO, and MR and atrial pacing can improve hemodynamics. Some mechanisms of SAM are related to geometric factors, kinetic factors, and structural abnormalities [3]. Geometric factors include annular undersizing, anterior mitral valve displacement, low anterior:posterior leaflet length ratio, reduced mitro-aortic angle, and distance reduction between the MV coaptation point and interventricular septum [4]. Hyperdynamic LV is a kinetic factor. Structural abnormalities include small LV, chordal anomalies, bulging interventricular septum, papillary muscle displacement, redundant posterior leaflet, and redundant anterior leaflet. Some authors reported that ventricular pacing or atrioventricular sequential pacing can affect the severity of

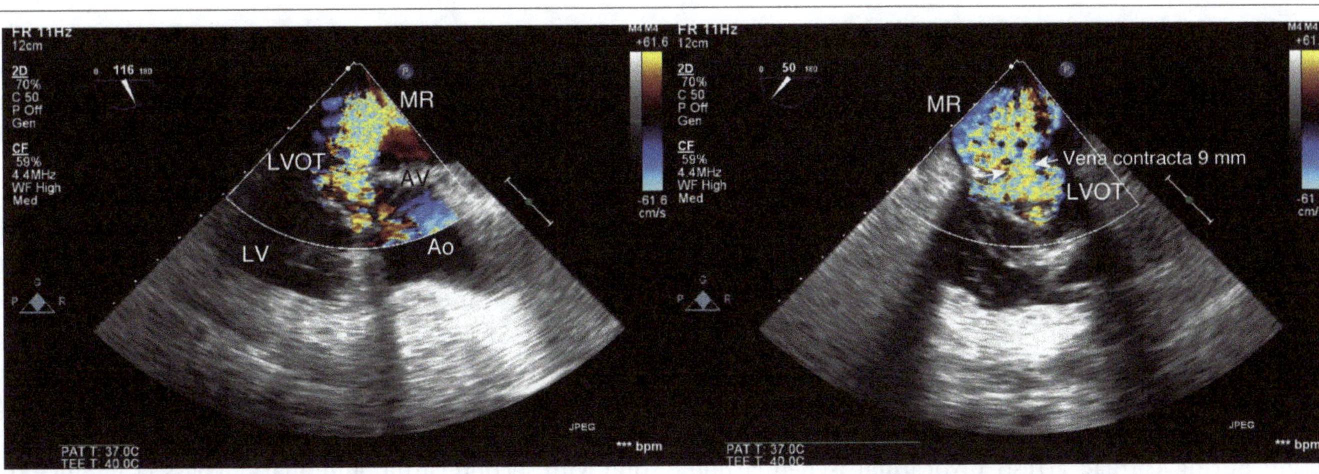


**Fig. 1** Massive mitral regurgitation and turbulent flow in the left ventricular outflow tract. *MR* mitral regurgitation, *LVOT* left ventricular outflow tract, *Ao* ascending aorta, *AV* aortic valve, *LV* left ventricle

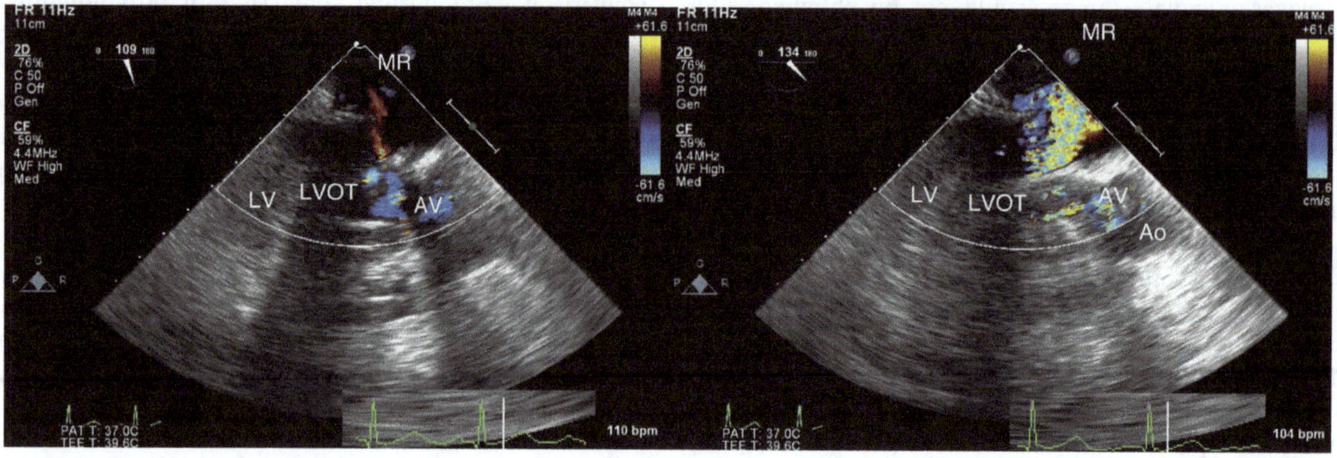


**Fig. 2** Mitral regurgitation in normal sinus rhythm (left) and junctional rhythm (right). *MR* mitral regurgitation, *LVOT* left ventricular outflow tract, *Ao* ascending aorta, *AV* aortic valve, *LV* left ventricle

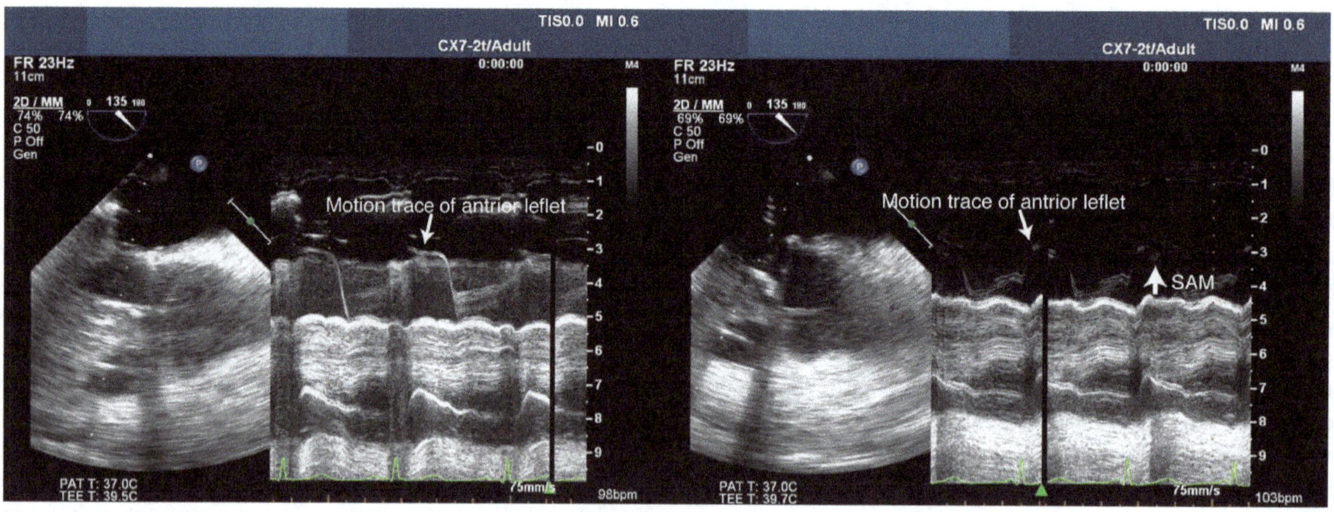


**Fig. 3** Motion tracing of the anterior leaflet in normal sinus rhythm (left) and junctional rhythm (right). Systolic anterior motion (SAM) is shown in junctional rhythm (large arrow)

SAM [5, 6]. In the present case, junctional rhythm caused deterioration of SAM. Junctional rhythm causes atrioventricular dyssynchrony and loss of atrial kick. These can contribute to decreases in mean arterial pressure and cardiac output by approximately 15% and the decreases can be accentuated in patients with heart disease [7, 8]. The mechanism by which junctional rhythm causes deterioration of SAM might be the impairment of LV filling due to atrioventricular dyssynchrony and loss of the atrial kick in junctional rhythm. In addition, underlying right ventricular dysfunction also plays a role in LV underfilling. There are some causes of RV dysfunction after cardiac surgery including inadequate myocardial protection during cardiac arrest, myocardial ischemia due to residual air, high pulmonary vascular resistance, and inadequate settings of mechanical ventilation [9]. In the present case, the right cause of RV dysfunction is unclear; however, long CPB, residual air, compression for control of bleeding by the surgeons might be related to RV dysfunction.

The management of SAM depends on the underlying mechanism and severity. In most cases, volume loading, discontinuation or reduction of inotropic drugs, and administration of beta blockers and vasopressors can resolve SAM [10–12]. It has been demonstrated that conservative hemodynamic maneuvers for intraoperative transient SAM are reliable and result in good clinical outcomes, although some cases require surgical correction with second cardiopulmonary bypass [13]. Since the present case had right ventricular failure, maintaining

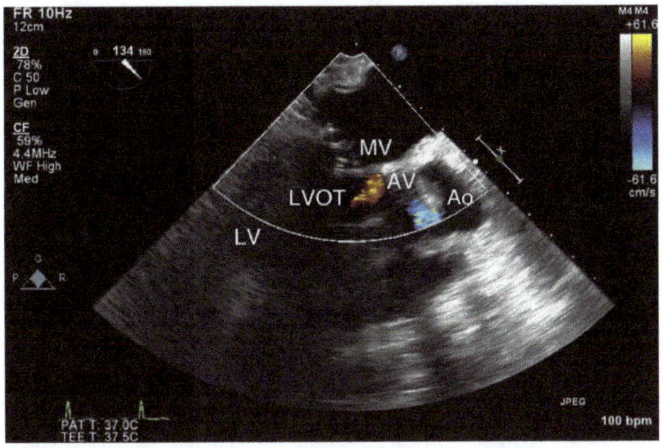


**Fig. 4** Mid-esophageal long axis view under atrial pacing on the sixth postoperative day. There is no mitral regurgitation and left ventricular outflow tract obstruction. *MV* mitral valve, *LVOT* left ventricular outflow tract, *Ao* ascending aorta, *AV* aortic valve, *LV* left ventricle

normal sinus rhythm seemed to be more important than in patients without right ventricular failure [14].

Second, TEE in the ICU is useful for the identification of causes of unstable hemodynamics after cardiac surgery. The usefulness of echocardiography for diagnosis and decision-making has been shown in the ICU, and basic echocardiography skills have become mandatory for all intensivists in some guidelines [15–17]. On the other hand, the use of TEE is reserved for instances in which diagnostic information for clinical decision-making cannot be obtained by TTE in a timely manner. However, TEE is considered an advanced skill and is not considered a minimum requirement for intensivists [17–19].

After cardiac surgery, obtaining useful images is sometimes difficult due to the narrowing of acoustic windows caused by the surgical incision, drapes, and drains. In addition, unclear images are insufficient for clinical decision-making in critical situations. Strengths of TEE include less dependence on operator skills and better spatial resolution compared to that of TTE [20]. In the present patient, the causes of recurrent hemodynamic exacerbation were different and could not be diagnosed without TEE. Basic hemodynamic assessment with TEE is not that difficult and training in basic TEE skills with simulators is evolving [21, 22]. Thus, the barrier to learning of basic TEE skills by intensivists can be overcome.

This case report shows that junctional rhythm can cause deterioration of SAM, LVOTO, and MR, and can lead to unstable hemodynamics in a patient with right ventricular failure after MVR. Atrial pacing can resolve SAM, LVOTO, and MR and can improve hemodynamics in a patient with unstable normal sinus rhythm. TEE in the ICU can play a pivotal role in clinical decision-making. Given that there are various causes of hemodynamic deterioration after cardiac surgery and some cannot be diagnosed without TEE, both TTE and basic TEE skills are required for intensivists.

## Additional files

**Additional file 1.** Mid-esophageal long axis view on the second postoperative day. Massive mitral regurgitation and turbulent flow is seen in the left ventricular outflow tract.

**Additional file 2.** Mid-esophageal long axis view in normal sinus rhythm.

**Additional file 3.** Mid-esophageal long axis view in junctional rhythm.

**Additional file 4.** Mid-esophageal long axis view in junctional rhythm (2-dimensional mode).

### Abbreviations

ICU: intensive care unit; LVOTO: left ventricular outflow tract obstruction; MR: mitral regurgitation; MVR: mitral valve repair; RVSWI: right ventricular stroke work index; SAM: systolic anterior motion; $SvO_2$: mixed venous oxygen saturation; TEE: transesophageal echocardiography; TTE: transthoracic echocardiography.

### Author contributions

YS performed ultrasound imaging, conducted the literature review, and wrote the manuscript. TN reviewed and edited the manuscript. MN, JI, NS, and KF reviewed and commented on the manuscript. All authors read and approved the final manuscript.

### References

1. Alfieri O, Lapenna E (2015) Systolic anterior motion after mitral valve repair: where do we stand in 2015? Eur J Cardiothorac Surg 48:344–346
2. Loulmet DF, Yaffee DW, Ursomanno PA, Rabinovich AE, Applebaum RM, Galloway AC, Grossi EA (2014) Systolic anterior motion of the mitral valve: a 30-year perspective. J Thorac Cardiovasc Surg 148:2787–2793
3. Ibrahim M, Rao C, Ashrafian H, Chaudhry U, Darzi A, Athanasiou T (2012) Modern management of systolic anterior motion of the mitral valve. Eur J Cardiothorac Surg 41:1260–1270
4. Maslow AD, Regan MM, Haering JM, Johnson RG, Levine RA (1999) Echocardiographic predictors of left ventricular outflow tract obstruction and systolic anterior motion of the mitral valve after mitral valve reconstruction for myxomatous valve disease. J Am Coll Cardiol 34:2096–2104
5. Milas BL, Bavaria JE, Koch CG, Troianos CA (2001) Case 8-2001. Resolution of systolic anterior motion after mitral valve repair with atrial pacing. J Cardiothorac Vasc Anesth 15:641–648
6. Ushijima T, Nishida T, Kan-O M, Tominaga R (2016) Left ventricular pacing can be a complementary solution for systolic anterior motion after mitral valve plasty. Eur J Cardiothorac Surg 49:1004–1005
7. Landesberg G, Hillel Z (2015) Electrocardiography, perioperative ischemia, and myocardial infarction. In: Miller RD (ed) Miller's anesthesia, 8th edn. Saunders, Philadelphia
8. Haldemann G, Schaer H (1972) Haemodynamic effects of transient atrioventricular dissociation in general anaesthesia. Br J Anaesth 44:159–162
9. Haddad F, Couture P, Tousignant C, Denault AY (2009) The right ventricle in cardiac surgery, a perioperative perspective: II. Pathophysiology, clinical importance, and management. Anesth Analg 108:422–433
10. Brown ML, Abel MD, Click RL, Morford RG, Dearani JA, Sundt TM, Orszulak TA, Schaff HV (2007) Systolic anterior motion after mitral valve repair: is surgical intervention necessary? J Thorac Cardiovasc Surg 133:136–143
11. Crescenzi G, Landoni G, Zangrillo A, Guarracino F, Rosica C, La Canna G, Alfieri O (2009) Management and decision-making strategy for systolic anterior motion after mitral valve repair. J Thorac Cardiovasc Surg 137:320–325

12. Varghese R, Anyanwu AC, Itagaki S, Milla F, Castillo J, Adams DH (2012) Management of systolic anterior motion after mitral valve repair: an algorithm. J Thorac Cardiovasc Surg 143:S2–S7
13. Kuperstein R, Spiegelstein D, Rotem G, Stein M, Kogan A, Sternik L, Raanani E (2015) Late clinical outcome of transient intraoperative systolic anterior motion post mitral valve repair. J Thorac Cardiovasc Surg 149:471–476
14. Haddad F, Doyle R, Murphy DJ, Hunt SA (2008) Right ventricular function in cardiovascular disease, part II: pathophysiology, clinical importance, and management of right ventricular failure. Circulation 117:1717–1731
15. Expert Round Table on Ultrasound in ICU (2011) International expert statement on training standards for critical care ultrasonography. Intensive Care Med 37:1077–1083
16. Expert Round Table on Echocardiography in ICU (2014) International consensus statement on training standards for advanced critical care echocardiography. Intensive Care Med 40:654–666
17. Levitov A, Frankel HL, Blaivas M, Kirkpatrick AW, Su E, Evans D, Summerfield DT, Slonim A, Breitkreutz R, Price S, McLaughlin M, Marik PE, ElBarbary M (2016) Guidelines for the appropriate use of bedside general and cardiac ultrasonography in the evaluation of critically ill patients-part II: cardiac ultrasonography. Crit Care Med 44:1206–1227
18. American Society of Anesthesiologists and Society of Cardiovascular Anesthesiologists Task Force on Transesophageal Echocardiography (2010) Practice guidelines for perioperative transesophageal echocardiography. An updated report by the American Society of Anesthesiologists and the Society of Cardiovascular Anesthesiologists Task Force on Transesophageal Echocardiography. Anesthesiology 112:1084–1096
19. Mayo PH, Narasimhan M, Koenig S (2015) Critical care transesophageal echocardiography. Chest 148:1323–1332
20. Mayo P, Mekontso Dessap A, Dessap AM, Vieillard-Baron A (2015) Myths about critical care echocardiography: the ten false beliefs that intensivists should understand. Intensive Care Med 41:1103–1106
21. Vignon P, Merz TM, Vieillard-Baron A (2017) Ten reasons for performing hemodynamic monitoring using transesophageal echocardiography. Intensive Care Med 43:1048–1051
22. Jelacic S, Bowdle A, Togashi K, VonHomeyer P (2013) The use of TEE simulation in teaching basic echocardiography skills to senior anesthesiology residents. J Cardiothorac Vasc Anesth 27:670–675

# 31

# Early abnormal transient hyperemic response test can predict delayed ischemic neurologic deficit in subarachnoid hemorrhage

Hosam Al-Jehani[1,2,3,4*], Mark Angle[1], Judith Marcoux[3] and Jeanne Teitelbaum[1]

**Abstract**

**Background:** Early detection of vasospasm is crucial to prevent significant delayed ischemic neurological deficit post subarachnoid hemorrhage. The standard methods of detection, including cerebral angiogram and computed tomography are invasive and not safe to be repeated, as is very often indicated clinically. Transient hyperemic response test has been previously used to predict autoregulation failure in traumatic brain injury and subarachnoid hemorrhage.

**Aims:** We investigate the usability of transient hyperemic response test as a predictor of clinical vasospasm in a cohort of patients with aneurismal subarachnoid hemorrhage.

**Methods:** A retrospective review of all THRT examinations done between January 2011 and July 2012 conducted at Montreal Neurological Institute and Hospital and the Montreal General Hospital. Patients diagnosed with aSAH in which the THRT was performed within the first 24–48 h of admission were included in the study. Two-dimensional transcranial Doppler images were obtained and velocities were recorded. A positive response was one in which the velocity was increased by more than 9% of the baseline systolic velocity, indicating an intact cerebral autoregulation. Lindegaard ratio > 3 is considered abnormal and in the context of elevated systolic velocity of the MCA, is highly suggestive of DIND.

**Results:** Fifteen patients met the inclusion criteria. A total of 6 patients developed clinical and radiological vasospasm. Out of these 6 patients, 5 (83%) had an abnormal THRT in the initial TCD assessment ($p = 0.0406$). We found that abnormal transient hyperemic response test readings are predictive of subsequent vasospasm development.

**Conclusions:** The results of this small retrospective study support the notion that transient hyperemic response test has predictive value in vasospasm development and may prove useful in patient monitoring and successful clinical management.

**Keywords:** Transient hyperemic response test (THRT), Delayed ischemic neurologic deficit (DIND), Vasospasm (VS), Subarachnoid hemorrhage (SAH)

## Background

Vasospasm (VS) and its clinical counterpart, delayed ischemic neurological deficit (DIND), are common causes of morbidity and mortality in patients suffering from subarachnoid hemorrhage (SAH). There are multiple causes of VS but the most frequent are traumatic brain injury and aneurysmal SAH [1, 2]. Aneurysmal SAH carries a significant risk of morbidity and high mortality rate. Survivors of SAH are often faced with sequelae of their hemorrhage and as many as 17–40% of SAH sufferers develop vasospasm and subsequent neurological deficits [1, 2]. As a result, only a small percentage of all survivors return to their premorbid “normal” condition.

DIND is a common complication clinically detected in 30–40% of patients with aneurysmal SAH, although it might be angiographically present in up to 70% of a SAH patients [3, 4]. It usually begins between day 4 and

*Correspondence: hjehani@iau.edu.sa
[1] Neurocritical Care Unit, Montreal Neurological Institute and Hospital, McGill University, Montreal, QC, Canada
Full list of author information is available at the end of the article

7 post aneurysmal SAH episode and is heralded by a new neurological deficit or worsening of an existing one. Other metabolic and homeostatic derangements such as inflammation, microvascular dysfunction, or cerebral edema have also been described [3, 5].

Although the gold standard for diagnosis of vasospasm and DIND is a cerebral angiogram [6], several non-invasive tests are available to clinicians to better detect vasospasm. These include, but not limited to TCD, [7, 8] and more recently improved application in CT perfusion [9, 10]. However, for the most part, these applications are non-diagnostic of DIND. Another major concern with these imaging modalities is that irrespective of how informative they are, the radiation doses and contrast material involved in their generation, limit their utility as dynamic tests to go along with the clinical evolution in the short-term or better still, in real time. This has major drawbacks for the very nature of the decision-making process required in a critical care setting. This raises the need for a test that can be safely repeated and is informative in the realm of parameters affecting clinical care decisions.

Here, we investigate the utility of THRT as a predictor of clinical DIND in a cohort of patients with aSAH. The results of this small retrospective study may shed some light on the initial autoregulatory mechanism in patients presenting with aSAH.

## Methods

### Study design and equipment

A retrospective review of all THRT examinations done between January 2011 and July 2012 conducted at the intensive care units of the Montreal Neurological Institute and Hospital and the Montreal General Hospital. Both of these hospitals are tertiary care neurology and neurosurgery centers. All the procedures were carried out after ethical review and according to the hospitals safety protocols. Patient consent was received prior to accessing retrospective data. All of the TCD examinations were performed by a single operator (HA). All examinations were performed on a Zonare TCD ultrasound machine using the modifiable range 2–4 m Hz P4-1c Phased Array probe (ZONARE Medical Systems, Inc., Mountain View, CA, USA).

### Sample selection

Twenty-one patients with a diagnosis of aSAH in which the THRT was performed within the first 24–48 h of admission were included in the study. Patients for whom the TCD examination was not possible, due to absent or suboptimal temporal insonation window, were excluded. Patients unable to tolerate the THRT due to induced bradycardia were also excluded. To harmonize the cohort, patients with severe carotid artery disease as well as with traumatic SAH associated with significant other traumatic intracranial lesions, such as contusions and diffuse brain swelling, were excluded from the sample.

### Data acquisition

Two-dimensional transcranial Doppler images were obtained and velocities were recorded. The THRT technique was used according to the method described previously [11]. In brief, while insonating the middle cerebral artery (MCA), the common carotid artery was occluded in the neck. The carotid artery was identified either by circulation arrest on the Doppler signal of the MCA or, to account for cross flow from the contributors of circle of Willis, more than 30% reduction of the systolic velocity of the middle cerebral artery. The compression was carried out for 5–9 s. Then, upon restoration of circulation, the first systolic peak was ignored and the following three systolic velocity peaks were kept for analysis and averaged. A positive response was one in which the velocity was increased by more than 9% of the baseline systolic velocity, indicating an intact cerebral autoregulation. The TCD was repeated every 48 h.

### Data analysis

Lindegaard ratio is defined as the ratio between the velocities in the MCA to that of the extracranial internal carotid artery. A ratio greater than three is considered abnormal, and in the context of elevated systolic velocity of the MCA, is highly suggestive of DIND. In some patients, a computerized tomography angiogram or a formal digital subtraction angiography was performed within the first 24–48 h of admission and this data was included in the analysis of our cohort. The statistical analysis of calculating the means, Fisher contingency tables, and the likelihood ratio were performed on Graph pad prism software (version 4.0, 2010).

## Results

### Patient data, demographics, and incidence of DIND

A total of 21 patients were initially reviewed. Three patients with traumatic SAH due to associated contusions and diffuse brain swelling, and two other patients with carotid artery disease in the form of fibromuscular dysplasia in one and severe atherosclerotic disease in the other were excluded. Two patients suffered a transient bradycardic response at the time of the first carotid compression and further testing was abandoned with no other adverse events reported due to the administration of the test. The remaining 15 patients were: 11 females and four males with an age ranging from 42 to 74 years with resulting sample mean age of 54.8 years. The distribution of these patients along the Hunt and Hess scale, location of aneurysms, and treatment offered to secure the aneurysms are presented in Table 1. The majority of the patients were grade 1–3 ($n = 10$) on the Hunt and Hess scale and the remainders were grade 4–5 ($n = 5$). Five patients were submitted to microsurgical clipping of the aneurysms and eight for endovascular coiling. Two patients were considered idiopathic SAH as no source of the SAH was identified on vascular imaging. Of the 15 patients treated in the NICU, six (40%) developed symptomatic DIND necessitating introduction of the Montreal Neurological Hospital's protocol. Two additional patients developed an asymptomatic vasospasm seen on vascular imaging with no treatment offered giving rise to a total incidence in vasospasm of 53.3%.

**Early abnormal THRT predicted development of DIND**

On initial TCD evaluations, five patients had MCA velocity greater than 120 cm/s. Of those patients, only one patient developed vasospasm in subsequent course. In comparing the group of patients with symptomatic vasospasm ($n = 6$) to those with asymptomatic or no vasospasm ($n = 9$), we found that five out of the six patients (83%) in the vasospasm group had an abnormal THRT ($p = 0.0406$, Fisher's exact test, two-tailed) (sensitivity 83%, specificity 78%, PPV 71%, NPP 88%) (Table 2).

Two patients with asymptomatic vasospasm showed an abnormal THRT, and with the global cohort incidence of vasospasm of 53.3% (8 out of 15 patients); there is a significant predictability of THRT to future development of vasospasm ($p = 0.0002$, Fisher's exact test, two-tailed, likelihood ratio 3.4) (Table 3). This is comparable to the predictability of the Lindegaard ratio for vasospasm in our cohort (50% with vasospasm and 22% with no vasospasm, $p = 0.0003$, *data not shown*).

**Table 1 Patient demographics**

| Patient no. | Age and gender | Location of aneurysms | Hunt and Hess grade | Treatment |
|---|---|---|---|---|
| 1 | 53, F | SAH, MCA | 1 | Clipping |
| 2 | 54, F | SAH, MCA, ICH | 4 | Clipping |
| 3 | 57, M | SAH, Acom | 2 | Coiling |
| 4 | 49, M | SAH, MCA, ICH | 5 | Clipping |
| 5 | 48, F | SAH, MCA | 1 | Coiling |
| 6 | 45, F | SAH, negative | 1 | None |
| 7 | 58, M | SAH, Pcom | 1 | Coiling |
| 8 | 42, F | SAH, ICA, HIE | 4 | Coiling |
| 9 | 49, F | SAH, negative | 3 | None |
| 10 | 74, F | SAH, Pcom | 1 | Coiling |
| 11 | 55, F | SAH, Acom | 3 | Clipping |
| 12 | 48, F | SAH, Basilar, IVH | 4 | Coiling |
| 13 | 74, F | SAH, Pcom | 1 | Coiling |
| 14 | 43, F | SAH, MCA | 3 | Clipping |
| 15 | 73, M | SAH, Pcom, IVH | 2 | Coiling |

The patients' age, gender, location of aneurysm, distribution along the Hunt and Hess scale and treatment performed to secure the aneurysm of the fifteen patients taking part on the study

*SAH* subarachnoid hemorrhage, *MCA* middle cerebral artery, *ICH* intracerebral hemorrhage, *Acom* anterior communicating artery, *Pcom* posterior communicating artery, *HIE* hypoxic ischemic encephalopathy, *IVH* intraventricular hemorrhage

**Table 2 Abnormal THRT is predictive of subsequent vasospasm development**

| | Vasospasm | Asymptomatic or no vasospasm | Total |
|---|---|---|---|
| Abnormal THRP | 5 | 2 | 7 |
| Normal THRP | 1 | 7 | 8 |
| Total | 6 | 9 | 15 |

As many as 83% patients who developed vasospasm had an abnormal THRP ($p = 0.0406$, Fisher's exact test, $n = 15$)

**Radiological imaging is moderately predictive of DIND**

In terms of radiological imaging, six patients had digital subtraction angiography (DSA), seven had computed tomography angiography (CTA), and computed tomography perfusion (CTP). Of the six patients with DSA, only two (33%) showed initial evidence of spasm and subsequently developed clinical DIND, with a similar percentage finding in the CTA group (*data not shown*).

When considering the CTP analysis, in the group with no vasospasm, none of the three patients showed any abnormality in the CTP maps including cerebral blood volume (CBV), cerebral blood flow (CBF), mean transit time (MTT), and time to peak (TTP). Of the remaining four patients who developed vasospasm, none of the patient showed abnormality neither in the CBV nor the CBF; while three patients (75%) showed prolongation of the MTT and TTP ($p = 0.14$, Fisher's exact test, two-tailed) (Table 4).

## Discussion

To prevent DIND related cerebral damage, it is recommended to commence a decisive treatment within 2 h of the onset of the symptoms [12]. This proves difficult to achieve in a clinical setting; firstly, due to the subtlety of the initial manifestation of DIND symptoms; and secondly, due to the difficulty of detecting a worsening neurological function in the presence of a major primary deficit. Therefore, this might not be a realistic endeavor in a lot of healthcare systems leaving many patients at a heightened risk of permanent deficits [2, 4].

The gold standard for the diagnosis of DIND is a cerebral angiogram [6]. It is an invasive procedure with inherent risk, including injury of the access artery and thromboembolic ischemic stroke [13]. Transcranial Doppler applications (TCD) have been used frequently as a

**Table 3 Abnormal THRT can predict asymptomatic vasospasm development**

| | Vasospasm | No vasospasm | Total |
|---|---|---|---|
| Abnormal THRP | 8 | 0 | 8 |
| Normal THRP | 0 | 7 | 7 |
| Total | 8 | 7 | 15 |

All patients including those who developed an asymptomatic vasospasm had an abnormal THRP prior to the event ($p = 0.0002$, Fisher's exact test, $n = 15$)

**Table 4 CTP analysis is moderately predictive of subsequent vasospasm development**

| | No vasospasm | Vasospasm | Total |
|---|---|---|---|
| Abnormal maps | 0 | 3 | 3 |
| Normal maps | 3 | 1 | 4 |
| Total | 3 | 4 | 7 |

Only MTT and TTP maps in the CTP measurements showed abnormal measurements in the patients who developed vasospasm ($p = 0.14$, Fisher's exact test, $n = 7$)

non-invasive diagnostic method of DIND. The measurements are based on trends of increased systolic velocities and increased Lindegaard ratio (mean velocity in the middle cerebral artery/mean velocity in ipsilateral extracranial internal carotid artery ratio (MCA/ICA) to improve the specificity of diagnosis) [7, 8]. TCDs are a popular method because of their non-invasive nature and the fact that they do not have the side effects associated with the use of contrast agents and radiation. Moreover, they are easily accessible and pose no risk to the patient in terms of transportation while critically ill [7, 8].

Another method frequently used in the clinics is computed tomography perfusion (CTP) [9, 10]. Improvement in the imaging capabilities of CTP does allow for a non-invasive assessment of the cerebral circulation dynamics, but it is liable to the inter-evaluator variability and lack of clear interpretation paradigms given the multiplicity of variables involved in generating and influencing these images [9, 10]. To add to the complexity of this issue, we frequently find areas of clinical deterioration that do not match the areas of vascular spasm detected on vascular imaging, a phenomenon called "clinico-radiological dissociation". Another early detection method is continuous electroencephalography (cEEG); able to detect changes suggestive of vasospasm [14]. However, for the most part, these applications are non-diagnostic of DIND. Another major concern with these imaging modalities is that irrespective of how informative they are, the radiation doses and contrast material involved in their generation limit their utility as dynamic tests to go along with the clinical evolution in the short-term or better still, in real time.

This has major drawbacks for the very nature of the decision-making process required in a critical care setting. This raises the need for a test that can be safely repeated and is informative in the realm of parameters affecting clinical care decisions.

An invasive cerebral blood flow monitoring has the ability to detect changes conducive of vasospasm 24–48 h earlier than the onset of clinical vasospasm. This is suggestive of a failure of an initial autoregulatory mechanism that, if detected early, can be valuable in identifying patients at risk of developing DIND [15–18]. Transient hyperemic response test (THRT), also known as carotid compression test, is a type of TCD examination of the cerebral vessels. It was described for the first time by Giller in 1991 as a bedside test for the assessment of cerebral autoregulation with the basic premise that, in the presence of an intact autoregulation, the cerebral vessels will be able to contract in response to a hyperemic challenge generated by a brief carotid occlusion [11]. This would be translated in the TCD signal as an increase in systolic velocity. In a normal response, the velocity should increase by a minimum of 9% from the baseline velocity. Any value less than that or reduction of the velocity denoted a global failure of autoregulation. Since then, several studies have confirmed this concept in animal models, human subjects as well as several diseases including traumatic brain injury (TBI) and SAH [19–21] THRT has been used to predict autoregulation failure in traumatic brain injury as well as the development of autoregulation failure conducive of DIND in patients with SAH [20–22].

In our study, THRT was performed in the first 24–48 h and was abnormal in 83% of patient who subsequently developed DIND. Of interest, the two patients with radiological vasospasm also exhibited an abnormal THRT. This raises the possibility that the stress of SAH can prime the cerebral circulation into a deregulatory process that leads to the development of vasospasm, whether clinically overt or silent. Moreover, this predictability was not influenced by the clinical grade of the SAH, an observation that can lead to an unbiased and more attentive attitude toward patients at theoretical risk of DIND and establish lower threshold for their investigation and escalation of therapy when necessary. Although not reported in this study results, we occasionally detected the resolution of the autoregulation failure by the return of the normal response despite the aggressive therapy for vasospasm. This at least in theory can guide the timing of weaning of DIND treatment with an aim to reduce treatment morbidity.

Lam et al. reported the use of THRT in post-clipping patients performed 0–5 days post bleed, with five out of six patients exhibiting abnormal THRT [20]. Another study compared three autoregulatory parameters: THRT, Sxa (based on TCD), and TOxa (based on near-infrared spectroscopy) and found equivalent reliability between the three parameters in predicting DIND, favoring THRT due to the time consuming nature of the latter two [22].

Another interesting observation emerging from our small retrospective cohort study is that the systolic velocity in the MCA was elevated in five patients from their ictus; however, it did not translate into the development of DIND. We hypothesize that this could be a secondary response to either aggressive initial management or to the systemic stress response seen in SAH patients.

The analysis and comparison of the data obtained from THRT and radiological imaging measurements suggests that the latter methods are only moderately predictive of subsequent DIND development. We found that of all the CTP maps the MTT and TTP were the most predictive. These observations will have to be validated in a larger cohort studies.

This study suffers from the inherent drawbacks of any retrospective review. Our sample size is small but illustrative to this test. Longitudinal THRT testing was not done in all patients and would be considered in future projects.

Our results suggest the utility of THRT in detecting patients at increased risk of DIND from the time of admission, which if supported by prospective trials, will allow supporting a watchful clinical approach to their clinical course of investigation and management. It can also lead us to better select patients for trials involving early interventions in SAH and DIND, as it might serve as discriminatory test to stratify high versus low risk candidates. Understanding the trend of THRT during the period of DIND and its resolution might prove useful as well.

## Conclusions

Early abnormal THRT can predict future development DIND in patients with SAH, independent of flow velocities or the clinical grade of the SAH.

### Authors' contributions

HA performed all the TCD examination and written the manuscript. MA provided clinical care and reviewed the manuscript. JM provided clinical care and reviewed the manuscript. JT provided clinical care and reviewed the manuscript. All authors read and approved the final manuscript.

### Author details

[1] Neurocritical Care Unit, Montreal Neurological Institute and Hospital, McGill University, Montreal, QC, Canada. [2] Department of Neurosurgery and Critical Care Medicine, King Fahad University Hospital, Imam Abdulrahman Bin Faisal University, Dammam, Saudi Arabia. [3] Department of Neurology and Neurosurgery, Montreal Neurological Institute and Hospital, Montreal General Hospital, McGill University, Montreal, QC, Canada. [4] Department of Neurosurgery, King Fahad Specialist Hospital in Dammam, Dammam, Saudi Arabia.

### References

1. Modi NJ, Agrawal M, Sinha VD, D'Andrea A, Conte M, Cavallaro M et al (2016) Post-traumatic subarachnoid hemorrhage: a review. Neurol India 64(Suppl:S1):8–13
2. Perrein A, Petry L, Reis A, Baumann A, Mertes P, Audibert G (2015) Cerebral vasospasm after traumatic brain injury: an update. Minerva Anestesiol 81(11):1219–1228
3. Brown RJ, Kumar A, Dhar R, Sampson TR, Diringer MN (2013) The relationship between delayed infarcts and angiographic vasospasm after aneurysmal subarachnoid hemorrhage. Neurosurgery 72(5):702–708
4. Dorsch NW, King MT (1994) A review of cerebral vasospasm in aneurysmal subarachnoid haemorrhage part I: incidence and effects. J Clin Neurosci 1:19–26
5. Rowland MJ, Hadjipavlou G, Kelly M, Westbrook J, Pattinson KT (2012) Delayed cerebral ischaemia after subarachnoid haemorrhage: looking beyond vasospasm. Br J Anaesth 109(3):315–329
6. Mills JN, Mehta V, Russin J, Amar AP, Rajamohan A, Mack WJ (2013) Advanced imaging modalities in the detection of cerebral vasospasm. Neurol Res Int 2013:415960
7. Schatlo B, Pluta RM (2007) Clinical applications of transcranial Doppler sonography. Rev Recent Clin Trials 2:49–57
8. Purkayastha S, Sorond F (2012) Transcranial Doppler ultrasound: technique and application. Semin Neurol 32(4):411–420
9. Wintermark M, Reichhart M, Thiran JP, Maeder P, Chalaron M, Schnyder P et al (2002) Prognostic accuracy of cerebral blood flow measurement by perfusion computed tomography, at the time of emergency room admission, in acute stroke patients. Ann Neurol 51(4):417–432
10. Murphy BD, Fox AJ, Lee DH, Sahlas DJ, Black SE, Hogan MJ et al (2006) Identification of penumbra and infarct in acute ischemic stroke using computed tomography perfusion-derived blood flow and blood volume measurements. Stroke 37(7):1771–1777
11. Giller CA (1991) A bedside test for cerebral autoregulation using transcranial Doppler ultrasound. Acta Neurochir 108(1–2):7–14
12. Chalouhi N, Ali MS, Jabbour PM, Tjoumakaris SI, Gonzalez LF, Rosenwasser RH et al (2012) Biology of intracranial aneurysms: role of inflammation. J Cereb Blood Flow Metab 32(9):1659–1676
13. Cloft HJ, Joseph GJ, Dion JE (1999) Risk of cerebral angiography in patients with subarachnoid hemorrhage, cerebral aneurysm, and arteriovenous malformation: a meta-analysis. Stroke 30(2):317–320
14. Rathakrishnan R, Gotman J, Dubeau F, Angle M (2011) Using continuous electroencephalography in the management of delayed cerebral ischemia following subarachnoid hemorrhage. Neurocrit Care 14(2):152–161
15. Werner C, Engelhard K (2007) Pathophysiology of traumatic brain injury. Br J Anaesth 99(1):4–9
16. Budohoski KP, Reinhard M, Aries MJ, Czosnyka Z, Smielewski P, Pickard JD et al (2012) Monitoring cerebral autoregulation after head injury. Which component of transcranial Doppler flow velocity is optimal? Neurocrit Care 17(2):211–218
17. Czosnyka M, Smielewski P, Piechnik S, Steiner LA, Pickard JD, Budohoski KP et al (2001) Cerebral autoregulation following head injury. J Neurosurg 95(5):756–763
18. Czosnyka M, Brady K, Reinhard M, Smielewski P, Steiner LA, Piechnik S et al (2009) Monitoring of cerebrovascular autoregulation: facts, myths, and missing links cerebral autoregulation following head injury. Neurocrit Care 10(3):373–386
19. Smielewski P, Czosnyka M, Kirkpatrick P, Pickard JD (1997) Evaluation of the transient hyperemic response test in head-injured patients. J Neurosurg 86(5):773–778
20. Lam JM, Smielewski P, Czosnyka M, Pickard JD, Kirkpatrick PJ (2000) Predicting delayed ischemic deficits after aneurysmal subarachnoid hemorrhage using a transient hyperemic response test of cerebral autoregulation. Neurosurgery 47(4):819–825 **(discussions 25–6)**
21. Lang EW, Mehdorn HM, Dorsch NW, Czosnyka M (2002) Continuous monitoring of cerebrovascular autoregulation: a validation study. J Neurol Neurosurg Psychiatry 72(5):583–586
22. Budohoski KP, Czosnyka M, Smielewski P, Varsos GV, Kasprowicz M, Brady KM et al (2013) Cerebral autoregulation after subarachnoid hemorrhage: comparison of three methods. J Cereb Blood Flow Metab 33(3):449–456

# Applicability of a modified EFAST protocol (r-EFAST) to evaluate hemodynamically unstable patients after percutaneous cardiac intervention

José Luis Vázquez Martínez[1,2*], Kary Leonisa Quiñones Coneo[1], Tomas Villen Villegas[3], María Sánchez Porras[1], Cesar Pérez-Caballero Macarrón[1], Ana Coca Pérez[1] and Luis Fernandez Pineda[4]

**Abstract**

Percutaneous cardiac intervention is an invasive diagnostic and therapeutic technique which carries a significant complication rate. Although the usefulness of EFAST protocol is widely recognised, this paper will attempt to explore a modified approach involving a focused examination on the retroperitoneal (r-EFAST). We have provided examples of 3 cases where r-EFAST was used to detect retroperitoneal bleeding in critical situations.

**Keywords:** Congenital heart defect, Cardiac catheterization, Retroperitoneal space, Hematoma

## Background

Ultrasound is widely regarded as being an accurate and reliable procedure to evaluate patients who have suffered an acute thoraco-abdominal trauma. Developed in late 1990s [1], the Focused Assessment with Sonography for Trauma (FAST) is one of the first ultrasound protocols for the rapid detection of free peritoneal and/or pericardial fluid. The term "Extended FAST" (EFAST) was adapted during the following decade [2] to include the addition of thoracic ultrasound views, encompassing a broader scope for diagnosis of other possible associated injuries, such as hemothorax or pneumothorax. Since its clinical implementation, EFAST has proven to be more reliable than the physical examination [3].

With the continued advancement of imaging equipment and surgical instruments, the application of interventional radiology techniques is becoming more widespread in the diagnostic and therapeutic management of vascular and cardiac diseases. As a result, however, complications related to this procedure have proportionally increased [4, 5]. Percutaneous cardiac interventions have been associated with the following complications; retroperitoneal hematoma, renal injury, aortic wall hematoma, inferior epigastric injury or local vascular complications (acute thrombosis, distal embolization, dissection, poorly controlled bleeding, pseudoaneurysm or arteriovenous fistula). Retroperitoneal bleeding is one of the more serious complications that can occur as the retroperitoneal space has the capacity to harbour large volumes of blood with no clinical signs and symptoms until hypovolemia occurs late in the clinical course [6]. Complications tend to occur in up to 8% of cardiac catheterization, being more frequently associated with therapeutic rather than diagnostic procedures (15.1% vs. 4.6%). The incidence of non-puncture related bleeding ranges from 0.9 to 1.2%, with the retroperitoneal hematoma being the most common finding (0.12–0.5%). Despite its unfamiliar etiology, the hematomas origin might be spontaneous or iatrogenic, which could be secondary to endovascular trauma or the use of anti-coagulation drugs during the procedure. Risk factors predisposing to retroperitoneal haemorrhage after percutaneous transfemoral cardiac intervention are the following: the female sex, low platelet count, sheath removal

*Correspondence: jvazquezm@salud.madrid.org
[1] Pediatric Intensive Care Unit, Ramón y Cajal University Hospital, Madrid, Spain
Full list of author information is available at the end of the article

protocol, the use of hydrophilic guide wire [7] and post-procedure anticoagulation, presenting the greatest risk [8].

The purpose of this paper is to explore the usefulness of a modified EFAST protocol (r-EFAST), including the bedside retroperitoneal clinician-performed assessment, to detect retroperitoneal hematoma or renal parenchymal injury in hemodynamically unstable patients after a percutaneous cardiac intervention without any suspected complications during the procedure in the catheterization laboratory.

## Cases presentation

We will present the cases of three patients with congenital heart disease without a previous medical history of hemorrhagic diathesis, family history of bleeding or lumbar trauma, who have been diagnosed with a retroperitoneal hematoma after percutaneous cardiac intervention using the r-EFAST protocol. r-EFAST is a bedside, rapid ultrasound protocol used to detect retroperitoneal hematoma or parenchymal renal injury. Once the standard EFAST has been performed in the supine position (scanning the upper right and left abdominal quadrants, pericardial, pelvis and anterior thoracic views), patients are adjusted, to a moderate degree, in a lateral decubitus position. This provides a clearer scan of the retroperitoneal space (Fig. 1), by sliding the probe for the upper right and left postero-lateral thoraco-abdominal junction zone, although the pararenal spaces are best shown transverse epigastric view (Fig. 2).

The examinations were carried out using a TOSHIBA with convex array transducer 3.5–5 MHz and a linear array transducer 6–8 MHz. The accesses were obtained on the common femoral artery (two patients left and one patient right), and long 5-French sheaths were advanced. Patients have given their consent for participation in this report.

### Case 1

A 16-year-old woman with a previous medical history of partial atrioventricular canal defect and subpulmonary membrane, which had been surgically corrected when she was 5 years old, underwent a percutaneous stent implantation in the pulmonary artery due to a residual stenosis. The patient was taken to the Cardiology Service without experiencing any problems during the procedure. Within 24 h upon admission, the patient developed a progressive left flank pain with positive fist percussion. Within 48 h, she experienced a sudden clinical deterioration with hypotension and a decreased haemoglobin level (12.8–8.3 g/dl), and was subsequently transferred to the Intensive Care Unit (ICU). EFAST result was positive), revealing a small amount of fluid in the Douglas' pouch. By performing r-EFAST, a left perirenal hematoma was found and identified as the likely origin of the hypotensive event. Abdominal CT scan with intravenous contrast revealed a left perirenal hematoma of 1.5 cms without signs of active contrast extravasations, with a small hematoma component open to the pararenal space (Fig. 3). The patient was successfully managed with conservative treatment. Serial r-EFAST showed no changes to the hematoma size or evidence of bleeding during the patient's stay in ICU.

### Case 2

A 16-year-old male with a previous medical history of aortic coarctation and isthmus hypoplasia operated in the neonatal period. Due to recoarctation, cardiac

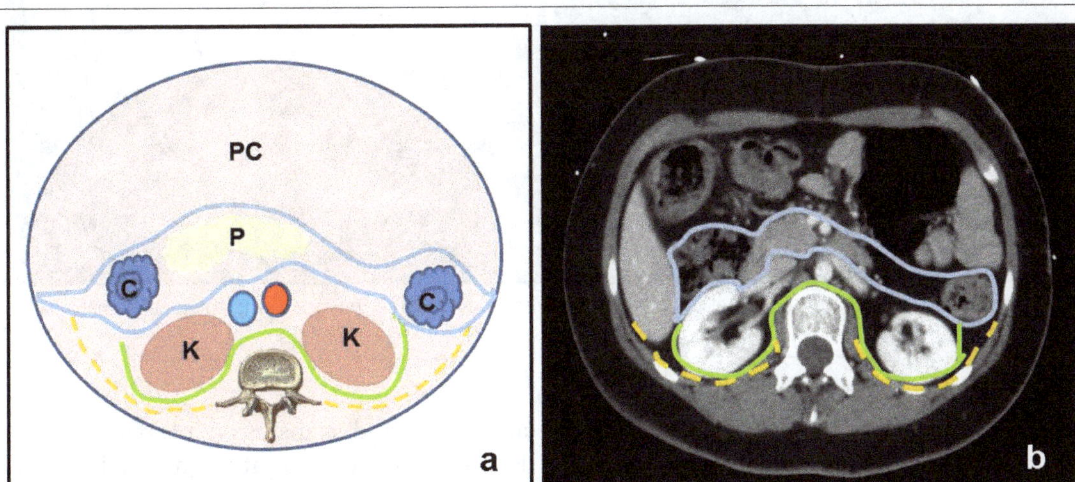


**Fig. 1** Retroperitoneal space anatomy. **a** Diagram shows the anterior pararenal space (*blue line*), the perirenal space (*green line*) and the posterior pararenal space (*yellow line*). Kidney (K), pancreas (P), colon (C) and peritoneal cavity (PC) **b** Perirenal and pararenal spaces in CT Scan with intravenous contrast

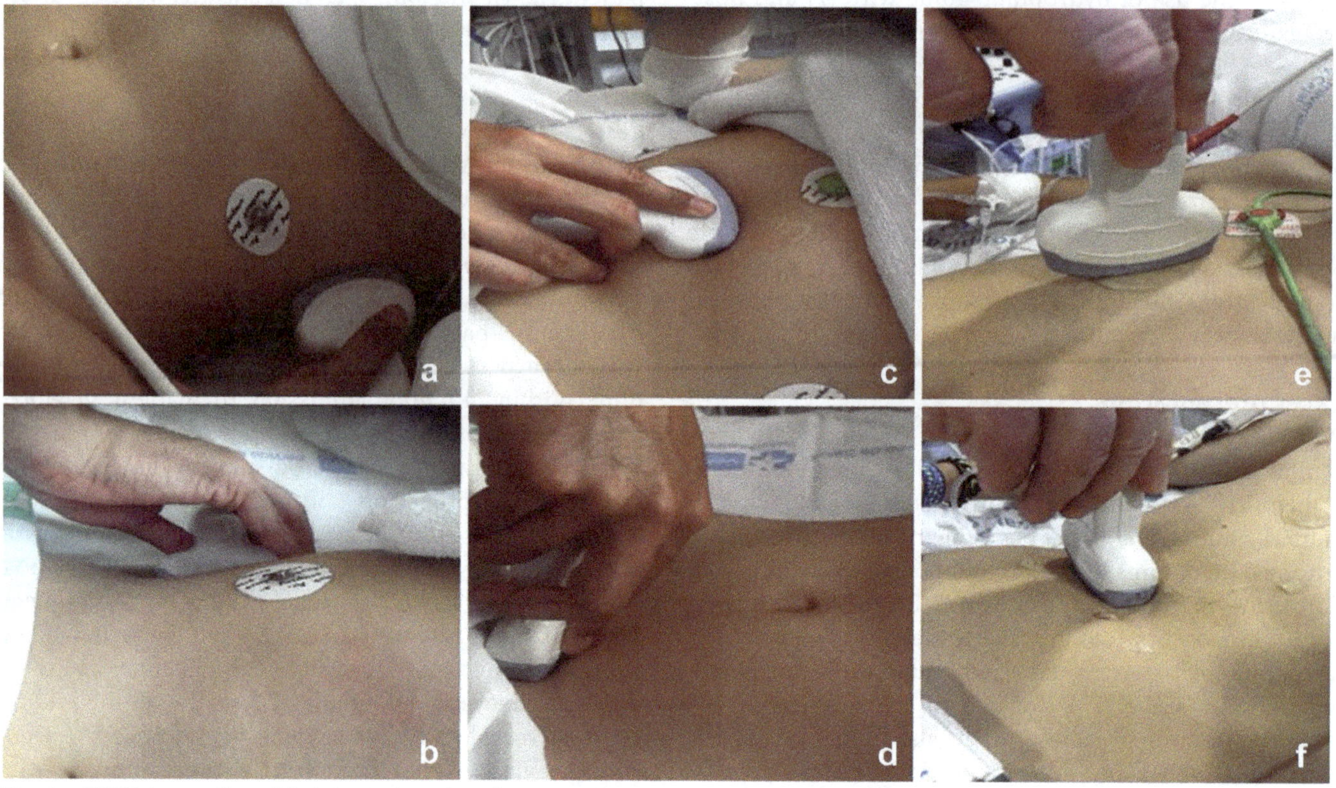

**Fig. 2** r-EFAST views: **a** *Upper left* abdominal quadrant. **b** *Upper right* abdominal quadrant. **c** Pericardial. **d** Pelvis. **e** Anterior thoracic. **f** Transverse epigastric

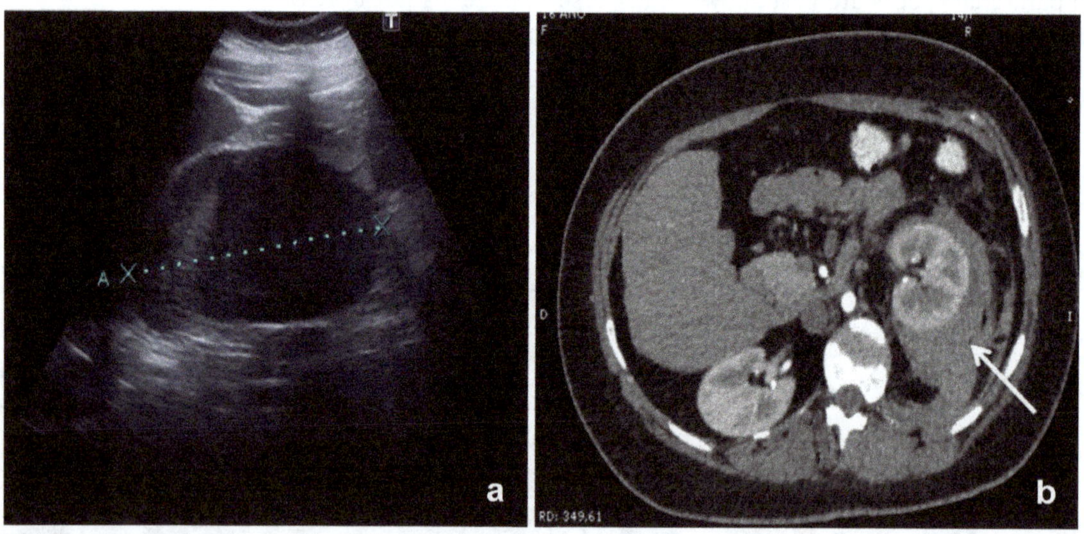

**Fig. 3** **a** r-EFAST: left perirenal hematoma of 1.5 cm (callipers). **b** CT Scan with intravenous contrast: peri- and pararenal hematoma (*arrow*) displacing anteriorly the left kidney

catheterization (balloon angioplasty) was performed. Forty-eight hours after the procedure, he developed a sudden left flank pain, abdominal distension, palpitations, sweating, hypotension, tachycardia, obnubilation and decreasing levels of haemoglobin, resulting in ICU admission and transfusion of packed red blood cells. EFAST result was negative (no air in pleural space and absence of free fluid in the pleural, pericardial or intraperitoneal space). The r-EFAST findings were however consistent with retroperitoneal bleeding revealing a collection of fluid measuring 14 × 2 cm in the right perirenal space extending to pararenal, paravesical and presacral spaces. The abdominal—CT scan with intravenous contrast confirmed retroperitoneal US findings with no active bleeding signs; the intraperitoneal space was free of any fluid collection (Fig. 4). The patient showed no further signs of bleeding episodes and was discharged after 8 days.

### Case 3

A 21-year-old-woman with a diagnosis of tricuspid atresia, ventricular septal defect and transposition of great arteries in the Fontan stage, underwent a percutaneous cardiac procedure for stenting the Fontan conduit and the left pulmonary artery; no incidents were described during the procedure. After 6 h, the patient presented symptoms of diffuse abdominal pain and a decrease in haemoglobin level from 12 to 5 g/dl. EFAST resulted positive (intraperitoneal free fluid) and r-EFAST demonstrated a retroperitoneal hematoma confirmed with the abdominal CT scan with intravenous contrast (left renal hematoma up to 6 cms open to intraperitoneal space with multiple foci of active bleeding) (Fig. 5). A selective embolization of the left renal artery medial segment was performed but finally, due to the persistent hemodynamically instability, a nephrectomy was required.

## Conclusions

Standard EFAST can be performed by physicians as a non-invasive bedside tool. It was strictly designed for the rapid detection of free peritoneal/pericardial/pleural fluid and free pleural air benefitting from diagnostic accuracy without a significant inter-operator variability, having a medium sensitivity but high specificity. Point-of-care

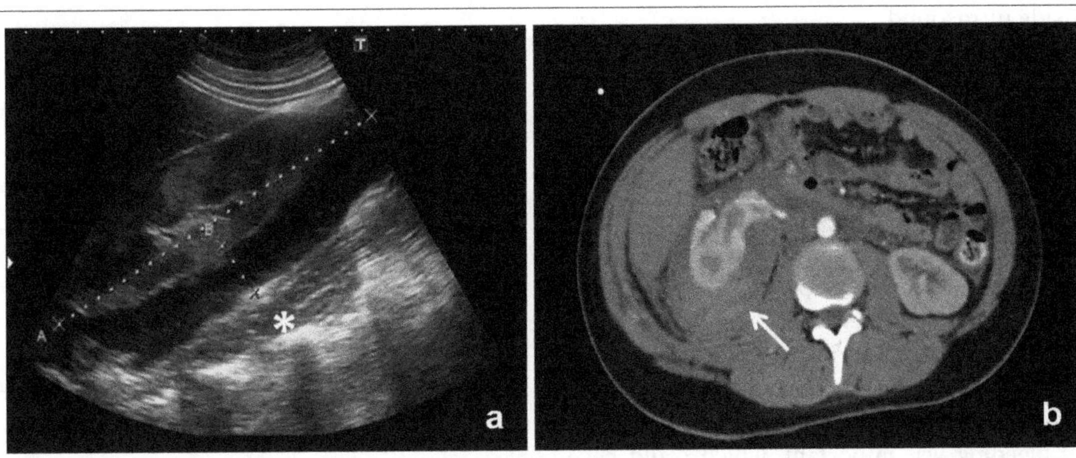


**Fig. 4** **a** r-EFAST: perirenal fluid collection anterior to psoas muscle (*asterisk*) measuring approximately 14 × 2 cms (callipers). **b** CT Scan with intravenous contrast: right perirenal hematoma with different densities that may correspond to active bleeding extending to pararenal space (*arrow*)

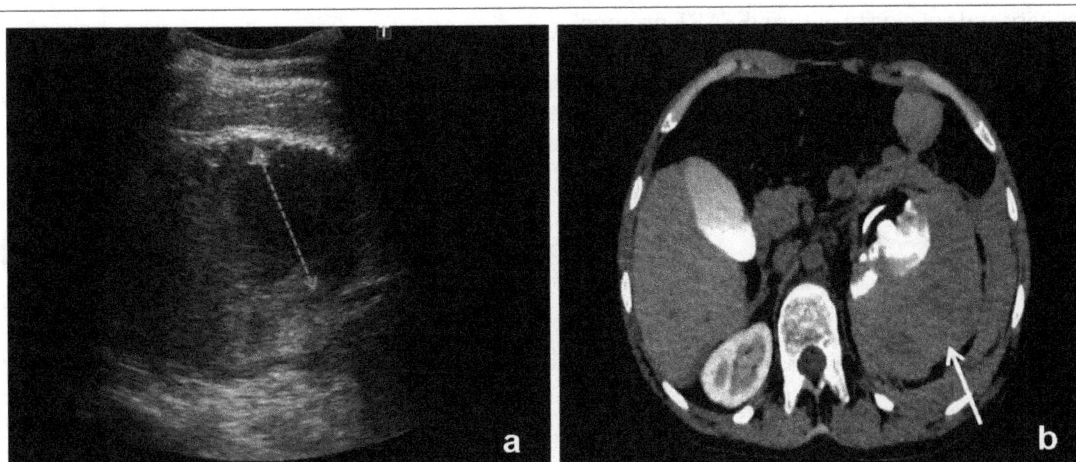


**Fig. 5** **a** r-EFAST: left renal hematoma of 6 cms (*arrow*). **b** CT Scan with intravenous contrast: perirenal hematoma (*arrow*), open to pararenal space. Also note the inhomogeneous distribution of intravenous contrast in the left kidney

ultrasound is a significantly more powerful tool when performed in a high prevalence population. The design of new protocols is important in different pathologies and situations such as the case of EFAST in blunt trauma. EFAST has been implemented in other clinical scenarios and ultrasound protocols, such as shocked adult patients (RUSH exam) [9]. In a similar approach, Heller et al. [10] focused the assessment with sonography on human immunodeficiency virus co-infected tuberculosis patients (FASH protocol) to diagnose extra-pulmonary tuberculosis.

The modification in the EFAST technique, r-EFAST, permits the detection of organ injury and/or free fluids in the retroperitoneal space when complications are suspected, such as, hematoma perirenal or kidney injuries in hemodynamically unstable patients after percutaneous cardiac intervention with abdominal pain and/or decreased haemoglobin level. This event is previously suspected by clinical examination and eventually confirmed by bedside ultrasound.

The r-EFAST extends beyond the EFAST for detecting source of bleeding in the retroperitoneum, not contemplated in the original EFAST. Although r-EFAST may likely require additional procedural time in comparison with EFAST, it is highly dependent upon the experience of the physician ("a good FAST exam takes only 30 s") [11]. We would therefore recommend including r-EFAST as part of training programmes for physicians who assist patients with congenital heart diseases.

Some limitations must be taken into account. Firstly, the reported series is small ($n = 3$). Secondly, all patients were hemodynamically unstable, so it must be assumed that the amount of bleeding was important, which could have improved the sensitivity of the protocol and partially compensate the inter-operator variability. In case of smaller losses of blood, the r-EFAST could fail. Further studies and researches in this field should be designed to establish the accuracy, sensitivity and specificity of the r-EFAST protocol.

**Abbreviations**

FAST: Focused Assessment with Sonography for Trauma; EFAST: Extended Focused Assessment with Sonography for Trauma; r-EFAST: Modified Extended Focused Assessment with Sonography for Trauma; ICU: Intensive Care Unit; CT: computed tomography; US: ultrasound.

**Authors' contributions**

JLVM developed the idea for the r-EFAST, wrote manuscript and provided figures. LFP and KLQC wrote the manuscript. TVV revised the manuscript critically for important intellectual content. ACP, CPCM and MSP identified the cases to make the r-EFAST. All authors contributed substantially to this work and all of them revised and agreed to the final version of the manuscript. They all agree to be accountable for all aspects of the work. All authors read and approved the final manuscript.

**Author details**

[1] Pediatric Intensive Care Unit, Ramón y Cajal University Hospital, Madrid, Spain. [2] Pediatric Intensive Care Unit, Crta Colmenar Viejo 9100, 28034 Madrid, Spain. [3] Emergency Department, Ramón y Cajal University Hospital, Madrid, Spain. [4] Pediatric Cardiology Department, Ramón y Cajal University Hospital, Madrid, Spain.

**Acknowledgements**

Not applicable.

**References**

1. Rozycki GS, Shackford SR (1996) Ultrasound, what every trauma surgeon should know. J Trauma 40(1):1–4
2. Kirkpatrick AW, Sirois M, Laupland KB et al (2004) Hand-held thoracic sonography for detecting post-traumatic pneumothoraces: the Extended Focused Assessment with Sonography for Trauma (EFAST). J Trauma 57(2):288–295
3. Rothlin MA et al (1993) Ultrasound in blunt abdominal and thoracic trauma. J Trauma 34:488–495
4. Fang CC, Ng Jao YT, Han SC, Wang SP (2007) Renal subcapsular hematoma after cardiac catheterization. Int J Cardiol 117(3):e101–e103
5. Kent KC, Moscucci M, Mansour KA, DiMattia S, Gallagher S, Kuntz R, Skillman JJ (1994) Retroperitoneal hematoma after cardiac catheterization: prevalence, risk factors, and optimal management. J Vasc Surg 20(6):905–910
6. Sanchez CE, Helmy T (2012) Percutaneous management of inferior epigastric artery injury after cardiac catheterization. Catheter Cardiovasc Interv 79(4):633–637
7. Edem E, Kilic H, Karacan A, Akdemir R (2016) Renal subcapsular hematoma caused by hydrophilic guide wire during patent ductus arteriosus closure. Heart Views 17(3):103–105
8. Peters S, Yazar A, Lemburg S, Cristoph H (2007) Renal perforation and retroperitoneal hematoma: an usual complication following cardiac catheterization. Int J Cardiovasc Imaging 23:805–808
9. Perera P, Maiholt T, Riley D, Mandavia D (2010) The RUSH exam: rapid ultrasound in shock in the critically ill patients. Emerg Med Clin N Am 28(1):29–56
10. Heller T, Wallrauch C, Goblirsch S, Brunetti E (2012) Focused assessment with sonography for HIV-associated tuberculosis (FASH): a short protocol and a pictorial review. Crit Ultrasound J 4(1):21
11. Dammers D, El Moumni M, Hoogland II, Veeger N, ter Avest E (2017) Should we perform a FAST exam in haemodynamically stable patients presenting after blunt abdominal injury: a retrospective cohort study. Scand J Trauma, Resusc Emerg Med 25:1

# Permissions

 Every chapter published in this book has been scrutinized by our experts. Their significance has been extensively debated. The topics covered herein carry significant findings which will fuel the growth of the discipline. They may even be implemented as practical applications or may be referred to as a beginning point for another development.

The contributors of this book come from diverse backgrounds, making this book a truly international effort. This book will bring forth new frontiers with its revolutionizing research information and detailed analysis of the nascent developments around the world.

We would like to thank all the contributing authors for lending their expertise to make the book truly unique. They have played a crucial role in the development of this book. Without their invaluable contributions this book wouldn't have been possible. They have made vital efforts to compile up to date information on the varied aspects of this subject to make this book a valuable addition to the collection of many professionals and students.

This book was conceptualized with the vision of imparting up-to-date information and advanced data in this field. To ensure the same, a matchless editorial board was set up. Every individual on the board went through rigorous rounds of assessment to prove their worth. After which they invested a large part of their time researching and compiling the most relevant data for our readers.

The editorial board has been involved in producing this book since its inception. They have spent rigorous hours researching and exploring the diverse topics which have resulted in the successful publishing of this book. They have passed on their knowledge of decades through this book. To expedite this challenging task, the publisher supported the team at every step. A small team of assistant editors was also appointed to further simplify the editing procedure and attain best results for the readers.

Apart from the editorial board, the designing team has also invested a significant amount of their time in understanding the subject and creating the most relevant covers. They scrutinized every image to scout for the most suitable representation of the subject and create an appropriate cover for the book.

The publishing team has been an ardent support to the editorial, designing and production team. Their endless efforts to recruit the best for this project, has resulted in the accomplishment of this book. They are a veteran in the field of academics and their pool of knowledge is as vast as their experience in printing. Their expertise and guidance has proved useful at every step. Their uncompromising quality standards have made this book an exceptional effort. Their encouragement from time to time has been an inspiration for everyone.

The publisher and the editorial board hope that this book will prove to be a valuable piece of knowledge for researchers, students, practitioners and scholars across the globe.

# List of Contributors

**Juan Carlos Ovalle and Mauricio Gómez Betancourt**
Emergency Medicine Specialist, Universidad del Rosario, Bogotá, Colombia

**José Moreno-Montoya and Ana-María Barragán González**
Epidemiology, Biostatistics and Public Health Research Group, EPIBIOS_UR, Escuela de Medicina y Ciencias de la Salud (EMCS), Universidad del Rosario, Bogotá, Colombia

**Yury Forlan Bustos Martínez**
Chief of the Department of Emergency Medicine and Director of the Simulation Center, Escuela de Medicina y Ciencias de la Salud (EMCS), Universidad del Rosario, Bogotá, Colombia

**Frederick A. Zeiler, Markus T. Ziesmann, Jason Park, Ashley Vergis and Lawrence M. Gillman**
Departments of Surgery, University of Manitoba, 409 Tache Avenue, Winnipeg, MB R2H 2A6, Canada

**Patrick Goeres**
Undergraduate Medical Education, University of Manitoba, Winnipeg, MB, Canada

**Bertram Unger**
Medical Education, University of Manitoba, Winnipeg, MB, Canada

**Dimitrios Karakitsos**
Departments of Internal Medicine, University of South Carolina, School of Medicine, Columbia, SC, USA

**Michael Blaivas**
Departments of Internal Medicine and Emergency Medicine, University of South Carolina, School of Medicine, Columbia, SC, USA

**Peiman Nazerian, Gabriele Cerini, Simone Vanni, Chiara Gigli, Stefano Grifoni and Maurizio Zanobetti**
Department of Emergency Medicine, Careggi University Hospital, Largo Brambilla 3, 50134 Florence, Italy

**Maurizio Bartolucci**
Radiology Department, Careggi University Hospital, Florence, Italy

**Giovanni Volpicelli**
Department of Emergency Medicine, San Luigi Gonzaga University Hospital, Orbassano, Turin, Italy

**Chiara Mozzini, Anna Maria Fratta Pasini, Ulisse Garbin and Luciano Cominacini**
Department of Medicine, Section of Internal Medicine, University of Verona, Piazzale L.A. Scuro, 10, 37134 Verona, Italy

**Devjani Das, Monica Kapoor, Cara Brown and Afoma Ndubuisi**
Department of Emergency Medicine, Northwell Health-Staten Island University Hospital, 475 Seaview Ave, Staten Island, NY 10305, USA

**Sanjey Gupta**
Department of Emergency Medicine, Northwell Health-Franklin Hospital, 900 Franklin Ave, Valley Stream, NY 11580, USA

**Alessandro Lamorte**
Emergency Department, San Luigi Gonzaga Hospital, Regione Gonzole 10 Orbassano, 10043 Turin, Italy

**Enrico Boero**
Anesthesiology and Intensive Care, Department of Surgical Sciences, University of Turin, Turin, Italy

**Paola Crida**
Turin University, Turin, Italy

**Abdul R. Conteh**
Holy Spirit Hospital, Makeni, Sierra Leone

**Marco Foletti and Paolo Narcisi**
Rainbow for Africa NGO, Via Zuretti 29, Turin, TO, Italy

**Saeed Ali Alzahrani**
King Saud bin Abdulaziz University for Health Sciences, Riyadh, Kingdom of Saudi Arabia

**Majid Abdulatief Al-Salamah**
Emergency Medicine, College of Public Health and Health Informatics, King Saud bin Abdulaziz University for Health Sciences, Riyadh, Kingdom of Saudi Arabia

**Wedad Hussain Al-Madani**
National & Gulf Center for Evidence Based Health Practice (NGCEBHP), King Saud bin Abdulaziz University for Health Sciences (KSAUHS), Riyadh, Kingdom of Saudi Arabia

**Mahmoud A. Elbarbary**
KSAUHS, Ministry of National Guard-Health Affairs, King Abdullah International Medical Research Center, Riyadh, Kingdom of Saudi Arabia

**Domagoj Damjanovic, Ulrich Goebel, Hartmut Buerkle and Axel Schmutz**
Department of Anesthesiology and Critical Care, Medical Center-University of Freiburg, Faculty of Medicine, University of Freiburg, Hugstetter Strasse 55, 79106 Freiburg, Germany

**Benedikt Fischer, Martin Huth and Hartmut Breger**
Information Technology Section, Department of Anesthesiology and Critical Care, Medical Center-University of Freiburg, Faculty of Medicine, University of Freiburg, 79106 Freiburg, Germany

**Fernando Pla, Leonardo Vera, Omar Cardillo and Lisandro Miguel Montorfano**
Department of Ultrasound, Clemente Álvarez Emergency Hospital, Av. Pellegrini 3205, 2000 Rosario, Santa Fe, Argentina

**Stefano Geniere Nigra**
Emergency Medicine Residency, University of Pavia, Strada Nuova 65, 27100 Pavia, Italy

**Thiago Thomaz Mafort, Rogério Rufino and Claudia Henrique da Costa**
Department of Pulmonology, Piquet Carneiro Policlinic, State University of Rio de Janeiro, Av. Mal. Rondon, 381, São Francisco Xavier, Rio de Janeiro 20950-003, Brazil
Postgraduate Programme in Medical Sciences, School of Medical Sciences, State University of Rio de Janeiro, Av. Prof. Manuel de Abreu, 444, 2° andar, Vila Isabel, Rio de Janeiro 20550-170, Brazil

**Mariana Soares da Cal, Laura Braga Monnerat, Patrícia Frascari Litrento, Laura Lizeth Zuluaga Parra and Arthur de Sá Earp de Souza Marinho**
Department of Pulmonology, Piquet Carneiro Policlinic, State University of Rio de Janeiro, Av. Mal. Rondon, 381, São Francisco Xavier, Rio de Janeiro 20950-003, Brazil

**Agnaldo José Lopes**
Department of Pulmonology, Piquet Carneiro Policlinic, State University of Rio de Janeiro, Av. Mal. Rondon, 381, São Francisco Xavier, Rio de Janeiro 20950-003, Brazil
Postgraduate Programme in Medical Sciences, School of Medical Sciences, State University of Rio de Janeiro, Av. Prof. Manuel de Abreu, 444, 2° andar, Vila Isabel, Rio de Janeiro 20550-170, Brazil
Rehabilitation Sciences Post-Graduation Programme, Augusto Motta University Centre (UNISUAM), Rua Dona Isabel, 94, Bonsucesso, Rio de Janeiro 21032-060, Brazil

**Christopher J. Smith and Tabatha Matthias**
Section of Hospital Medicine, Division of General Internal Medicine, Department of Internal Medicine, University of Nebraska Medical Center, 986430 Nebraska Medical Center, Omaha, NE, USA

**Abdulrahman Morad and Christopher Balwanz**
Division of Cardiology, Department of Internal Medicine, University of Nebraska Medical Center, Omaha, NE, USA

**Elizabeth Lyden**
Department of Biostatistics, University of Nebraska Medical Center, Omaha, NE, USA

**Vincent Issac Lau and Robert Thomas Arntfield**
Department of Medicine, Division of Critical Care, Schulich School of Medicine and Dentistry, Western University, London, ON, Canada
London Health Sciences Centre, Victoria Hospital Rm, D2-528, 800 Commissioners Road East, London, ON N6A 5W9, Canada

**Fehmi Ferhi, Khalil Tarmiz and Khaled Benjazia**
Department of Anaesthesiology and Critical Care Medicine, Farhat Hached University Hospital Center, 4002 Sousse, Tunisia
The Research Unit on Maternal Morbidity and Mortality UR17SP08, Sousse, Tunisia
Ibn Jazzar Medical School Sousse, Avenue Mohamed El Karoui, 4002 Sousse, Tunisia

**Abdeljalil Khlifi and Feten Hachani**
Ibn Jazzar Medical School Sousse, Avenue Mohamed El Karoui, 4002 Sousse, Tunisia
Department of Obstetrics and Gynaecology, Farhat Hached University Hospital Center, 4002 Sousse, Tunisia

**Francesco Corradi**
Servizio di Anestesia e Rianimazione, Ente ospedaliero Ospedali Galliera, Genoa, Italy

**Chiara Robba**
Anaesthesia and Intensive Care, IRCSS S. Martino Hospital, Genoa, Italy
Neurocritical Care Unit, Addenbrookes Hospital Cambridge, Cambridge, UK

**Guido Tavazzi**
Emergency Department, Anaesthesia and Intensive Care Unit, Fondazione IRCCS Policlinico S. Matteo, Pavia, Italy
Department of Clinical, Surgical, Diagnostic and Paediatric Sciences, Anaesthesia, Intensive Care and Pain Therapy Unit, University of Pavia, Pavia, Italy

**Gabriele Via**
Cardiac Anesthesia and Intensive Care, Cardiocentro Ticino, Via Tesserete, 48, Lugano, Switzerland

**Nova L. Panebianco**
Department of Emergency Ultrasound, Emergency Medicine, Hospital at the University of Pennsylvania, Philadelphia, PA, USA

**Elizabeth A. Hall**
Department of Emergency Ultrasound, Emergency Medicine, Hospital at the University of Pennsylvania, Philadelphia, PA, USA
Ashtabula, OH 44004, USA

**Ibrahim Showaihi**
Department of Emergency Ultrasound, Hospital at the University of Pennsylvania, Philadelphia, PA, USA

**Frances S. Shofer**
Epidemiology & Biostatistics, Department of Emergency Medicine, Hospital at the University of Pennsylvania, Philadelphia, PA, USA

**Anthony J. Dean**
Division of Emergency Ultrasonography, Hospital at the University of Pennsylvania, Philadelphia, PA, USA

**Eva Tenza-Lozano, Ana Llamas-Alvarez and Enrique Jaimez-Navarro**
Intensive Care Unit, Department of Intensive Care Medicine, Elche General University Hospital, Camino de la Almazara 11, 03203 Elche, Spain

**Javier Fernández-Sánchez**
Department of Clinical Medicine, Miguel Hernandez University, Sant Joan d'Alacant, Spain

**Mirko Zanatta, Piero Benato, Sigilfredo De Battisti, Concetta Pirozzi, Renato Ippolito and Vito Cianci**
Emergency Department of Arzignano Hospital, AULSS 8 Berica, Via Parco 1, 36071 Arzignano, Vicenza, Italy

**Jesper Weile and Anders Broens Moellekaer**
Emergency Department, Regional Hospital Herning, Herning, Denmark
Research Center for Emergency Medicine, Aarhus University Hospital, Aarhus, Denmark

**Jacob Brix**
Department of Learning & Philosophy, Research Group for Evaluation & Capacity Building, Aalborg University, Aalborg, Denmark

**R. Ketelaars and G. J. van Geffen**
Department of Anesthesiology, Pain and Palliative Medicine, Radboud University Medical Center, Radboud Institute for Health Sciences, Geert Grooteplein-Zuid 10, 6525 GA Nijmegen, The Netherlands
Helicopter Emergency Medical Service-Lifeliner 3, Radboud University Medical Center, Radboud Institute for Health Sciences, Geert Grooteplein-Zuid 10, 6525 GA Nijmegen, The Netherlands

**E. Gülpinar, T. Roes and M. Kuut**
Department of Anesthesiology, Pain and Palliative Medicine, Radboud University Medical Center, Radboud Institute for Health Sciences, Geert Grooteplein-Zuid 10, 6525 GA Nijmegen, The Netherlands

**Elena Bignami**
Anesthesiology, Critical Care and Pain Medicine Division, Department of Medicine and Surgery, University of Parma, Parma, Italy

**Antonio Anile and Giacomo Castiglione**
Intensive Care Unit, Ospedale Vittorio Emanuele, AOU Policlinico–Vittorio Emanuele, Catania, Italy

**Jole Russo**
Department of Anesthesia and Intensive Care, Ospedale Vittorio Emanuele, ASP Caltanissetta, Gela, Italy

**Ahmed Najjar and Michel W. Bojanowski**
Department of Neurosurgery, Centre Hospitalier de l'Université de Montréal, Montreal, QC, Canada

**André Y. Denault**
Division of Critical Care, Centre Hospitalier de l'Université de Montréal, Montreal, QC, Canada
Department of Anesthesiology, Montreal Heart Institute, Université de Montréal, 5000 Belanger Street, Montreal, QC H1T 1C8, Canada

**Søren Helbo Skaarup and Anders Løkke**
Department of Respiratory Diseases and Allergy, Aarhus University Hospital, Nørrebrogade 44, 8000 Aarhus C, Denmark

**Christian B. Laursen**
Department of Respiratory Medicine, Odense University Hospital, Odense, Denmark
Department of Clinical Research, University of Southern Denmark, Odense, Denmark

**Rossella Sassanelli, Lisa Mattuzzi and Sara Scapol**
Anesthesia and Intensive Care Clinic, Department of Medicine, University of Udine, Via Colugna 50, 33100 Udine, Italy

**Teresa Dogareschi and Alessandra Spasiano**
University-Hospital of S. M. Misericordia, Udine, Italy, 33100, P.le S. Maria della Misericordia n 15, Udine, Italy

**Ludmilla Seremet**
Hospital S. Vito al Tagliamento, Pordenone, Italy, Via della Vecchia Ceramica 1, 33170 Pordenone, Italy

**Angelo Cagnacci**
Gynecologic and Obstetric, Department of Medicine, University of Udine, Via Colugna 50, 33100 Udine, Italy

**Jeremy S. Faust**
Department of Emergency Medicine, Harvard Medical School, Brigham and Women's Hospital, 10 Vining Street, Neville House, Boston, MA 02115, USA

**James W. Tsung**
Department of Emergency Medicine and Division of Emergency Ultrasound, Icahn School of Medicine, Mount Sinai Hospital, New York, NY, USA

**Miguel Angel Montorfano**
Department of Ultrasound, Clemente Álvarez Emergency Hospital, Rosario, Argentina
AREU EMS Public Regional Company, Niguarda Ca' Granda Hospital, Milan, Italy
Present Address: Av. Pellegrini 3205, 2000 Rosario, Santa Fe, Argentina

**Federico Perez Quirante and Federico Rodríguez**
Department of Ultrasound, Clemente Álvarez Emergency Hospital, Rosario, Argentina

**Luca Neri**
AREU EMS Public Regional Company, Niguarda Ca' Granda Hospital, Milan, Italy

**Irene W. Y. Ma**
Division of Emergency Ultrasound, Department of Emergency Medicine, Massachusetts General Hospital, 326 Cambridge Street, Suite 410, Boston, MA 02114, USA
Division of General Internal Medicine, Department of Medicine, University of Calgary, 3330 Hospital Dr NW, Calgary, AB T2N 4N1, Canada

**Andrew S. Liteplo and Christina Wilson**
Division of Emergency Ultrasound, Department of Emergency Medicine, Massachusetts General Hospital, 326 Cambridge Street, Suite 410, Boston, MA 02114, USA

**Joshua D. Caplin and Michael A. Fifer**
Cardiology Division, Department of Medicine, Massachusetts General Hospital, 15 Parkman Street #800, Boston, MA 02114, USA

**Aftab Azad**
Division of Emergency Ultrasound, Department of Emergency Medicine, Massachusetts General Hospital, 326 Cambridge Street, Suite 410, Boston, MA 02114, USA
Department of Emergency Medicine, Hamad Medical Corporation, Doha, Qatar

**Aranya Bagchi**
Department of Anaesthesia, Massachusetts General Hospital, 55 Fruit Street, Boston, MA 02114, USA

**Vicki E. Noble**
Division of Emergency Ultrasound, Department of Emergency Medicine, Massachusetts General Hospital, 326 Cambridge Street, Suite 410, Boston, MA 02114, USA
Department of Emergency Medicine, University Hospitals, Cleveland Medical Center, Case Western Reserve University, 11100 Euclid Ave, Cleveland, OH 44106, USA

**Federico Barbariol, Ilaria Toretti, Giovanni Maria Guadagnin, Daniele Orso, Livia Pompei and Giorgio Della Rocca**
Anesthesia and Intensive Care Medicine-Department of Medical and Biological Sciences, University of Udine, P.le S. M. della Misericordia 15, 33100 Udine, Italy

**Luigi Vetrugno and Tiziana Bove**
Anesthesia and Intensive Care Clinic, Department of Medicine, University of Udine, Via Colugna 50, 33100 Udine, Italy
University-Hospital of S. M. Misericordia, Udine, Italy, 33100, P.le S. Maria della Misericordia n 15, Udine, Italy

**Francesco Forfori**
Anesthesia and Intensive Care Medicine IV, Pisa University Hospital, Pisa, Italy

**Duraid Younan and Jeffrey Richey**
Department of Surgery, Division of Acute Care Surgery, University of Alabama at Birmingham, Birmingham, AL, USA

**T. Mark Beasley**
Department of Biostatistics, University of Alabama at Birmingham, Birmingham, AL, USA
Birmingham/Atlanta VA Geriatric Research, Education, & Clinical Center, Department of Veteran's Affairs, Birmingham, AL, USA

**David C. Pigott, C. Blayke Gibson and John P. Gullett**
Department of Emergency Medicine, University of Alabama at Birmingham, Birmingham, AL, USA

**Jean-Francois Pittet and Ahmed Zaky**
Department of Anesthesiology and Perioperative Medicine, University of Alabama at Birmingham, Birmingham, AL, USA

**Yusuke Seino, Nobuo Sato, Kimiya Fukui, Junya Ishikawa, Masahi Nakagawa and Takeshi Nomura**
Department of Intensive Care Medicine, Tokyo Women's Medical University, 8-1, Kawada-cho, Shinjuku-ku, Tokyo, Japan

**Mark Angle and Jeanne Teitelbaum**
Neurocritical Care Unit, Montreal Neurological Institute and Hospital, McGill University, Montreal, QC, Canada

**Hosam Al-Jehani**
Neurocritical Care Unit, Montreal Neurological Institute and Hospital, McGill University, Montreal, QC, Canada
Department of Neurosurgery and Critical Care Medicine, King Fahad University Hospital, Imam Abdulrahman Bin Faisal University, Dammam, Saudi Arabia
Department of Neurology and Neurosurgery, Montreal Neurological Institute and Hospital, Montreal General Hospital, McGill University, Montreal, QC, Canada
Department of Neurosurgery, King Fahad Specialist Hospital in Dammam, Dammam, Saudi Arabia

**Judith Marcoux**
Department of Neurology and Neurosurgery, Montreal Neurological Institute and Hospital, Montreal General Hospital, McGill University, Montreal, QC, Canada

**José Luis Vázquez Martínez**
Pediatric Intensive Care Unit, Ramón y Cajal University Hospital, Madrid, Spain
Pediatric Intensive Care Unit, Crta Colmenar Viejo 9100, 28034 Madrid, Spain

**Kary Leonisa Quiñones Coneo, María Sánchez Porras, Cesar Pérez-Caballero Macarrón and Ana Coca Pérez**
Pediatric Intensive Care Unit, Ramón y Cajal University Hospital, Madrid, Spain

**Tomas Villen Villegas**
Emergency Department, Ramón y Cajal University Hospital, Madrid, Spain

**Luis Fernandez Pineda**
Pediatric Cardiology Department, Ramón y Cajal University Hospital, Madrid, Spain

# Index

www.ingramcontent.com/pod-product-compliance
Lightning Source LLC
LaVergne TN
LVHW082146200926
848484LV00008B/2113